TORTURED SCIENCE

Health Studies, Ethics, and Nuclear Weapons in the United States

Compiled and Edited by:
Dianne Quigley, Amy Lowman, and Steve Wing
Collaborative Initiative for Research Ethics and Environmental Health (CIREEH)

Critical Approaches in the Health Social Sciences Series
Series Editor: RAY H. ELLING

Routledge
Taylor & Francis Group
LONDON AND NEW YORK

First published 2012 by Baywood Publishing Company, Inc.

Published 2017 by Routledge
2 Park Square, Milton Park, Abingdon, Oxon OX14 4RN
711 Third Avenue, New York, NY 10017, USA

Routledge is an imprint of the Taylor & Francis Group, an informa business

Library of Congress Catalog Number: 2011009813
ISBN 13: 978-0-89503-395-6 (hbk)
ISBN 13: 978-0-89503-777-0 (pbk)

Library of Congress Cataloging-in-Publication Data

Tortured science : health studies, ethics, and nuclear weapons in the United States / compiled and edited by Dianne Quigley, Amy Lowman, and Steve Wing ; Collaborative Initiative for Research Ethics and Environmental Health (CIREEH).
p. cm. -- (Critical approaches in the health social science series)
Includes bibliographical reference and index.
ISBN 978-0-89503-395-6 (cloth : alk. paper) - - ISBN 978-0-89503-777-0 (pbk. : alk. paper) -- ISBN 978-0-89503-461-8 (epub) -- ISBN 978-0-89503-462-5 (epdf) 1. Environmental health--United States. 2. Nuclear weapons--Moral and ethical aspects. 3. Radiation--Physiological effect. I. Quigley, Dianne, 1955- II. Lowman, Amy, 1977- III. Wing, Steven. IV. Collaborative Initiative for Research Ethics and Environmental Health.
RA566.3.T665 2011
362.196'98--dc22

2011009813

Cover Photo: Photographed by Doug Brugge
Courtesy of the Navajo Nation Museum, Window Rock, Arizona
Catalog Number URC-028.F5 (Kathleen T. Tsosie, 1996)
Detail: cover photo was cropped 1/8" from bottom of photo.

Table of Contents

Tribute

We dedicate this book to Alice M. Stewart (1906-2002), the British physician and epidemiologist who, in the 1950s, discovered the link between prenatal x-rays and childhood cancer. In the 1970s she became involved in studies of radiation exposures among U.S. nuclear workers (see Chapter 9). Throughout her career Dr. Stewart integrated brilliant scientific inquiry with a deep sense of the dignity of patients, workers, and communities exposed to industrial and environmental hazards. She persisted in the pursuit of knowledge in radiation epidemiology, sometimes under great duress, as she suffered the ire of the medical and nuclear industries responsible for the exposures she studied. Always committed to increasing public understanding of science and community involvement in civic life, she supported efforts to prevent the hazards of nuclear weapons and nuclear production around the world. Dr. Stewart's technical knowledge and charisma made her equally adept at a scientific conference, in a court of law, or in a community meeting. Through her courage and determination she inspired many to work for a more ethical and inclusive scientific practice oriented toward the prevention of disease and promotion of health and democracy.

We also dedicate this work to the community groups around U.S. nuclear weapons facilities who have worked tirelessly to protect public health from the risks of low-level radiation and other hazards resulting from nuclear weapons production and use.

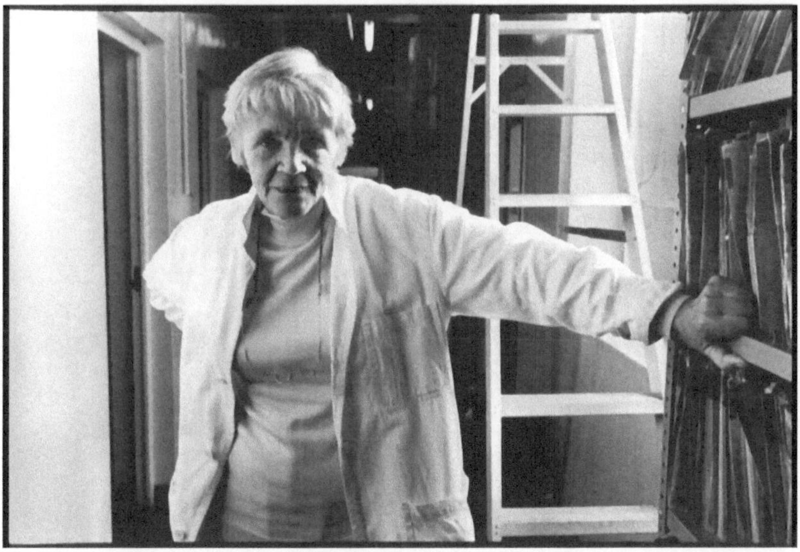

Dr. Alice Stewart, Birmingham Regional Cancer Registry, England, September 13, 1981.
Photo: Robert Del Tredici/The Atomic Photographers Guild.

Foreword: Class, Race, and Research on Health Impacts of Nuclear Weapons Production

Beginning with the Manhattan Project in WWII, the United States created a vast new industrial complex devoted to nuclear weapons. Mines, research labs, reactors, enrichment facilities, fabrication plants, and test sites were located from South Carolina to the Niagara Frontier, from California to Alaska and the Marshall Islands [1]. Nuclear weapons destroyed two Japanese cities. These activities contaminated land, air, water, and wildlife, and have sickened and killed people all over the world.

While this broad statement is undisputable, there is a lack of reliable research into radiation hazards in general and the impacts of the weapons complex on specific places and people in particular. The lack of documentation about the ecological effects of nuclear weapons programs, including their impact on human health, is due in part to the fact that most of the research has been conducted under the aegis of the governments and industries that have promoted nuclear weapons [2]. Financial and political conflicts of interest have prevented the development of an adequate research base not only due to technical problems in the design and conduct of studies [3], but due to the lack of an ethical framework that affirms human rights, social responsibility, and respect for the ecosystem. Development of more ethical research practices could help address these problems by transforming science and society in ways that promote self-determination, health and well-being.

Science usually presents itself as a disinterested quest for knowledge, an objective method that leads us inexorably toward truth. According to this view science is an autonomous practice that is unaffected by culture, economics, and politics. Ethics are of concern only in avoiding harm and promoting justice in the conduct of research, not in the framing of questions or decisions about what should be known and who should know it [4]. The myth of a value-free science unaffected by economic and social pressures allows the scientific community to fend off questions about social responsibility, who controls the production of scientific knowledge, who benefits, and who suffers from scientific inquiry [5]. By excluding the choices of research questions from scrutiny, scientists limit their investigations to the empirical tasks of hypothesis testing, data collection, analyses, and interpretation of measurable phenomena. Therefore, in the science of health impacts of nuclear weapons production, we need to recognize the perspectives and needs of human populations under investigation and the social responsibility of scientists involved with the nuclear weapons complex.

By considering the ethics of research on the health impacts of nuclear weapons production in the context of the role of science in society, we could strengthen organized efforts to reduce the impacts of production on workers and communities, compensate exposed populations, and convert military production into activities that satisfy human needs. We must relentlessly critique the objectivity myth while we avoid the trap of dismissing the rational and materialist traditions of science that are needed for understanding and changing the world in ways that can promote health and environmental sustainability [6]. We must distinguish those aspects of the dominant scientific culture that give science its strength and utility from forces in science that can create domination, exploitation, and justification of social inequalities.

Nuclear weapons production in the United States was undertaken by an alliance between the federal government and large corporations, some with familiar names like DuPont, Westinghouse, and Union Carbide. Secret facilities were created during World War II, many in rural areas inhabited disproportionately by low income people and people of color: Native Americans in the western states (Hanford, Los Alamos, the Nevada test site), low-income white populations in Appalachia (Oak Ridge), and the Black Belt of the South (Savannah River) [1]. Although contamination from these operations was by no means limited to local areas (the most prominent example being global fallout from weapons testing in Nevada) [7], host communities have borne the brunt of off-site pollution. Failure of officials to adequately inform populations about off-site releases; to conduct research into contamination of their land, air, water, and food; and study the health consequences of exposures [8], may be understood, in part, as a result of the low levels of political power, wealth, and education in these communities. Rural populations downwind from Hanford, Washington were exposed to massive uncontrolled experiments such as the deliberate releases of large amounts of radioactive iodine and other radionuclides at the Hanford plutonium production facility during times when winds were blowing toward the Yakima territory [9].

The new nuclear weapons labs and manufacturing sites drew on local labor pools and also attracted highly trained scientific staff from across the country and the world. Workplace protection, monitoring of workers' exposures, and conducting health studies often followed the class and race divisions within the workforce. Of the three large facilities built in Oak Ridge, Tennessee during World War II, one (X-10) was a scientific laboratory and two were production facilities [10]. Dosimeters for monitoring workers' radiation exposures were developed at X-10 during its first months of operation, and programs of widespread monitoring were instituted shortly afterward [11]. In contrast, little monitoring was conducted at production facilities where more jobs were held by local Appalachian mountain people [12]. At Los Alamos, employees of the University of California, which operated the laboratory, were monitored for exposures to radiation and other hazards, while the disproportionately Hispanic and Native American employees of the maintenance contractor, who worked in the same areas, were largely unmonitored [13].

Differences in worker protection and monitoring later translated into inequities in conducting health research. Epidemiologic studies that depend on good historical records focus on groups of workers who were best monitored. At Oak Ridge, X-10 has been studied far more than the production facilities. Within X-10, white males with no history of employment at the other facilities have received the most attention [14].

Although occupational protection, monitoring of exposure to hazards, and inclusion in epidemiologic studies have depended on race and class, secrecy and hostility toward workers compensation have been pervasive throughout the weapons complex [18]. This secrecy has made workers fearful of telling even their own medical care providers about their occupational exposures, and has limited monitoring and access to records needed for health studies. Company towns had formed around the nuclear weapons plants which made it difficult to question practices of industry. The military industries dominated employment and influenced politics, local schools, and medical care. Workers and residents were also affected by needs for secrecy and fears that information about production and exposures would interfere with the general public's support for the nuclear weapons program.

Employers have a unique responsibility for workplace safety, including reduction of unsafe conditions, provision of access to protection and training, the monitoring of hazardous agents, and the follow-up of injuries and exposures. However, there is little economic incentive for this protection when it is more profitable to replace workers than protect individual workers from injury, and when the consequences of exposures are delayed until after termination of employment. When workers organize for hazard pay or file suit to obtain compensation for occupational disease and injury, a neglect of these protections can be more severe. Corporations are responsible for maximizing returns to their shareholders, not for protecting workers, families, and communities.

CONTROL OF THE PRODUCTION OF SCIENTIFIC KNOWLEDGE

The U.S. Department of Energy and its predecessor federal agencies have been responsible for promoting nuclear technology as well as for assessing health effects of exposure to radiation [16]. Populations exposed to radiation and other hazards are affected by this control because research on the biological effects of radiation is used to justify exposure limits for workers and the public and to make decisions on eligibility for compensation and on liability for damages. The parties that control collection and sharing of exposure and health records work closely with the agencies that fund them and set exposure limits, as well as with the scientists that conduct research under agency funding. These groups share interests and have been hostile to independent researchers and exposed communities.

The initial program to develop nuclear weapons was created under a veil of secrecy. The culture that developed under the military priorities of World War II continued after the war and became more hostile toward the people of the United States as public relations problems developed with nuclear weapons testing and nuclear power. The report of the Advisory Committee on Human Radiation Experiments produced clear documentation that scientists working for the Atomic Energy Commission were fearful that workers and the public would learn about the extent of their exposures, would seek compensation for illness related to nuclear weapons production, and that the program would lose public support. These attitudes became entrenched in the culture at national laboratories and academic institutions [8].

Many scientists who exhibited independence from the radiation research establishment experienced hostility and difficulties with access to data and research funding. These include John Gofman, Alice Stewart, Thomas Mancuso, Karl Morgan, Edward Martell, Carl Johnson, Joseph Lyon, and Gregg Wilkinson [17-19]. Structural problems with the Department of Energy's research into health effects of the nuclear weapons program were investigated by the U.S. Congress, the DOE's Secretarial Panel for Evaluation of Epidemiologic Research Activity (Secretarial Panel for the Evaluation of Epidemiologic Research Activities, 1990), and an independent committee of the Physicians for Social Responsibility [16]. Conflicts of interest uncovered by these investigations led to the transfer of much of DOE's research to the Department of Health and Human Services in the early 1990s; however, the DOE maintained control of many records needed for research as well as the DHHS's energy-related research budgets.

ORGANIZING FOR ETHICAL SCIENTIFIC RESEARCH

Financial and political conflicts of interest in research on health impacts of nuclear weapons production create both ethical and scientific problems, aspects of the research process that cannot be separated. For example, constraints on epidemiologic studies have discouraged collection of data on exposures and diseases that could be used to investigate hazards and discouraged investigations when data do exist. Furthermore, constraints have distorted knowledge produced in epidemiologic studies by conditioning investigations and analyses on inappropriate assumptions and research methods [2]. Although the conflicts of interest (and the resulting body of knowledge skewed toward the interests of radiation industries) are in some ways unique to the history of nuclear weapons development, they are in other ways general problems that derive from control of science by undemocratic institutions [21]. The creation of more ethical and more reliable science depends on enfranchisement of people who have been excluded from the creation of scientific knowledge.

A movement for ethical research must strive to meaningfully involve workers, downwinders, and other affected populations in the research process. Meaningful involvement requires that exposed populations do not fear job loss or harassment by employers or government authorities. Meaningful involvement requires that they have access to education about science and research design, access to technical support from independent experts, and the right to organize to protect their interests. Creating this level of involvement is difficult because industry and government institutions have more resources and power than do workers and downwinders. Safeguards to protect whistleblowers and other activists as well as the provision of labor rights and funding for environmental and worker groups are essential. These safeguards and resources for workers and downwinders are especially needed because research may require collaboration with institutions, corporate and governmental, that create the hazards, monitor exposures, and maintain health records. Safeguards can help ameliorate the imbalance of power between those who create the hazards and those who are exposed.

CONCLUSION

War is an old plague, one of the horsemen of the apocalypse. Given the lack of ethics in preparing for and conducting war, it is not surprising that research on the health consequences of preparing for war has had ethical deficiencies. In this way nuclear war is not unique. However, as a uniquely modern technology (even biowarfare is centuries old), nuclear weapons have brought about their own special culture and problems.

The legacy of popular involvement and independent research in the environmental and health consequences of nuclear weapons production is a hopeful sign that, even in company towns and scientific institutions funded by the weapons establishment, people investigate problems, organize for healthful working and living conditions, fight for the public's right to know, and demand their rights to self-determination. Local groups have formed at nuclear weapons plants across the nation. Many of them seek to prevent environmental and workplace exposures to hazards, to provide compensation and care for the ill and injured, educate the public, and transform the weapons program itself to peaceful uses instead of preparation for war.

These U.S. organizations are part of a global movement that reflects the global reach of nuclear weapons production from uranium mining to enrichment, assembly, storage, and testing sites. The international movement includes the Japanese survivors of the atomic bombs the United States dropped on Hiroshima and Nagasaki, as well as their descendants. These groups demand a socially responsible science that is transparent and serves the needs of the exposed as well as the needs of the governments and industries responsible for the exposures. In some countries, including the United States and Japan, there has been some success in bringing compensation to victims. A most notable achievement of the work of activist organizations, nuclear worker advocacy groups, and public health professionals is the passage in 2000 of the Energy Employees Occupational Illness Compensation Act, a legislative package designed to provide health care and compensation to certain nuclear weapons workers who were injured from occupational exposure to radiation, beryllium, or silica [22]. Unfortunately, this program has been plagued by lack of records documenting worker exposures and a system of radiation risk assessment that has resulted in denial of many claims [23]. For all populations affected by production, testing, and use of nuclear weapons, much remains to be done to provide reparations to survivors.

As worker organizations and community groups prepare for the future, they can help to create the processes for public involvement and institutional accountability that will help produce a body of research on the health effects of nuclear weapons that is more ethical and more valid.

NOTES

1. Makhijani, A., Hu, H., and Yih, K. 1995. *Nuclear wastelands: A global guide to nuclear weapons production and its health and environmental effects.* Cambridge, MA: MIT Press.
2. Nussbaum, R. H., and Köhnlein, W. 1994. Inconsistencies and open questions regarding low-dose health effects of ionizing radiation. *Environmental Health Perspective* 102(8):656-667. Sterling, T. D. 1980. The health effects of low-dose radiation on atomic workers. A case study of employer-directed research. *International Journal of Health Services* 10(1):37-46. Wing, S., Richardson, D. B., Wolf, S., Mihlan, G., Crawford-Brown, D., and Wood, J. 2000. A case control study of multiple myeloma at four nuclear facilities. *Annals of Epidemiology* 10(3):144-153. Wing, S., Department of Epidemiology SoPHUoNCCHNCUSAswue. 2003. Objectivity and ethics in environmental health science. *Environmental Health Perspective* 111(14):1809-1818.
3. Nussbaum, R. H. 2007. Manipulating public health research: The nuclear and radiation health establishments. *International Journal of Occupational Environmental Health* 13(3):328-330.

4. Harding, S. 1991. *Whose science? Whose knowledge?: Thinking from women's lives.* Ithaca, NY: Cornell University Press.
5. Fox-Keller, E. 1995. Science and its critics. *Academe* 10-15.
6. Levins, R., and Lewontin, R. C. 1985. *The dialectical biologist.* Cambridge, MA: Harvard University Press.
7. National Cancer Institute. 1997. Estimated exposures and thyroid doses received by the American people from iodine-131 in fallout following Nevada atmospheric nuclear bomb tests NIH Publication No. 97-4264. Washington, DC: U.S. Department of Health and Human Services, National Institutes of Health, National Cancer Institute.
8. Advisory Committee on Human Radiation Experiments. 1995. Final report, Advisory Committee on Human Radiation Experiments. Washington, DC: U.S. Government.
9. HHIN, 2008: http://www.doh.wa.gov/hanford/publications/history/release.html
10. Johnson, L., and Schaffer, D. 1994. *Oak Ridge National Laboratory: The first fifty years.* Knoxville, TN: University of Tennessee Press.
11. Wing, S., West, C. M., and Wood, J. L., and Tankersley, W. 1994. Recording of external radiation exposures at Oak Ridge National Laboratory: Implications for epidemiological studies. *Journal of Exposure and Analysis of Environmental Epidemiology* 4(1):83-93.
12. Watkins, J. P., Reagan, J. L., Cragle, D. L., Frome, E. L., West, C. M., Crawford-Brown, D., et al. 1993. Data collection, validation, and description for the Oak Ridge Nuclear Facilities mortality study. Oak Ridge, TN: Oak Ridge Associated Universities/DOE.
13. Wing, S., Richardson, D. B., Wolf, S., Mihlan, G., Crawford-Brown, D., and Wood, J. 2000. A case control study of multiple myeloma at four nuclear facilities. *Annals of Epidemiology* 10(3):144-153.
14. Wing, S., Shy, C. M., Wood, J. L., Wolf, S., Cragle, D. L., and Frome, E. L. 1991. Mortality among workers at Oak Ridge National Laboratory. Evidence of radiation effects in follow-up through 1984. *Journal of the American Medical Association* 265(11):1397-1402.
15. Wing, S., Richardson, D. B., and Stewart, A. 1999. The relevance of occupational epidemiology to radiation protection standards. *New Solutions* 9(2):133-151.
16. Geiger, H. J., Rush, D., and Michaels, D. 1992. Dead reckoning: A critical review of the Department of Energy's Epidemiologic Research. Washington, DC: Physicians for Social Responsibility.
17. Lyon, J. L. 1999. Nuclear weapons testing and research efforts to evaluate health effects on exposed populations in the United States. *Epidemiology* 10(5):557-560.
18. Wilkinson, G. S. 1999. Seven years in search of alpha: The best of times, the worst of times. *Epidemiology* 10(3):340-344.
19. Greenberg, M. 1991. The evolution of attitudes to the human hazards of ionizing radiation and to its investigators. *American Journal of Industrial Medicine* 20(6):717-721.
20. Greene, G. 1999. *The woman who knew too much: Alice Stewart and the secrets of radiation.* Ann Arbor, MI: University of Michigan Press.
21. Huff, J. 2007. Industry influence on occupational and environmental public health. *International Journal of Occupational Environmental Health* 13(1):107-117.
22. Eligible workers or their survivors will receive a lump sum payment of $150,000. Those eligible include certain Department of Energy (DOE), DOE contractor, and

DOE vendor employees who were injured from exposure to radiation, beryllium, or silica while working in DOE nuclear weapons related programs. Survivors can make claims on behalf of covered employees. The federal government will provide medical benefits to eligible workers for their occupational illness.

23. Frank, L. 2009. Plan to pay sick nuclear workers unfairly rejects many, doctor says. pro publica: Journalism in the public interest. http://www.propublica.org/feature/plan-to-pay-sick-nuclear-workers-unfairly-rejects-many-doctor-says-731 accessed August 5, 2009.

Acknowledgments

This work was funded by a grant from the National Institute of Health, National Heart, Lung and Blood Institute Grant Program for "Short Courses in Research Ethics" (T15HL069792) as a report for the Collaborative Initiative for Research Ethics on Environmental Health sponsored by Syracuse University, Department of Religion from 2006-2007. This collection of narratives does not necessarily reflect the views of the sponsors of this report: the National Institute of Health, Syracuse University, its affiliated departments; the University of North Carolina, Chapel Hill, NC; or the collaborators of the Collaborative Initiative for Research Ethics and Environmental Health. Continued ethics research and training of the Collaborative Initiative for Research Ethics www.researchethics.org is now underway at Brown University Center for Environmental Health, Providence, RI.

We thank Carol Williams, Syracuse, NY, for all her administrative support in the development of this book.

Introduction

Federal health agencies conducted a major health study on people in the Hanford, Washington area who were potentially exposed to 740,000 curies of radioactive iodine in the 1940s and 1950s. The Hanford Thyroid Disease Study involved an extensive attempt to reconstruct doses of people born in areas potentially exposed to radiation from the Hanford plutonium production facility in the 1940s and 1950s. Many of these people studied were those who were offered screening for thyroid problems [1]. The accuracy of the scientific study was a function of a large number of assumptions including the magnitude and timing of releases, modeling of weather conditions, dispersion of fallout through the food chain, and individual behaviors. In the year 1999, the HTDS researchers reported that these radioactive releases were not related to excess thyroid diseases in the Hanford downwind area. Many of the affected people in the area could not believe these findings, felt very strongly that the study was flawed, and saw that there would be no further public health assistance for them from these negative findings. This Hanford study is a critical case example for examining the ethics and fairness of health studies and how scientific studies can benefit or harm researched communities.

Other community groups and their members who were organized for resolving health concerns about impacts from the massive radioactive contamination around their nuclear weapons production facilities (Rocky Flats, CO; Fernald, OH; Livermore Labs, CA) were similarly disappointed with the outcomes of government health research investigations conducted in the 1990s. Health studies that were conducted at these sites did not lead to any meaningful public health follow-up on major health concerns of the community members represented in public participation processes. No studies have yet resulted in a need for reparations to the communities with high radiation exposures that may have caused thyroid, bone, lung, or other relevant diseases. Many federal health researchers were leaving some affected study areas believing that their job in assessing health impacts was done. The September 11th, 2001 terrorist attacks were an urgent crisis that drew many federal health researchers away from continued studies of radiation health impacts from nuclear weapons experiments. Many community members affected by this contamination felt betrayed and deeply disappointed with these scientific research experiences.

The Collaborative Initiative for Research Ethics and Environmental Health (CIREEH), a small collaboration of university-based, public health scientists, and research ethics professionals, received funding in 2003 from the National Institute of Health (NIH) program on "Short Courses for Research Ethics" to assemble a collection of reviews of ethical issues in environmental and occupational health studies of populations exposed to Cold War nuclear experiments. Several CIREEH collaborators have been involved in health promotion and research activities with community groups near nuclear weapons labs and nuclear workers at those labs through the 1990s. The CIREEH requested ethical reflections on several health assessments conducted since 1990, when responsibility for etiologic epidemiology (but not surveillance) was transferred from the Department of Energy (DOE) to the Department of Health and Human Services (DHHS). These health research funds were administered primarily through the National Center for Environmental Health (NCEH) of the Centers for Disease Control (CDC) and the Agency for Toxic Substances and Disease Registry (ATSDR). In this time, DOE also funded several state health departments (i.e., in California and Colorado) to conduct health assessments of community and worker populations. The health assessments were most relevant to policy issues and plans for future research. In an ethical reflection of these health assessments, the CIREEH sought a focus on research relationships that involve community and worker participation. In this collection, we have also included an ethical reflection of Navajo mining studies in order to evaluate the environmental justice and cultural implications of nuclear activities, including Cold War nuclear experiments.

CIREEH collaborators were concerned with ethical issues related to (1) methodological approaches that are criticized in the field for their incomplete assessments of exposures; (2) research findings and study designs that have created distrust of scientific research, particularly among exposed populations; (3) research approaches that create unethical practices by failing to recognize community approval/consent; and (4) research and public health barriers that limit the potential for research to contribute to public health policy. The quality of radiation-risk research can be adversely affected by failure to establish respectful and democratic scientific partnerships involving radiation researchers and exposed populations. The lack of detailed knowledge about the life styles of populations downwind of many DOE facilities, as well as lack of consideration for work practices at the weapons production facilities that are not part of the official record, have led not only to poor science but to distrust on the part of residents and workers whose knowledge has not been represented in official studies. Poor science and low trust limit policy contributions.

In all, eleven ethical reviews have been written and compiled in this collection. The CIREEH contacted community health leaders from around the DOE weapons sites where major research studies were conducted. These community health leaders were directly involved in public participation efforts with those studies and bring a collective ethical assessment from their community to this book. They were also involved at national levels, having appointments with the CDC-ATSDR for national research agenda oversight. Four community-based narratives were written from Hanford, Washington (Trisha Pritikin), Rocky Flats (LeRoy Moore), Livermore Labs (Patricia Sutton, Marylia Kelley, Tracy Barreau, and Jackie Cabasso), and the Fernald Feed Materials Production Center (Edwa Yocum). Three narratives were written from nongovernmental researchers who have published in the radiation research field and have expressed concerns about the ethical adequacy of certain research methods and public involvement in health studies. These narratives include ethical reflections on the National Cancer Institute (NCI) nationwide fallout study by Seth Tuler, who assisted in coordinating public participation in that study. Researchers from Tufts University—Bindu Pannikar, Esther Yazzie, and Doug Brugge, a Navajo community health leader—provide a narrative about ethical issues pertaining to Navajo uranium miner health studies. Bob Alvarez, a policy analyst, focuses his narrative on research conducted on nuclear workers and the compensation awarded to them several years ago. Don Austin, an epidemiologist who conducted a state health department health assessment of workers, provides an ethical analysis of his research experience. Three ethical reviews of the challenges of health research of nuclear weapons impacts are provided by Sheldon Krimsky from Tufts University and Dianne Quigley and Ernest Wallwork of Syracuse University. These ethical analyses provide moral reflections on the conduct of these studies that can assist with improving future research or public health interventions.

The overall purpose of this book is to improve health research and public health programs among populations affected by nuclear weapons activities by incorporating the broader expertise of research ethics: new regulatory guidelines, ethical theories, and applied ethics case studies in community research. Usually the design and conduct of exposure assessments, epidemiologic studies, and risk assessments are developed only from the distinct technical perspectives of each discipline. These narratives and ethical analyses underscore the reality that these technical fields provide an incomplete framework for understanding the potential for research to benefit or harm human populations and their natural environments.

Scientific researchers often have lacked adequate training in public health ethics and may not approach their empirical research investigations with broader considerations for how to maximize benefits, minimize harm, and protect affected communities and workers. Evidence of this problem runs through the reflections of community and nongovernmental researchers assessing these health studies and is strongly criticized in the ethical review analyses. With more training and analysis from research ethics, the integrity of studies conducted by government and academic scientists can be improved. With more understanding of ethical research approaches for affected communities and worker populations, these collective research subjects can be given more beneficence and respect than is provided in standard public participation processes. Research ethics as its own discipline will prioritize protection of individuals/groups; the provision of community agreements/approvals; the mitigating of potential research harms; and a vigilance against forms of scientific contrivance, denial, and suppression of findings. Trained ethicists can bring expertise and experience to complex research issues, particularly those that can affect the multiple interests of diverse stakeholders. Ethical reviews can also contribute to democratic processes and help guard against control of research by institutions that have responsibility for exposing people to hazards.

While these community health studies were underway, the Advisory Committee on Human Radiation Experiments (ACHRE) was compiling recommendations for the federal government concerning research harms and abuses that had occurred to human radiation victims, including atomic veterans, downwinders, as well as Marshall Islanders and Navajo uranium miners. Many of their recommendations focused on the harms to individual research subjects with only several recommendations focused on group harms. Two major areas of their recommendations are priority issues in these ethical reflections. The ACHRE was not supportive of expensive dose-assessment studies in the absence of adequate measurements and recommended that funds be allocated for direct aid to survivors and their families, particularly atomic veterans [2]. The narratives provide evidence of the consequences of dose-assessment studies conducted around the named facilities that often had poor exposure measurements. The cost of these studies was well over $60 million, paid mostly to researchers and their institutions. A second major recommendation of the ACHRE was to increase research-ethics training among researchers due to the committee's grave concern over a lack of research-ethics training and the cultural ignorance of researchers.

With this book, we begin an initial effort to expand understandings of ethical issues involved with the collective risks from human radiation experiments: those to nuclear workers, downwind populations, Native Americans, and other affected cultural groups. Other research-health assessments were conducted at the DOE sites that are not included here. Savannah River, Oak Ridge, the Nevada Test Site, Los Alamos, Mound Laboratories, Piketon, Ohio, and Paducah, Kentucky are areas where there has been a great deal of community health organizing to understand health impacts from nuclear weapons testing and production. A few of these sites have had major health assessments during the past decade [3]. The CIREEH could not include more narratives at this time but would like to expand these ethical assessments. The CIREEH seeks to promote more assistance to these affected groups and communities with the support of research ethics. Such support is needed by many community groups working for health protection from contaminating facilities across the country.

NOTES

1. National Academy of Sciences. 2000. *An assessment of Centers for Disease Control and Prevention Radiation Studies: Review of Hanford Thyroid Disease Study Final Results and Report.* Washington, DC: National Academy Press.
2. Advisory Committee on Human Radiation Experiments. 1995. Chapter 18, Rec. V. Washington, DC: U.S. Government Printing Office.
3. For further information about all these health assessments, please go the website of the Centers for Disease Control and its link to "Radiation Studies," www.cdc.gov/nceh/radiation

http://dx.doi.org/10.2190/TORC1

CHAPTER 1

Commentary on Ethics and Community-Based Research: Responsibility, Precaution, and Transparency

Sheldon Krimsky

The narratives about the "downwinders" at the Hanford nuclear site describe communities stricken with grief from their experiences of elevated thyroid cancer and other diseases, which they attribute to radiation exposures from plutonium and uranium processing facilities [1]. Closure has not come after 50 years of uncertainty about the nature and causes of the disease patterns.

The Manhattan Project, a national priority effort to develop the atomic bomb, was supported by a culture of secrecy, which was deemed necessary to prevent the Germans from winning the race with the allies to unleash the power of nuclear fission. Ironically, the first use of the atomic bomb on civilians was not on Germany but on Japan, which did not have an active program for developing an atomic weapon of mass destruction.

The secrecy surrounding the development of the A-bomb extended to every aspect of its production and the hastily created communities that were formed around research and production facilities to support its development. It is even reported that Vice President Truman was not aware of the A-bomb project when it was initiated [2]. Similar examples of secrecy can be found with testing of atomic weapons in Nevada and more recently with the exposures American soldiers received from drugs and environmental chemicals during the first Gulf War period in the early 1990s [3].

A veil of secrecy hung over the radiation exposure soldiers received in the 1940s and 1950s as they observed atmospheric atomic testing. For decades government agencies (Atomic Energy Commission and the Department of Energy) refused to follow up on the illnesses of the atomic vets, who in later life felt they were treated like guinea pigs and abandoned after they participated in the early tests [4]. After the first Iraq Gulf War, returning veterans complained of a variety of neurological symptoms [5]. Initially, there was little or no transparency about the chemicals and vaccines soldiers might have been exposed to. The complex and diverse set of symptoms they reported during and after their military service did not comprise an easily recognizable pattern of disease. Their symptoms were like those of people who have been diagnosed with "multiple chemical sensitivity," a syndrome few medical practitioners believe is the result of environmental exposure.

In each of these cases (atomic testing, Gulf War exposures, and emissions from nuclear production facilities), the affected parties sought redress or validation from their government of the health claims of citizens and the need for continued health monitoring, and compensation to the families who had to deal with a close relative's protracted health problems.

SECRECY AT FEDERAL NUCLEAR SITES

At the Hanford nuclear weapons facility, the U.S. Government's initial secrecy conditions can be understood because of the strict national security requirements in effect during World War II. After the war, the global leadership in nuclear energy of the United States was no longer in question. New secrecy considerations were imposed in response to the arms race between the United States and the USSR, but there were no longer any secrets about the *function* of Hanford and its plutonium processing facilities. And there was no longer an overriding state interest in keeping people who worked at Hanford and who lived in Richland, Kennewick, Pasco, and other communities from understanding their exposures to radionuclides as well as to the importance of monitoring their risks from radiation disease.

The reason for continued secrecy and for the repression of any inquiry into health effects from radiation exposure is more likely the result of the government's effort to maintain weapon's production, minimize the expense or personnel effort needed to prevent exposures, and to avoid having to compensate workers or private citizens for radiation illness.

Yocum's report describes how government secrecy played itself out in the Fernald, Ohio communities where state and federal agencies continued to stay in the background and not communicate with the affected community [6]. As a consequence, the agencies lost their credibility with the community.

The atomic vets who were exposed to fallout radiation in the Nevada desert from the early atomic testing in the late 1940s and early 1950s wore exposure badges. When they retired from the military they were supposed to submit their badges to the military command. By the 1970s and 1980s, when the growing concern about the radiation disease of atomic vets influenced Congress to request health effects studies, it was learned that many of the radiation badges were lost or consumed by fires [7]. Thus, health-effects studies based on dosimetry measurements were constrained by missing information describing the exposure received by those serving in the military during the 1940s and 1950s.

Ms. Pritikin's account of the Hanford communities' thyroid disease explains the functionality of "compartmentalization" (restricting each person's knowledge to their own specific tasks) in the culture of atomic secrecy [8]. The concept of compartmentalization applied to the public health effects of radiation also functioned to protect the production system from being questioned. By treating each health effect as an isolated "monad" without tying it to the whole system, government bodies would not have to face the problem that the risks of the post-war production facility, which manufactured weapons grade uranium and plutonium, might outweigh the benefits, or that people were treated not as ends-in-themselves but as a means to an end, violating an important ethical principle that is essential for human dignity. The secrecy and compartmentalization that was emblematic of the post-war production at Hanford reduced the possibility of learning what the health risks could be.

COMMUNITY-INFORMED CONSENT

During the 1950s and 1960s the ethics of informed consent in human experiments had not yet been developed. It wasn't until the publication in 1979 of the Belmont Report on the ethical principles for the protection of human subjects that informed consent was codified for federally-sponsored experiments with human subjects. After reports appeared in the national press on the abuse of human research subjects, especially in poor communities, in prisons, and in state mental health facilities, Congress passed legislation that established our current regulations on the protection of human subjects. The Hanford experience speaks out for another form of informed consent; we can call it "community-informed consent." This form of informed consent has not been institutionalized in the United States with one exception. The courts have recognized the concept of community-informed consent for addressing issues of pornography. The term "community standards" is a legal concept that helps to resolve contested claims pitting free speech against offensive speech. Adult published materials and the sex trade must meet community standards. This is a new concept of informed consent at the community scale.

Informed consent applied to research and industrial facilities that carry risks involves both an "informed" component, namely, transparency about the risks including uncertainties in measurement, and once the risks are communicated properly, a requirement of community consent. Both of these components were missing for communities in the vicinity of the Hanford site.

A contemporary example of the application of community-informed consent can be found in a controversy over the siting of a research laboratory in Cambridge, Massachusetts in the mid-1980s. The respected consulting firm Arthur D. Little signed a contract with the Department of Defense (DOD) to develop more effective military defenses against chemical warfare agents like VX and soman. Secrecy about the laboratory was part of the contract negotiations [9]. Elected officials were told nothing about the research and the purpose behind the construction of the new state-of-the-art laboratory, which was situated near a bowling alley and a daycare center. Local fire department officials were advised of the chemicals being stored in the facility so that they could be prepared in the case of a fire. One of the fire officials leaked the information to elected officials in an adjoining town whereupon the siting of the DOD-funded laboratory became a public issue [10]. The City of Cambridge convened a commission consisting of sixteen individuals including public health experts and community residents. The commission met for several months to determine the risks of a worst-case scenario and then reached a decision over whether the risks were acceptable on "community standards." It is important to note that the Cambridge citizens' commission did not base its decision on balancing the risks of the research on chemical warfare agents with national security interests. If any balancing took place it was between the risks and benefits of the research to the community.

In its report to the city, the commission's unanimous decision was that the risks of the chemical warfare research were not justified when measured against the benefits to the community [10]. The decision was supported by the city's chief health officer and in subsequent litigation upheld by the Supreme Judicial Court of Massachusetts. This is one of a growing number of cases where the concept of community standards is being applied to risk assessment [10].

RESPONSIBILITY TO INFORM AND INVESTIGATE

The courts have consistently recognized the responsibility of corporations to inform consumers about the dangers of their products. When corporations intentionally withhold information about the risks, dangers, or adverse effects of chemicals or consumer products, they are liable for fines or formidable product-liability settlements. DuPont agreed to pay $16.5 million in a settlement of an EPA lawsuit challenging the company for withholding information on the toxicological effects of Perfluorooctanoic Acid (PFOA), a chemical used in the manufacture of nonstick pans. The obligation to inform runs deeply in American jurisprudence. Because government agencies can be shielded from liability suits by individuals and organizations, one can argue that its responsibility to inform is missing a powerful incentive.

The Hanford nuclear weapons production facility provides a useful case for discussing the government's role and responsibility for informing communities of potential hazards from toxic substances that are the byproducts of federal weapons production facilities and its responsibility for investigating claims. Elevated risk levels of a disease related to by-products of a government facility is *prima facie* evidence, albeit circumstantial, of a connection between the emissions and the disease. If the evidence is corroborated (elevated thyroid disease), then the government's responsibility to inform and to investigate becomes clear. If the evidence remains circumstantial, there may still be government responsibility to continue investigating the claims until there is a semblance of closure in the minds of the communities at risk.

Closure is a key element in a community's social psychology of perceived health effects from toxic chemicals. Health experts may reach a conclusion that a locally desired health study is not a good use of public funds or that it is unlikely to yield results. But like a parent looking for a lost child, turning over every stone is part of the process of reaching closure and peace of mind. Community residents at Fernald, Ohio, wanted the Centers for Disease Control to investigate the groundwater pathway for radionuclide and toxic chemical release from the Nuclear Feed Material Production Center. But according to Yocum, their request was ignored by the CDC [6]. Yocum's account depicts a community that received no closure on the issues of concern. For example, the health report was issued four years late and failed to respond to many questions still being asked by the residents.

It is of course possible that some studies requested by the community might be methodologically difficult or impossible to carry out. In such cases, it would seem that an equitable approach is for government to explore possibilities with the community and work out alternative studies that might bring the community to closure.

In the case of Hanford, another ethical concern is conflicts of interest. Historically, the research and development and safety functions of the Atomic Energy Commission were eventually divided between the Department of Energy and the Nuclear Regulatory Commission. Eventually Congress acknowledged that one agency should not have the responsibility for both promoting the development and evaluating the safety of nuclear energy. The same standards should apply to investigations of the health effects of nuclear production facilities. When the federal government became apprised of the public concerns over elevated rates of thyroid diseases in towns surrounding the Hanford facility, the responsibility for investigating, evaluating, and monitoring the health effects should have been assigned to an agency or independent research center that was neither administratively nor financially connected to the DOE.

The decision to call upon the Centers for Disease Control and the Fred Hutchinson Cancer Research Center to conduct the Hanford Thyroid Disease Study, looks on the surface to be a good model. The CDC is not under the DOE.

The fact that the selection was congressionally mandated also distinguishes it from a DOE initiative. However, Pritikin's chapter discusses how the recommendations of the Agency for Toxic Substances Disease Registry (ATSDR), a subunit of the CDC, for medical monitoring were dependent on funding from the DOE [8]. This situation could be construed as a conflict of interest, as one might argue that the agency responsible for producing radioactive contamination should not be the same party sponsoring an investigation into the health risks associated with said contamination. Even the remote appearance of conflict of interest can weaken the community's confidence in the process.

Given that there was a special interest in the study by the community, by virtue of its unique relationship to the Hanford facility, an argument can be made that the CDC and Hutchinson had a responsibility to communicate with the community during the planning phase and upon release of the results of the thyroid study. Community residents who were experiencing thyroid abnormalities or diseases potentially had valuable information that could have informed the investigation. I have argued elsewhere that there are categories of technical problems where nontrivial contributions can be made by nonexperts in the investigations and solutions. The neglect of these types of contributions I call "folk wisdom" may result in inferior outcomes or lost opportunities [11]. The reason for this is that the socialization of experts and their restricted cognitive structures can neglect some important components of knowledge. The highly specialized and reductionist nature of scientific inquiry can be aided by more intuitive, personal, and holistic approaches to problem solving.

Members of the team investigating thyroid disease in communities exposed to radionuclides from the Hanford facility have a responsibility for doing dependable, independent, and disinterested science. But they also have a responsibility for reflecting on and reporting the limitations of their measurements including the sensitivity of the measuring instrument. Epidemiological studies are much more valuable when they show a correlation than when they do not show a correlation. The reason for this is in the nature of epistemology. Epidemiology is a blunt instrument for measuring the correlation between exposure and disease. Blunt instruments underreport health effects. Typically, epidemiological studies yield more false negatives than false positives. Therefore, a positive result is more significant in epistemic terms than a negative result. As an example, if a scientist is looking for a bacteriological agent as the cause of a disease but has a low-powered microscope, failure to see a bacterium under the microscope is not a good reason to discard the hypothesis that there is an infectious agent. Negative findings are not conclusive. But a positive finding may be. "No evidence of an effect is not the same as evidence of no effect." Moreover, the failure to demonstrate causality or a dose-response effect for humans does not relinquish responsibility for responding to community needs. This point is made in Seth Tuler's discussion of seeking justice in the face of radioactive iodine releases [12]. Tuler cites the community advisory board's advice to the DHHS:

"The difficulties in identifying individuals whose injuries are caused by fallout exposure does not absolve the federal government of its civil and moral responsibility to aid the injured."

Because of these epistemological conditions, authors of dose response studies have a responsibility to discuss the power of the study, to report error bars on measurements, and to explain how these factors affect the confidence level of the conclusions. An instrument of low power with high measurement errors will have low confidence. Applying error bars on measurements can be used to calculate different outcomes based on low, medium, and high values of a dose.

Those in the affected communities who have credible circumstantial evidence of an adverse environmental health effect will undoubtedly not find closure when a blunt instrument uses dose estimates that are subject to large errors. The Hanford Thyroid Disease Study (HTDS) reached the conclusion that for the communities surrounding Hanford, there was no dose-response relationship between exposure to radioactive iodine and thyroid disease. Based on studies of endocrine disruptors, we now know that chemicals can exhibit an inverted "U-shaped" dose-response curve. These chemicals can produce adverse biological effects on mammals despite their nonmonotonic dose-response characteristics. A mistake would be made if failure to find a monotonic dose-response function for these chemicals led one to the conclusion that the chemicals did not cause an adverse effect [13].

PLUTONIUM SLUDGE

It sounds like a bad joke: plutonium sludge used to fertilize people's vegetable gardens. What were people thinking at the time? Was this sludge considered a good source of plant nutrients? Did they assume that small amounts of radioactivity in the sludge was not unsafe and that adopting the sludge was a sign of being patriotic? Had the homeowners who brought the sludge into their vegetable gardens thought about the risks? Was it a time when people did not ask any questions about radiation?

Sutton and colleagues describe the efforts of communities to acquire information on the human effects of plutonium sludge used in community gardens [14]. How did people justify the use of plutonium sludge as a "soil conditioner in parks, landscaping around public buildings, and in home lawns and gardens?" Was this all an honest mistake or was this a devious way for the Livermore Water Reclamation Plant (LWRP) to save the expense of landfilling radioactive sludge?

Radiation hazards have been known since the 1940s, but extensive studies began in the 1950s and 1960s. Tolerance levels for radiation were reduced in the 1970s and 1980s as more knowledge of the health effects, especially effects from lower doses, became available. The levels of acceptable X-ray doses for dentistry, mammography, and CAT scans were reduced to conform to new health information as the technology improved. The new X-ray technology made it possible to get good photos with better resolution and lower doses of radiation.

Once it became known that the health effects of radiation exposure were more hazardous than originally believed, what responsibility did government have to those who were given plutonium-laced sludge?

Under current environmental standards, there is support for the idea that the government's responsibility for plutonium risks should be covered "from cradle to grave." In other words, the government's oversight should include every aspect of production, distribution, storage, and disposal until the plutonium is out of sight and out of mind as a potential hazard to current or future populations. If science's understanding and knowledge of plutonium risks changes after the sludge is distributed to communities, a reasonable expectation would be for the government to reexamine the false negatives or its original policy and continue to track the exposed population for health effects.

PSYCHO-SOCIAL ASPECTS OF CLOSURE

Members of the public who were told the sludge was entirely safe may justifiably feel deceived by their government. They may ask, What did the government know and when did they know it? Or did government officials responsible for public safety initially ask the right questions before distributing the sludge? Did they take account of the uncertainties? What is the proper response of government when a community is seeking closure while at the same time trying to grasp its own vulnerability to plutonium hazards.

Loss of confidence by the community can only be regained if the community is brought into the process of assessing the risks. Government-community collaborations become important for several reasons. First, it sends a message to the residents that whatever mistakes might have been made in the past, the investigative agency intends to discover the truth about the health risks. Second, it acknowledges that members of the community who were exposed to higher levels of radiation have valuable knowledge about the historical events that can be useful to an investigative body. Including community members on advisory committees or health study teams can make the tacit and phenomenological knowledge more accessible.

It is unlikely that closure in this case could be attainable from a single study. More probable, however, is that closure (if it comes at all) will arise as the result of a continuing process of monitoring health effects and community-agency interactions. People have become dubious and inured to government claims that "the community is not at risk" or that "the plaintiff's sufferings have nothing to do with popular views about causation." This was said about Gulf War vets and the communities exposed to the contaminated air from the World Trade Center catastrophe. In both cases, initial claims of the health risks were premature and eventually proven false [15].

Concerns about risk from a serious exposure to toxic substances, especially but not only mixtures, must be taken through the life of those exposed and in some cases to the next generation. From epigenetic studies of mice, we have learned that imprinting from the exposure of a pregnant mouse (F_0) can be carried through two generations (F_1 and F_2), even as we fail to see any gross genetic abnormalities. This imposes a transgenerational responsibility on agencies investigating environmental contamination that may have been caused by governmental policies.

The Rocky Flats case study by Moore discusses the tireless efforts by Carl J. Johnson, who served as the chief public health office for Jefferson County, Colorado. Johnson brought to the public's attention the plutonium contamination from the government's nuclear bomb factory [16]. Moore's narrative describes the extent to which a government agency will go to protect its image or avoid taking responsibility for untoward events. Ironically, agencies of a government by the people exercise many of the tactics we have come to expect from corporations who seek to protect their image and power for the sake of their bottom line. Some would argue that an agency such as DOE, which took over some of the responsibilities of the Atomic Energy Commission, should not have been given the responsibility to oversee the safety of the facility or to set the standards for safe soil. Moore's example that DOE paid a contractor to refute Johnson's studies illustrates its interest in assuring the public that it had acted appropriately in the face of allegations that the public was endangered by plutonium contamination.

In Moore's account of Rocky Flats, one of the protagonists involved in the investigation into health hazards was quoted as saying: "For more than 40 years, assessment of health risks of radionuclides has been controlled by a vested interest establishment that has contrived to minimize or ignore adverse effects of all sources of human exposure to ionizing radiation." Why are government agencies so recalcitrant to engage in honest and open investigations of federal facilities, in particular, federal nuclear facilities? There are probably several reasons. First, government agencies do not like the negative publicity that arises from embarrassing congressional investigations and media spotlights on their practices. And while they might be called unresponsive or insensitive to community concerns by the local press, that might appear less worrisome to the agency than the disclosure of evidence of serious health hazards for which it has a role.

Second, while it might not be easy to sue a government agency, Congress can put pressure on agencies to pay compensation for health injury to the community. Alternatively, Congress can pass legislation to address compensation awards. In either case, agencies become defensive when they are faced with allegations of government-related activities that were responsible for illness. It took 30 years for a sitting president to apologize for the country to the people of Tuskegee, Alabama for the unethical experiments performed by government employees on black patients who had acquired sexually transmitted diseases [17].

People who take leadership roles in government agencies somehow become self-identified with the agency and are likely to take on a protective role defending the agency against any malfeasance rather than a role that is empathetic to community concerns. The third factor that could explain the behavior of federal agencies toward community health concerns (whether those agencies develop nuclear power or weapons or they evaluate the health risks of nuclear technology) has to do with the politics of that technology. Agency officials are hesitant to provide the grist in the form of health-effects data that will afford citizens greater reason to oppose further development of nuclear power. Federal health agencies typically set the bar high for demonstrating causality. While they do not make it impossible to accept cause and effect, the bar is much higher than "circumstantial evidence" from elevated disease rates or occupational illness.

Deception was a theme raised by community residents at the Rocky Flats, Hanford, and Livermore sites. When residents feel deceived about the safety of a facility, it is *prima facie* evidence that informed consent was not satisfactorily implemented. The community residents either felt that the high-level administrators knew things about the potential hazards that they did not communicate or they downgraded the importance of the uncertainties.

In clinical trials, if human subjects feel deceived then something is deficient about the informed-consent process. Perhaps the subjects were not adequately informed about the magnitude of the risks or their probability. In one highly publicized case at the University of Pennsylvania, the subject was not adequately informed about the conflicts of interest held by the institution and the clinical investigator [18]. Similarly, without a clear disclosure statement to the community, there can be no informed consent regarding a potentially hazardous facility.

Panikkar and colleagues have written an informative and stimulating chapter on uranium mining and the Navajo people [19]. The chapter documents the incidence of lung disease among Navajo miners, the beginnings of a government response to occupational and community illness from the uranium tailings and radon gas, the desecration of land from open-pit mining, and the growth of research on the health effects of uranium mining on the Navajo community. There is consistency between the findings of these authors and those who have written about Lawrence Livermore and Hanford on the fact that corporations involved in uranium mining, as well as the Atomic Energy Commission, the major federal agency responsible for uranium processing, turned a blind eye to the concerns of occupational sickness of uranium miners. They write ". . . from 1948–1969, no federal occupational standards kept miners safe from the harms of radiation and such intense mining" [19, p. 143]. This is another case in which a community of workers and their families have not felt that there has been satisfactory closure to their grievances which stem from the long period during which workers' health and safety were compromised. After many decades of filing claims, Congress finally acted by passing the Radiation Exposure Compensation Act, which gave workers and their families 20 years to file claims after 1990.

When some scientists were prepared to speak out about the hazards, they were told by their superiors to limit their speech. What is the ethical responsibility of public health researchers, who in the process of studying miners learned of their endangerment in the mines? Do they have a responsibility to warn the workers immediately? Should they get permission from superiors before informing workers about their risks? Should they remain completely neutral and simply produce research results that others can use to inform workers? These issues remain no less resolved today than they were 50 years ago. There are recent cases of physicians involved in clinical trials who felt that they had a moral obligation to warn patients about the risks of a drug therapy before a clinical trial was completed, despite legal warnings from their private sponsor [18]. That is a responsibility they bear from the Hippocratic Oath in their role as a doctor. But they also have a legal responsibility, by virtue of a contract or grant, to the company or government agency sponsoring the trial [20]. Their legal responsibility may be in conflict with informing the patient—at least before the trial was completed. Physicians working within government agencies are also obligated to follow agency protocols on making public declarations. Usually important risk communications are made through the agency director and not through individual researchers. The Supreme Court has recently ruled on public versus private speech of agency personnel arguing that an employee of an agency must follow the agency rules and protocols when they are under the aegis of making "public speech" [21]. According to a 5-4 decision of the Supreme Court "public employees' free-speech rights are protected when they speak out as citizens on matters of public concern, but not when they speak out in the course of their official duties" [22] Thus, the current ruling is consistent with the head of the Public Health Service's statement in its 1952 study. "We did not want to rock the boat . . . We had to take the position that we were neutral scientists trying to find out what the factors were, that we were not going to make any public announcements until the results of the study were published" [19]. Of course the head of the agency, like the principal investigator of any clinical trial, can decide to inform the participants that they are at risk and can advise them to minimize or avoid that risk. Panikkar and colleagues ask "At what point is it ethically incumbent upon researchers to 'go public' or even commit civil disobedience by disobeying orders to protect the lives of affected workers" [19].

The responsibility to inform human subjects of their risks during the progress of a clinical trial is well established in the aftermath of the Tuskegee experiments. But suppose the research is an epidemiological study. Do the investigators bear the same responsibility? Social and public health scientists cannot hide behind the premise that they are passive observers and that because they are not testing a drug or medical device on a population they are excused from informing research subjects of risks that they are facing. Let us assume, for example, that an epidemiological team is studying a group of workers who are exposed to vinyl chloride. If the team finds unambiguous evidence that there is an elevated risk of liver cancer in this occupational cohort compared with workers who are not exposed to the chemical, then it would seem irresponsible not to report this result and not to make recommendations for reducing or eliminating the risk. Similarly, under current standards, if miners are found to have higher risks of lung cancer, public health scientists bear a moral responsibility to inform them of the risks. Like the bystander who watches an assault and who is capable of informing the police to take action, the public health scientist cannot morally disengage from subjects when he or she has specialized knowledge that they are endangered from their workplace exposures. According to Panikkar and colleagues, at least one court concluded that physicians examining miners did not have a legal responsibility "to advise the miners voluntarily appearing for examinations of potential hazards in uranium mines . . ." [19]. Since that time ethical standards in research have changed. Institutional Review Boards (IRB) may set a high ethical bar on the fiduciary responsibility of researchers. A high moral standard for researchers is to (1) report; (2) inform; and (3) advise. This means that researchers should not hide valuable public health information because of political expedience. They should be responsible to inform the vulnerable populations of their risk. Beyond that, as knowledge bearers, they have a fiduciary responsibility to advise human subjects about reducing their risks. But the standards are not uniform and depend on the local conditions of the IRB.

COMMUNITY-BASED PARTICIPATORY RESEARCH

Community-Based Participatory Research (CBPR) can take several forms. At the minimum it can mean that researchers consult with and draw knowledge from members of the community in designing or executing the research protocol. It can also mean that researchers partner with members of the community by including them in the research team and as authors in a subsequent study. Luz Claudio, a public health scientist at the Mount Sinai School of Medicine, worked with community leaders in New York City to study the effect on residents of the air pollution from a power-generating plant. Her model of CBPR also included co-authorship of publications by Mt. Sinai scientists and community leaders involved in the study [18].

During the early 1980s, the Harvard School of Public Health conducted a study of the potential health effects of drinking water contamination from two town wells in Woburn, Massachusetts. Over three-hundred volunteers trained by Harvard scientists surveyed Woburn residents about abnormal pregnancies and childhood disorders. According to Brown and Mikkelsen,

> The most common objections to the study were directed against the very concept of public participation in science. All the critics charged that the

> study was biased because volunteers had conducted the health survey and because the study had a political goal [23, p. 26].

There are many other instances in which corporate-funded health studies and/or government-funded studies neglect the valuable perspective of community residents resulting in a biased outcome [24]. Research objectivity is an important ethical norm in science that must be protected whether or not the research is community-based, government-funded, or industry-funded.

ACCEPTABLE RISK

In the framework of risk management, the term "acceptable risk" is, on the surface, a normative idea. It means "What risk ought we (I) accept?" It is easy for people to conclude that "acceptable risk" is a subjective idea. Panikkar and colleagues state:

> There is always the problem of what level of risk is considered "acceptable." There is no scientific answer to the question of acceptable risk because it depends heavily on the personal values of each individual and communities and various moderating factors, such as income and employment that may be taken into consideration [19, p. 157].

For many normative or aesthetic judgments, there is certainly no scientific solution or empirical evidence to resolve the issue. But there is one thing to consider in the realm of public health. If a biological organism is under significant threat from an environmental exposure, then we can conclude that the risk is "unacceptable." Biological health is the bridge that crosses the normative and empirical realms. Biological health is the grounding for taking a moral position on deadly toxic exposures. It is still logically possible to say: "The exposure is killing the organism" and "The risk to the organism is acceptable." From a practical standpoint, rational beings would not accept these two statements unless your goal is to do harm or the organism is engaged in a higher good by being exposed. Of course there are circumstances where people expose themselves to deadly risks in time of war. But these are extraordinary times and people fighting in battle must set aside personal safety and rationality by following orders.

The case study by Robert Alvarez on the occupational health hazards of the nuclear weapons program shows us what happens to ethics during periods of national exigency [25]. But there are different time periods represented in the case. National exigency cannot be applied to all the periods. During the war, one can imagine the focus of the federal government toward one end and one end only, namely the production of the atomic bomb. The conventional explanation is that there was not time to both take a precautionary approach and get the job done—at least that's how most narratives of that period are written. This was, after all, wartime. But there is, even in war, an effort to account for and document the wounded. Documenting wartime casualties and helping the wounded is an important part of the government's responsibility. Ironically, more data were collected about combat soldiers than there were about the civilian "soldiers" at home producing the weapons and invariably exposed to the dangers of atomic radiation.

How do we account for the government's effort to cover up the occupational illnesses from radiation that were occurring after the war and through the 1950s and 1960s? The most prevalent story is that federal agencies (primarily but not exclusively the U.S. Atomic Energy Commission) were still engaged in a war, we called the "cold war," and just as feverishly driven to produce weapons of mass destruction to compete with the Soviet threat. After World War II we weren't just producing one or two atomic bombs. The nuclear production system was in the business of producing thousands of nuclear warheads, expanding the number of workers exposed to radiation. Thus, the impulse to turn a blind eye to radiation hazards was part of the same tunnel vision that occupied the agencies during wartime. When individual radiation health experts began to leak out data, the agency saw itself as wanting to protect its mission; everything else was secondary. Thus, they asked what the impact of releasing risk information and health data would be to the radiation workers. The value system in which they operated was that all decisions must be viewed in terms of whether they will support or detract from the primary mission. It was a time when cancer was kept quiet in families. No one talked about cancer in the media. Alvarez encapsulates these ideas in this statement "Fears over liability and lack of public trust that might result from disclosure of workplace hazards was of dominant concern." It took many years for the government to finally adopt a position that any person in the street would have acknowledged from the outset. "An agency whose mission it is to promote the development of nuclear weapons should not be responsible for studying the risks to workers or the general population of its production facilities" [25]. The AEC had its blinders on when there were debates over atmospheric testing. Until independent scientists from other agencies and universities were able to assess the data of radiation hazards, the public only received public relations notices designed to keep the manufacturing process on course and to protect the budgets from paying out compensation to workers who were stricken with radiation disease and ancillary medical problems. Releasing health information that might affect the agency mission was heretical to those who had but one missionary zeal—to keep up the flow of weapons.

PUBLISHING PRELIMINARY FINDINGS

One of the ethical dilemmas raised by the Alvarez case relates to the publication of preliminary findings. Early release of preliminary results may either exaggerate the risks (false positives) or understate the effects (false negatives). Complex public health assessments of environmental or occupational exposures often require iterative analyses, peer review, reanalysis of data, and additional or multiple data sources before consensus can be reached about the findings. There is no consensus among scientists or bioethicists on the ethics of publishing preliminary findings. The decision about whether to publish preliminary data or to wait for additional studies and more data can be made on scientific grounds, but is often guided by political or legal considerations. Journal editors may decide that the analysis is premature and not ready for publication. Investigators usually want to publish quickly so they will have standing in the scientific community on the subject matter. Or there may be competition among investigators over who will be first to publish on the subject matter. However, scientists must weigh the ethical consequences of publishing preliminary results. Will the release of the preliminary data bring anxiety and stress to a population at risk? Will the release create negative publicity for a public agency? Will the publication of preliminary data yield results that the investigator later will have to retract, potentially diminishing his or her stature in the field? However, I would make a distinction between withholding publication based on the quality of the science versus doing so out of concern for the political fallout of the results. Alvarez quotes Samuel Milham, an epidemiologist at the Department of Social and Health Services, Washington State who said "I felt that publication of my findings at this time might disturb the continuity of the study in progress and might cause undue concern in workers" [25].

There are some ethical considerations with regard to publishing preliminary data that *should* enter into decision making. If people can be helped, in a precautionary way, from the communication of preliminary results of a health study, then, it can be argued; there is an ethical responsibility to get the data out early. For example, if the preliminary data suggest a continuing health risk and one for which there is some action that can be taken to prevent further injury, then releasing preliminary data can be a duty. As a general norm, knowledge that can prevent harm should be communicated to the appropriate audience. The debate gets more complex if the data are released through the press rather than through a scientific journal. It is the responsibility of the individual investigator to balance the interests of science with the interests of public health. The scientist may decide that the preliminary data, while suggestive of health risks from an occupational exposure, is not sufficiently reliable to impel a "responsibility to inform." The scientist is not solely acting on his or her own. Journal editors make their own determination over whether the preliminary results should be reported in their journal. The journals may be hesitant to publish a paper based on preliminary and possibly incomplete data, yet the author may feel an obligation to warn people who, he or she believes, are currently at risk.

Public agencies are generally much more cautious about releasing preliminary findings than individuals or journals because if they misguide action by a premature release, they will be severely criticized by stakeholder groups, the media, and politicians. On the other hand, if they remain quiet and do not release their findings, they are unlikely to get criticized, but will probably be viewed as being cautious. By acting conservatively on the release of early findings, the agency is protecting its image foremost but may also be responding to political winds that do not want to create public angst or foster litigation against the government or "responsible" corporate parties.

In one respect, independent scientists have autonomy over when and how they publish their results. Journals, as the gatekeepers of certifiable knowledge, act as a control agent against premature publications. On occasion, scientists have been known to report their data to the press prior to or in lieu of getting it published. There has been a serious ethical critique of such practices, known as "science by press conference." Some journals have adopted policies against publishing original articles if the data were released to the press prior to publication.

INSTITUTIONAL CONFLICTS OF INTEREST

Alvarez reports that former Secretary of Health, Education and Welfare Joseph Califano declared that "DOE had a potential conflict-of-interest between its missions of military and civilian nuclear energy development and assessing their health risks." The definition and standards for institutional conflict of interest have been slow to emerge even as Congress has acted legislatively on setting standards of conflict of interest for government employees and issued guidelines to universities on academic conflicts of interest. The USDA is often cited as an agency that regulates and promote agricultural products—an inherent conflict of interest in meeting the public interest. It is difficult for an agency to resolve these conflicts without separating the functions in different agencies. The Environmental Protection Agency was created so that one agency wouldn't be regulating pesticides while simultaneously promoting them for use in agriculture. Eventually, that is what happened to the Atomic Energy Commission and the Department of Energy. The safety assessment function of nuclear weapons and energy production was placed with an agency that was not promoting or funding its development, namely the Nuclear Regulatory Commission. But for agencies that still operate under competing or potentially conflicting missions, accountability for potential conflicts of interest comes only from the oversight by Congress, the General Accounting Office, or from the independent Inspector General, who will report on how effective the balance in these missions is carried out.

CONCLUSION

Community-based research, in contrast to "research on communities," is a process through which science and citizens are symbiotic to the research mission. Sometimes it means that the research protocols or hypotheses are driven by community interests. Or it could mean that citizens and scientists are partners in the research process. The cases reported in this commentary describe how community values and ethical considerations enter into public and occupational health research from past negligence by federal and state agencies from lack of oversight, failure to respond to grievances, or neglect of compensation for illnesses. Many of the cases refer to events that took place around nuclear weapons production and testing. But the issues are not simply of historical interest. The ethical problems are recurring. In 2001 when fireman, forensic experts, police and cleanup crews were sent to the World Trade Center in the aftermath of its destruction by acts of terrorism, they were exposed to extremely unhealthy air that was filled with the fine granular remains of plastics, glass and concrete that pulverized during the collapse of two 100-story buildings. These individuals, known as first responders, were advised that the air in downtown Manhattan was safe—many therefore did not use safety masks. Five years later, medical and public health scientists were investigating the etiology of lung diseases and leukemia reported in this population. No clear accountability has been established for the incomplete and poor science that contributed to the misinformation about air quality post 9-11. Because precautionary action was not taken at the time, many more lives were shortened beyond those affected directly by the unconscionable acts of terrorism associated with a day that will live in infamy.

NOTES

1. D'Antonio, M. 1993. *Atomic harvest: Hanford and the lethal toll of America's nuclear arsenal.* New York: Crown Publishers.
2. Bernstein, B. J. 1975. Roosevelt, Truman, and the atomic bomb, 1941-1945: A reinterpretation. *Political Science Quarterly* 90:23-69.
3. Kang, H. K., Natelson, B. H., Mahal, C. M., et al. 2003. Post-traumatic stress disorder and chronic fatigue syndrome-like illness among Gulf War veterans: A population-based survey of 30,000 veterans. *American Journal of Epidemiology* 157:141-148.
4. Uhl, M., and Ensign, T. 1980. *GI Guinea Pigs.* New York: Wideview Books.
5. McCauley, L. A., Rischitelli, G., Lambert, W. E., et al. 2001. Symptoms of Gulf War veterans possibly exposed to organophosphate chemical warfare agents at Khamisiyah, Iraq. *International Journal of Occupational and Environmental Health* 7:79-89.
6. Yocum, E. 2011. *A community's experience with environmental health research at the Fernald feed production plant.* In this volume, pp. 53-67. Amityville, NY: Baywood.
7. Johnson, J. C., Thaut, S., and Page, W. F. 1996. *Mortality of veteran participants in the Crossroads Nuclear Test.* Washington, DC: National Academy of Sciences.
8. Pritikin, T. 2011. *Insignificant and invisible: The human toll of the Hanford Thyroid Disease Study.* In this volume, pp. 25-52. Amityville, NY: Baywood.

9. Krimsky, S. 1986. Local control of research involving chemical warfare agents. In *Governing science and technology in a democracy*, ed. M. L. Goggin, 194-217. Knoxville, TN: University of Tennessee Press.
10. Krimsky, S. 1986. Research under community standards: Three case studies. *Science, Technology & Human Values* 11(3):14-33.
11. Krimsky, S. 1984. Epistemic considerations on the value of folk-wisdom in science and technology. *Policy Studies Review* 3(2):245-262.
12. Tuler, S. 2011. *Institutional preferences for justice, avoiding harm, and expertise in public health policy making about the health consequences of iodine-131 nuclear weapons testing fallout.* In this volume, pp. 121-142. Amityville, NY: Baywood.
13. Krimsky, S. 2000. *Hormonal chaos*. Baltimore, MD: Johns Hopkins University Press.
14. Sutton, P., Cabasso, J., Barreau, T., and Kelley, M. 2011. *A collaborative effort to address the distribution of plutonium-contaminated sludge in Livermore, California.* In this volume, pp. 99-119. Amityville, NY: Baywood.
15. Haughney, C. 2003. Health effects at World Trade Center debated. *Washington Post,* January 7, p. A03.
16. Moore, L. 2011. *Democracy and public health at Rocky Flats: The examples of Edward A. Martell and Carl J. Johnson*. In this volume, pp. 69-97. Amityville, NY: Baywood.
17. Harter, L. M., Stephens, R. J., Japp, P. M. 2000. President Clinton's apology for the Tuskegee syphilis experiment: A narrative of remembrance, redefinition and reconciliation. *Howard Journal of Communications* 11:19-34.
18. Krimsky, S. 2003. *Science in the private interest.* Lantham, MD: Rowman & Littlefield, 132-135.
19. Pannikar, B., Yazzie, E., and Brugge, D. 2011. *Ethics of uranium mining research and the Navajo people*. In this volume, pp. 143-163. Amityville, NY: Baywood.
20. Canadian Association of Teachers. 2001. *The Olivieri Report.* Toronto: James Lorimer and Co. Ltd.
21. Stout, D. 2006. Justices set limits on public employees' speech rights. *New York Times,* May 30.
22. *Garcetti v. Ceballos*, 547 U.S. 410 (2006).
23. Brown, P., and Mikkelsen, E. J. 1990. *No safe place.* Berkeley, CA: University of California Press, p. 26.
24. Krimsky, S. 1986. Private sector science and the community: The Morris Township-Bellcore Case. In *The regulatory environment for science: Social restraints and legal controls of research,* ed. Marcel LaFollette. Washington, D.C.: Office of Technology Assessment.
25. Alvarez, R. 2011. *The risks of making nuclear weapons.* In this volume, pp. 181-198. Amityville, NY: Baywood.

http://dx.doi.org/10.2190/TORC2

CHAPTER 2

Insignificant and Invisible: The Human Toll of the Hanford Thyroid Disease Study

Trisha Thompson Pritikin

THERE'S A JOB FOR YOU AT HANFORD

The Hanford nuclear site in the arid expanse of southeastern Washington State was home to the world's first full-scale plutonium production facility. The frigid waters of the mighty Columbia River and the isolation of this vast desert region drove Lt. Col. Franklin Matthias [1] to target the area as the future location of a secret atomic city—part of the Manhattan Project launched in 1942 to develop and build atomic bombs [2].

Hanford needed thousands of workers in order to succeed in this immense, top-secret effort. Government recruiters went across the country [3] offering high salaries, free transportation, and promotional stories of the "beauty" of the Hanford region, home to immense dust storms and desert extremes. Notices were posted in union halls and community centers across the country stating "There's a job for you at Hanford." Thousands of workers responded to the recruiting effort, including my father.

My dad was a highly patriotic U.S. Navy survivor of the attack on Pearl Harbor and graduate of UC Berkeley in mechanical engineering. He was drawn to Richland—the town nearest to the Hanford facility—eager to get in on the new science of the atom. In 1947 he moved his family into one of the Atomic Energy Commission's (AEC) alphabet-lettered homes, built to house engineers, physicists, chemists, and a smattering of pathologists who came to inhabit Richland and work at the Hanford nuclear site [4].

Richland

Richland was a peaceful town when the fierce desert sandstorms were at bay. As a child, I recall attending countless productions of *South Pacific* at the Richland community theater and coming away singing childlike renditions of "I'm gonna wash that man right outta my hair." My parents and many of our neighbors spent weekend evenings tuned in to Don Ho's *Hawaii Calls*, dreaming that they could recreate a little corner of Hawaii and the Pacific in the desert heat of southeastern Washington State. My favorite childhood haunt at the time was the Tahitian Room at the Uptown Mall, where tropical paradise came in the form of plastic palm trees and birds of paradise. The Uptown Mall, to this day, sports its original atomic symbol, rising proudly above store roofs. My City of the Atom expressed its pride through businesses such as "Atomic Bowling," "Atomic Foods," "Atomic Lawn Care," and a high school athletics team called the "Bombers," represented by an "R" outlined by a mushroom cloud. One writer noted that the people of Richland were "so proud of being citizens of America's 'atomic city' that when Richland finally became an independent municipality, the town fathers included a mock atomic explosion in the celebration" [5].

Hanford's gigantic nuclear reactors produced fissionable, man-made plutonium, a basic component of nuclear weapons. Hanford's location was far from other communities, so that, in case of reactor malfunction, any resulting accident would expose only a limited number of people to potentially massive radiation releases [6]. A declassified AEC memo referred to populations around nuclear weapons production sites like Hanford as ". . . low use segment[s] of the population" [7]. The towns of Richland, Kennewick, and Pasco, built to house project scientists, construction crews, and their families, would be the only nearby communities within the radiation contamination zone. Those of us who lived in this "sacrifice zone" would have had no chance of escape had one of the reactors malfunctioned. It is truly tortuous to understand now that the tranquil rows of government homes with their picket fences and well-manicured lawns of my hometown could have become killing grounds at any time, radiation-contaminated for decades to come.

Plutonium Production and Risk to Surrounding Communities

The first reactor, a huge graphite cylinder used in the production of plutonium, started up on September 27, 1944. Hanford's initial plutonium shipment left for Los Alamos by caravan on February 3, 1945 [8]. The first atomic bomb in the world was detonated at the Trinity Site in central New Mexico on July 16, 1945, relying on Hanford plutonium. Three weeks later, an almost identical plutonium bomb, called "Fat Man," was dropped on Nagasaki, also triggered by Hanford plutonium.

Back at the production site, Hanford secretly released hundreds of harmful radioactive substances into the environment through a chemical process used to separate plutonium and uranium from fuel rods [9, 10]. Some of these releases were intentional and some accidental [11, 12]. In 1944, Hanford released its first several hundred curies of radioiodine-131 (I-131) [13]. I-131 is one of many short-lived radionuclides of iodine produced in large quantities during nuclear fission. I-131 very easily becomes airborne and can travel long distances [14]. People can be exposed to I-131 through inhalation and/or ingestion. In general, radioiodine is primarily uptaken by the thyroid gland and parathyroids at the base of the neck. If enough radioiodine reaches the thyroid, thyroid disease or thyroid cancer can result. If left untreated, hypothyroidism (underactive thyroid) can lead to loss of mental function and physical energy, and can even lead to coma and death. Hyperthyroidism (overactive thyroid) can cause a range of disabling conditions, including heart arrhythmias. Thyroid cancer, while often treatable, can kill; living with it can be a nightmare.

When the Hanford facility released radioiodine, it deposited in pastures downwind from the site where dairy cows and goats grazed. As a result, milk from the local dairies and backyard cows and goats contained radioiodine. This is of particular concern to children who often drink more milk than adults and are therefore at a greater risk of contracting thyroid diseases. Furthermore, compared with adults, children have smaller thyroid glands and receive a larger dose per unit of radioiodine ingested [15]. For example, a newborn's thyroid dose is about 16 times higher than an adult's dose, per ingested micro-curie of I-131 [16]. In addition to being exposed to I-131 through milk consumption, some members of communities surrounding the Hanford site were exposed by eating contaminated fruits and vegetables and breathing contaminated air.

Culture of Secrecy

During World War II, Hanford and the other Manhattan Project sites operated under a culture of secrecy. They adopted a security system known as "compartmentalization" where workers were told only what was necessary to perform their jobs [17, p. 3]. This compartmentalization continued after the end of World War II, as Hanford was transferred to civilian control.

The culture of secrecy was nearly a total preoccupation with Hanford workers and their families. The Federal Bureau of Investigation (FBI) maintained an ominous presence in the workplace and the neighborhoods of Hanford workers. One worker commented that, "We know there are a lot of FBI men working in the areas. There have been cases of men talking or telling their wives more than they should. We all know when a guy starts getting careless. And it isn't very long until he isn't around any more." To share concerns about Hanford's operations means dismissal and ostracism [17, p. 4].

My dad never talked about his work to anyone. In fact, before my mother passed away of aggressive cancer in 1999, she insisted to me that my dad's job at Hanford was merely to "produce power" through nuclear means. She reacted in disbelief when I explained to her that the primary purpose of Hanford's reactors was production of plutonium, not power.

Worker and Community Concerns about Safety

Many scientists and Hanford officials claim that the large radiation releases from Hanford were allowed due to incomplete understanding among early Hanford scientists of the dangers from radiation. Yet, while Hanford officials' early knowledge of radiation harm may have been "incomplete," these same officials established guidelines early on for the amount of radiation they felt they could release into the environment without causing harm to workers or surrounding communities:

> Hanford officials knowingly exposed workers and the public to levels of radiation exposure which they considered dangerous. For example, for the atmospheric releases of radioactive iodine (I-131), the guidelines were routinely ignored from the beginning of plutonium separation in December 1944 into the early fifties [18, p. 3-4].

Furthermore, "reports declassified in 1986 show that health specialists at Hanford recognized the risks of releasing so much radiation and were aware that the emissions could endanger residents of the region" [19].

Once the first atomic bomb was dropped on Hiroshima and Hanford workers learned about the nature of their work, workers started to worry that building atomic bombs might not be safe. Two weeks after the bombings of Hiroshima and Nagasaki in August 1945, Herb Parker and another top health official, Dr. Simeon Cantril, wrote a memo to workers, responding to questions about Hanford's effect on surrounding communities. Parker and Cantril reassured workers that "the amounts [of radioactive iodine in Richland] are entirely innocuous" [20].

Public Suspicions Grow: Death Mile

Members of surrounding communities had reasons to be concerned. On a high plateau east of Hanford, outside of the small town of Mesa, there is a stretch of highway known as Glade Road. According to townspeople, of the 108 people who lived in 28 homes within a mile of the highway, 24 men, women, and children have become ill or died from cancer since the mid-1960s [21].

> Further east, in the cafes of Basin City, Eltopia, Connell, and Cunningham, men and women raise their chins to show visitors scars on their throats where surgeons removed diseased thyroids. In this region, the white slashes are called "downwinder scars." Mothers describe the horror of losing infants to unexplained illnesses. Husbands grow tearful remembering young wives who died from cancer, blood disorders, and other diseases [21].

As people began to talk about cancers and thyroid disease in their neighborhoods, near the Hanford plant, and as far away as Spokane and Walla Walla, Washington, public concern grew over the possibility that Hanford had secretly released radiation onto an unsuspecting population. It was known that disease sometimes takes decades to develop after exposure to environmental toxins such as radiation [22]. Could so much disease be the delayed effect of Hanford exposures?

Release of DOE Classified Information

The Hanford Education Action League (HEAL) [23] in Spokane made repeated Freedom of Information Act (FOIA) requests to get answers to these public concerns [24]. In February 1986, after mounting pressure, the Department of Energy (DOE) released the first 19,000 pages of previously classified Hanford historical documents. Journalist Karen Dorn Steele of the Spokesman Review in Spokane, Washington, educated the public about the contents of those documents. Her articles described Hanford's radiation releases and confirmed concerns among government officials, health officials, and the public living both near to and far from the Hanford facility about the extent of those releases. The public learned that between 1944 and 1972, Hanford released large quantities of radionuclides into the air [25]. The radionuclide released in the greatest amounts and the one for which the best documentation is available is I-131. Between 1944 and 1957, an estimated 750,000 [26] curies of I-131 were released into the atmosphere [27-29]. Furthermore, for the first 6 months of 1955, Hanford exceeded the permissible release amounts [17, 30]. In fact, the radioactive emissions from Hanford are the largest ever documented from an American nuclear plant [19].

According to Jerry Leitch, regional radiological representative for the U.S. Environmental Protection Agency in Seattle, off-site radiation exposures to releases from Hanford were "without precedent in terms of the number of people affected and the magnitude of the doses received" [31]. In addition to the magnitude of doses, the duration of exposure to radiation put people in the Hanford region at even greater risk. A DOE publication states that "the risks of adverse health effects are higher when exposure is spread over a long period than when the same dose is received at one time" [32]. Furthermore, health physicists have predicted that the kind of exposures that people potentially received from Hanford, such as beta-emitting I-131, would cause more serious long-term health effects than other exposures, such as gamma ray exposures [33, 34].

TWO STUDIES

The governors of Washington and Oregon made requests to study if and how these levels of radiation from the Hanford facility affected surrounding communities. In March 1986, the CDC established an independent panel of scientists, the Hanford Health Effects Review Panel (HHERP), to evaluate the Hanford documents released by DOE. The panel recommended two studies:

- to estimate radiation doses received by area residents, the Hanford Environmental Dose Reconstruction Study (HEDR),
- to examine the feasibility of studying the potential health effects of iodine-131 among exposed populations. This led to the Hanford Thyroid Disease Study (HTDS) [35].

Hanford Environmental Dose-Reconstruction Study

The U.S. Department of Justice opposed a dose-reconstruction study as useless "public relations," but quickly changed its mind once the first suit for Hanford radiation damages was filed [36]. The DOE proposed that Batelle Pacific Northwest Laboratories, a long-term Hanford contractor, and Hanford Historical Documents Review Committee (HHDRC) conduct a joint dose-reconstruction study [37]. However, when the DOE refused to provide funding for the study, the effort was abandoned. This resulted in major public outcry. In response, the DOE insisted it would carry out its *own* dose-reconstruction study and formed the Technical Steering Panel (TSP) to direct Batelle in the HEDR study [38]. The aim of HEDR study was to estimate radiation doses from offsite releases during the 1940s, 1950s, and 1960s [39]. Preliminary results of the HEDR suggested that some infants and children were exposed to enough I-131 to destroy their thyroids [40].

Hanford Thyroid Disease Study

In September 1988, President Reagan signed legislation authorizing the CDC to conduct a thyroid disease study to look at whether children exposed to Hanford's offsite I-131 releases were at increased risk of developing any of 12 categories of thyroid disease [41, 42]. The Fred Hutchinson Cancer Research Center (FHCRC) in Seattle was chosen to carry out the study, with the CDC to oversee and administer its work. The HTDS began in 1989 [43]. The study population was a sample of people born between 1940 and 1946 to mothers who lived in seven counties in eastern Washington State: Benton, Franklin, Adams, Walla Walla, Okanogan, Ferry, and Stevens [44]. Researchers identified birth certificates for 5,199 people born between 1940 and 1946, of which ninety-four percent was located. Of these, 4,350 were still living and 527 were deceased, for which 502 death certificates were obtained. A total of 3,400 people of the original 5,199 were willing and able to participate fully in the study [45].

Participants provided information, based upon their best recollection, about where they lived during 1944-1957 and the amounts of foods and milk they consumed during that period [46]. Each participant had a complete diagnostic evaluation for thyroid disease in a medical clinic [47]. If the participant had a history of thyroid disease, medical records regarding that disease were sought. Each participant's radiation dose to the thyroid was then estimated using HEDR software [48].

HTDS FINAL REPORT AND COMMUNITY REACTION

> The US Centers for Disease Control and Prevention deserves an "F" for its presentation of the results of the Hanford thyroid study, a chorus of critics in the Northwest say [49].

This was the tone of much of the media coverage following the release of the HTDS draft final results on January 28, 1999. The HTDS draft Executive Summary claimed:

> [HTDS provides] rather strong evidence that exposure at these levels does not increase the risk of thyroid disease. These results should consequently provide a substantial degree of reassurance to the population exposed to Hanford radiation that the exposures are not likely to have affected their thyroid or parathyroid health [50, p. 18].

Just 3 years before this statement was released, I held my beloved father's hand as he lay dying from aggressive thyroid cancer. A tracheotomy tube protruded from a hole cut into his windpipe, allowing him to breathe, at least minimally, with an airway closed off by tumor growth. Tumors spread like wildfire to his lungs and brain. Just weeks after the FHCRC and the CDC declared that Hanford radiation exposures were not likely to affect thyroid health, I cradled my mother in my arms as she too died, having suffered from thyroid disease and hyperparathyroidism, wanting so much to live, but defeated by rapidly metastatic malignant melanoma.

It is very difficult to be *reassured*, as the HTDS summary suggested, when family members have died of thyroid cancer, and when one's whole family has developed thyroid disease, with no history of the disease anywhere in the extended family. To many of us who were children in the Hanford downwind region during I-131 releases, these "reassurances" were worthless, even insulting, to the memory of loved ones dead of thyroid cancer or suffering with thyroid and parathyroid disease. To place such a statement in public materials, knowing that many of those who were children in the Hanford region during I-131 releases were currently suffering from thyroid cancer, thyroid disease, or had lost family members to these diseases, was at best an exercise of very poor judgment and, at worst, just plain callous.

A *Seattle Times* article reported the following reactions to the HTDS results:

> We're 10 years older and $18 million poorer, but we still don't know whether Hanford downwinders were harmed by its radioactive emissions. We do know that 20 percent more of them are dead than expected. And we do know that eastern Washingtonians were found to have two to three times more thyroid disease than other populations generally.
>
> But those seemingly alarming findings may not mean a thing, according to researchers at the Centers for Disease Control in Atlanta and Seattle's Fred Hutchinson Cancer Research Center that studied downwinders.
>
> Then again, maybe the findings do mean something. No one, it seems, can say for certain.
>
> The Hanford downwinder thyroid disease study is one of the most maddening chapters in the annals of epidemiology [51].

An epidemiological study, by nature, is the study of populations. Populations, by definition, are composed of individuals, each with a very real-life experience. Suddenly, the HTDS and its results, released after months of hushed and restrictive secrecy, reflected not life as it was for those of us who grew up in the Hanford downwind area during release years, but as a funhouse mirror, distorting our lives, and denying our experience. I felt myself becoming deeply angered, yet I knew that angry outbursts would accomplish nothing with HTDS scientists. They needed to understand that too many of us—too many of the people I had grown up with—now had thyroid disease, and/or thyroid cancer. They needed to know that I, that *we,* were *not* reassured by the HTDS's purported "no harm" findings. It was up to us to let the world know that this epidemiologic study, for some reason, did not reflect our reality. This study had made us insignificant and invisible.

I had believed that the HTDS would finally show the world what had happened to all of us who lived in the shadow of Hanford. Yet, here we were, being fed a story of a reassuring, happy, healthy life next to a plutonium production facility, in spite of more than 750,000 curies of I-131 wafting through the air, landing on everything we touched or ate, and saturating my baby milk and ice cream. Those of us who had followed the progress of the HTDS and held out so much hope that it would reflect our reality concluded that something was amiss with either the data or the methodology on which HTDS was based [52]. We wanted to get to the bottom of this.

Fighting Back

And so the critiques began, by citizens and scientists alike. Articles and letters to the editor were appearing in regional papers from members of the American Nuclear Society and their allies, portraying these conclusions of the HTDS as final, irrefutable evidence that Hanford's I-131 had caused no harm to those exposed [53]. It was through the efforts of Dr. Owen Hoffman and his colleagues at SENES Oak Ridge, Inc. Center for Risk Analysis that we were able to begin to understand what had gone wrong and how to discuss the scientific fallacies of this study publicly. Dr. Hoffman and his colleagues at SENES were able to translate complex statistical concepts into understandable terms, thus enabling us to raise these important issues with the HTDS researchers and the media.

Thus empowered, my colleague Tim Connor, an investigative journalist and Hanford activist, and I, armed with a letter of protest co-signed by more than 22 representatives of citizen groups from around the country, went to meet with Dr. Richard Jackson, then director of the National Center for Environmental Health at the CDC. This letter we hand-carried raised serious concerns with a number of scientific issues within the HTDS, and with the communication and interpretation of the findings of this study by FHCRC and CDC to the public, Congress, and the media. The concerns included:

- FHCRC scientists' presentation of this study as if it were conclusive proof of no thyroid or parathyroid harm from Hanford's I-131 releases,
- FHCRC's blatant exaggeration of the statistical power of the study, and
- the uncertainties in dose estimates and confounding Nevada Test Site atomic tests and global fallout I-131 dose were not specifically addressed for the HTDS cohort.

The letter went on to discuss significant problems created by the information blackout that kept even those citizens who had been following the study throughout its history from learning about the results of the preliminary draft of the study until we read about it in the *New York Times* on the morning of January 28, 1999.

Tim and I met with Dr. Jackson in a small conference room, down a long hallway, past empty cubicles and deserted copy machines in an underused area of the Humphrey Building of the Department of Health and Human Services Building in Washington, DC. We asked Dr. Jackson to support a precedent-setting extended review of the HTDS by the National Academy of Sciences (NAS), National Research Council (NRC) a review that would address both the scientific and communications aspects of HTDS. This would be far more extensive and public than the normal NAS review of CDC's studies [54]. Dr. Jackson, to his credit, listened to the anguish in our voices and quickly understood the importance of this review to those of us whose lives had been so impacted by Hanford [55].

EXPERT REVIEW

The Experts Look at What Went Wrong

The NRC Subcommittee concluded that while the study itself was well-designed, HTDS scientists reported the study's findings as more conclusive than they really were purported to be [56]. "Shortcomings in the analytical and statistical methods used by the study's investigators overestimated the ability to detect radiation effects, which means the study results are less definitive than had been reported" [57, p. 1].

There were several important reasons why the HTDS was limited in its ability to detect radiation effects. The NRC Subcommittee saw the study's weakest link as the estimation of individual radiation doses from the 1940s and 1950s. The doses, which were being correlated to incidence of thyroid and parathyroid disease within the HTDS study group, were estimated based on assumptions about participants' milk consumption, their mother's milk consumption during periods when participants were breastfed, and the radioiodine levels of the milk and fresh food they consumed during the periods of greatest radioiodine releases from Hanford. These estimates depended on the accuracy of study participants' (or other informants') memories of the sources and quantity of milk intake decades in the past, as well as on estimates of how much radioiodine was released at specific times, where it was dispersed by wind and rain, how much was ingested or inhaled by dairy animals grazing on pasture or eating stored feed, and where the resulting milk (and other fresh food) was distributed [58]. Since records about these factors were not collected at the time downwinders were exposed, researchers used mathematical models, which have large uncertainties, to estimate HTDS participants' doses [59].

Computer-assisted telephone interviews (CATIs) were used within the HTDS to collect information about cohort members' early dietary habits, including times and durations of breastfeeding period, if any. Many of the HTDS cohort members reported being breastfed for part of their infancy. But, for some 1,212 participants in the HTDS, for whom there was no CATI data, a default diet of cows' milk was assigned. If any of these participants had actually consumed fresh sources of milk or breast milk, their doses could have been underestimated.

In addition, the technical review of the HTDS found evidence that the estimation of the amount of radioiodine that is passed into mothers' milk (the milk transfer coefficient) assumed in the HEDR was underestimated. This would also lead to an underestimate of true dose for cohort members who were breastfed as infants—particularly those born in 1945, during the highest I-131 releases from Hanford [59, p. 8]. If a subgroup of the HTDS cohort, such as this subgroup, received systematic overestimation or underestimation of dose, this would diminish the ability of the study to detect a relationship between radioiodine and thyroid disease, and lead to an overestimation of the study's ability to detect an effect.

Another possible explanation for uncertainty in dose estimates for HTDS cohort members is referred to as *inter-individual stochastic variability*. Some of the factors that may cause true dose to vary from the estimated dose include where the I-131 actually deposits, how much lands on vegetation, how much gets into the food chain, how much people actually ingested or inhaled, individual variation in size of the thyroid mass, and uptake from blood to the thyroid gland. Individual variability in dose estimates may also be influenced by radiosensitivity differences or intake levels of iodized table salt (consumption of iodized table salt may reduce the levels of radioiodine taken up by the thyroid), as well as other individual factors. HTDS researchers only considered some of these factors, but they may help explain why, on a street in my town of Richland, it was possible for two families to live the same length of time during the same period and be exposed to the same I-131 releases, yet one family developed thyroid disease and the family next door had no thyroid health impact at all.

The technical review of the HTDS also found that certain factors in the study led to an underestimation of uncertainty of HTDS doses which would contribute to lowering the statistical power of the HTDS [59, p. 9]. Overall, the NRC Subcommittee found that the statistical power of the HTDS to detect an association between radioiodine and thyroid disease was not as high as claimed by the HTDS researchers due to inadequate allowance for imprecision in the dose estimates [60, 61].

Another source of uncertainty in the HTDS cohort dose estimation arises from the fact that, during the 1950s and early 1960s, two other environmental sources of I-131 contributed to the thyroid doses received around Hanford. The first of these was fallout from nuclear weapons tests detonated at the Nevada Test Site (NTS) during the 1950s. The second source was fallout from nuclear weapons tests ("global fallout") conducted by the United States and other countries outside of the U.S. mainland in the 1950s and 1960s, including Test Bravo in the Marshall Islands (1954), which deposited I-131 and other radionuclides within the Hanford downwind region. The issue raised by the NRC Subcommittee in its review of HTDS was that, if NTS or global fallout could have resulted in significant I-131 exposures in the HTDS study area, and if the variation within the area was large, then it was very important to take both global and NTS fallout into account in the HTDS [60, p. 8]. Rather, the HTDS analysis of NTS I-131 doses was based upon a median dose for all subjects, causing them to be essentially disregarded [62]. The expert review concluded that HTDS could not rule out the possibility that dose-response relationships were actually present, but not able to be seen due to the fact that these confounding exposures from global and NTS fallout were not explored thoroughly [62, p. 11]. The uncertainty in dose due to the fact that doses were, of necessity, modeled and possibly confounded by global and NTS fallout, should have been communicated at the HTDS public briefing on January 28, 1999.

In a letter transmitted to the CDC just 10 days before HTDS results were made public, the NRC Committee on the Assessment of CDC's Radiation studies raised and emphasized problems with the uncertainties of individual doses calculated with the HEDR methods used in conjunction with the HTDS:

> It should be noted that the inherent uncertainty associated with the individual doses will decrease the likelihood of determining a meaningful risk coefficient for the effects of radioiodine on the target population [63].

Scott Davis, the principal HTDS investigator, is reported to have said that "he couldn't agree more" that there should have been a more thorough scientific review of the study before it was released [64]. A citizens' letter to the director of the NCEH stated, "It is appalling that CDC would go forward with the release of the HTDS under such circumstances, and so quickly after its NRC review committee had identified such major problems" [65].

Loss of High Percentage of the HTDS Study Group

Of particular concern to experts and public alike was the failure of HTDS scientists to account for uncertainty due to deaths and nonparticipation. An original 5,199 people were identified as possible HTDS participants based on time and location of birth. Of these, approximately two-thirds (3,447) completed the HTDS clinical exam and some withdrew after the exam. The other one-third of the originally identified potential subject group had either died before the study began or didn't wish to participate. This is considered a rather high rate of cohort loss [59, p. 17], and this level of cohort loss can seriously bias study results, even if the losses were of equal proportions with regard to exposure or disease categories [66].

Experts reviewing the HTDS felt that the loss of one-third of the cohort was probably not random in ways that were relevant to the study [59, p. 17]. Those who knew or suspected that they had been exposed to Hanford radiation or who had thyroid disease may have been more likely to participate in the HTDS. Deaths may have been exposure related. (Sometimes this is called *selective survival.*) The review concluded "that this uncertainty was not addressed analytically is another reason why the HTDS report overstates the strength of conclusions with regard to the size of effect that may be present in light of the data" [59].

An Important Finding Overlooked

> The [study] population also had a surprising amount of thyroid disease although its prevalence was not dose related. The overall incidence of almost 19 percent autoimmune thyroiditis with this number reaching 24 percent for women in the study is more than might be expected from results of normal population studies. The numbers for hypothyroidism (19% of the total population, 27.5 percent of the women) is also higher than one might expect from other epidemiological studies of presumably normal populations [67, p. 6].

HTDS conclusions were focused entirely upon the lack of any correlation between estimates of the participants' thyroid doses and the subsequent occurrence of thyroid illness. There was no recognition of the excess rates of thyroid disease found within the study group as compared with what would be expected from an unexposed group. Although the comparison of thyroid disease rates of HTDS participants to rates in other populations is made difficult due to the study's protocol for thyroid screening, something that does not occur in other populations, the observation of excess occurrence of thyroid disease in the HTDS was not seriously considered when study conclusions were drawn.

The importance of attending to diverse and conflicting findings in epidemiological studies was emphasized by Alice Stewart, the epidemiologist who discovered the link between obstetric x-rays and childhood cancer:

> The epidemiologist is like a conductor—you must hear every note, you must be able to detect a false note anywhere. If you hear a false note, you don't send the violins away: you try to work with them. You must include all types of seemingly extraneous data in the collection process, it might be the key to unraveling a mystery. Handling the noise is the greatest thing in epidemiology [68, p. 216].

Had this been a thyroid disease prevalence study rather than a dose/incidence comparison, high prevalence of thyroid disease would have been found. As Stewart said, "The best way not to find something is not to look for it" [68, p. 193].

While looking at estimated dose and levels of thyroid disease among the study group, the HTDS found 20 thyroid cancers out of a participating study group of 3,441 (.58 percent). Based upon the amounts of I-131 released from Hanford, the Agency for Toxic Substances and Disease Registry had predicted that its medical monitoring program would find 90 thyroid cancers out of a study group of 14,000 (.64 percent) [69].

The Connecticut Tumor Registry (CTR) is the oldest population-based tumor registry in the country and is similar to the HTDS in that both require histological confirmation of thyroid cancer diagnosis. There would be 5.3 cancers projected by the CTR for a group of 3,441 (probability of thyroid cancer, $0.00153983 \times 3441 = 5.3$). The ratio of observed cancer *found* by the HTDS is nearly four times the rate of residents in Connecticut.

Hypothyroidism occurs in approximately 2 percent of the population [70]. The HTDS found 7.8 percent confirmed hypothyroid prevalence. Benign thyroid nodules occur in 2-4 percent of the general population. Over 7 percent prevalence was found in the HTDS. In the final HTDS report, under the "second alternative" of diagnosis, there were 297 cases of nodules (8.6 percent). Goiter and other disorders of the thyroid are reported to occur in 2.6 percent of the population, according to the National Health Interview Statistics data. The HTDS found autoimmune thyroiditis, alone, was 18.9 percent. Eight hundred and six (23.4 percent) were found to be antibody positive, although this was not discussed in the summary report.

Strength of the HTDS Findings Overstated

> The subcommittee is concerned that the results of the study were reported—and interpreted—in black and white terms of whether a statistical test was passed or failed. It recommends that confidence limits be provided throughout the report to allow the readers to judge how large a radiation effect might be consistent with the data. It feels that the HTDS investigators probably overstated the strength of their finding that there was no radiation effect [60, p. 81].

The expert technical review of the HTDS commended HTDS authors for responding to the NRC Subcommittee's recommendation to include confidence intervals [59]. Yet, the final report failed to make full use of the confidence intervals in interpreting study results. Had confidence intervals been used as counterpoint to HTDS authors' reliance on statistical significance in drawing conclusions, HTDS authors' results would have demonstrated inconclusiveness [59, p. 18].

Correct interpretation of lack of significance in the HTDS report

> . . . is simply that, when examined using the models and methods of the authors, the data do not overwhelmingly favor any alternative over the null. This correct interpretation leaves open the possibility that the evidence favors the alternative (that there is an effect) albeit not very strongly when using the authors' approach [59, p. 18].

HTDS researchers' statements such as "the results of the HTDS provide no evidence of a statistically significant association" conflate absence of statistical significance with absence of evidence [59, p. 18; 72]. The two concepts must be separated, at which point, it can be seen that there is a lack of significance, but that some of the evidence provides weak support for the possibility of small effects [59, p. 18].

The problems that have been discussed regarding power and dosimetry uncertainty in HTDS require more thorough analysis, which would have had a "serious impact on the interpretation of the study, leading to even more ambiguous results, which in turn should lead to even more cautious and limited interpretation" [59, p. 19].

HTDS: Consistent With Other I-131 Studies Showing Risk

The HTDS final report stated, "There is little evidence in the literature to suggest that people exposed to I-131 at the levels found in this study over a period of months or years would experience higher rates of thyroid or parathyroid disease as a result of their exposure" [59, p. 19; 71, p. 543].

Technical reviewers challenged this statement and found no studies published in the scientific literature that study protracted exposures at the levels found within the HTDS. The reviewers concluded that "The reason that there is little evidence is due to the absence of evidence, not to the existence of studies that actually show no risks from protracted exposures" [59, p. 20]. Furthermore, the technical reviewers concluded that

> The results and conclusions of the Final Report of the Hanford Thyroid Disease Study (HTDS) . . . cannot be used to rule out important risks for thyroid cancer, neoplasms, or hypothyroidism from exposures to iodine-131 (I-131) from the Hanford nuclear facility [73].

Considering the HTDS limitations in measurement and resulting uncertainties, expert review of the study found that even though HTDS findings did not show statistically significant elevations in risk, HTDS results are not inconsistent with other published studies supporting risks for certain thyroid diseases from I-131 exposures, if the upper bounds of the reported confidence intervals are considered [74].

HTDS authors used three different approaches to analyze whether their results were inconclusive because of dose uncertainties in the primary analyses [71, p. 603]. They found similar results in each of their analyses, which the technical review found to be consistent with low statistical power in each of the three approaches, rather than consistent with a hypothesis that there is no relation between exposure and disease [59, p. 20].

The final sentences of the HTDS report state:

> These findings do not definitively rule out the possibility that Hanford radiation exposures are associated with an increase in one or more of the outcomes under investigation. However, it does mean that if such associations exist, they were likely too small to detect using the best epidemiologic methods available [72, p. 21].

HTDS findings do not rule out the possibility that Hanford I-131 exposures are associated with an increase in thyroid health outcomes [75]. HTDS findings are compatible with significant increase in health risk from these exposures as well as with no increase. "Even the best epidemiologic methods are not enough to compensate for a study population that is too small and measurements too uncertain to detect even large risks" [59, p. 21].

HTDS ETHICAL ISSUES

Poor Communication of Results

The NRC Subcommittee found that in media and public briefings on HTDS, the investigators failed to pay sufficient attention to the health concerns of the public, and that HTDS investigators and CDC officials should have offered more balanced, and possibly alternative, interpretations of the findings and discussed their implications for individuals [60, p. 13]. The public's disapproval of the researchers' conclusions and interpretations was reflected at the public briefing in Hanford on January 28, 1999, when, throughout the entire several-hour briefing, an exposed Hanford resident held up a hand-painted sign, reading "I DON'T BELIEVE YOU."

NRC Subcommittee members identified significant risk communication problems with the release of the report [76], including the way HTDS investigators overstated the certainty of their results in the media by claiming that the study findings were "clear and unequivocal" [77] and that the HTDS was "a very powerful study" [78] with "sufficient statistical power" [79] and "a very high probability of detecting relationships between Hanford radiation dose and diseases under study if such relationships exist" [80].

The HTDS Sounds the Death Knell for Hanford Public Health Programs

In addition to disappointment and confusion, the inappropriate communication with the public concerning the HTDS draft results harmed people exposed to Hanford's I-131 emissions in other ways. Prior to the release of the HTDS draft final report, the federal Agency for Toxic Substances and Disease Registry (ATSDR) determined that a medical monitoring program was merited for people exposed as children to I-131 released from Hanford between 1945 and 1951:

> ATSDR has determined that about 14,000 children who lived in areas downwind of Hanford from 1945 to 1951 received high exposure to I-131 through drinking contaminated milk, and are at risk of having thyroid and parathyroid abnormalities, including thyroid cancer and hypothyroidism, as a result [81].

The proposed medical monitoring program would have been the first concrete assistance offered to downwinders after years of scientific studies and legal battles [82].

The ATSDR also proposed an I-131 subregistry for Hanford to include people exposed as children during the years of highest releases of I-131 from Hanford. Specifically, the subregistry was to include people born in Adams, Benton, or Franklin counties between 1940 and 1951, and people who lived in these counties who were 5 years of age or younger and lived there more than 30 days during 1945-51. I was very relieved that, finally, there would be data collected on people like me, who were too young to be included within the HTDS cohort, but who had developed thyroid disease or thyroid cancers and had lived within the Hanford downwind area during childhood. The subregistry would track the health of approximately 17,000 people to take a look at illnesses they may have developed. Finally, the world would begin to get a better picture of what had happened to those of us exposed as children to Hanford's radiation releases.

However, the FHCRC's claim that the HTDS was evidence of "no harm" from Hanford sounded the death knell for both of these programs [83]. At the public meeting on HTDS on January 28, 1999, the CDC announced that they would recommend a change in plans for medical monitoring [84]. We were to receive no help in the form of medical monitoring and there would be no gathering of information on our current health. This was not the fault of the ATSDR, whose officials had tried valiantly to secure funding for these programs after a multitude of planning meetings with significant expert advice and public involvement. This was a case of the proverbial fox guarding the henhouse. The DOE, the source of our involuntary exposures, refused to fund these programs to finally help us in spite of the recommendation to do so by the ATSDR. Hanford downwinders' attempts to appeal to the legal system was spectacularly unsuccessful in resolving the DOE's refusal to fund these needed programs for the very people it exposed [85]. Based on the draft results of the HTDS and a report from the Institute of Medicine questioning the value of medical monitoring [86], the CDC denied Hanford's downwinders the only concrete help they had ever been offered.

There is something both intrinsically wrong and ethically abhorrent in a system that allows the wrongdoer, in this case, DOE, successor to the Atomic Energy Commission—the power to decide whether public health programs recommended by the ATSDR for populations that the DOE itself exposed and injured, should be funded. The experience at Hanford illustrates that this structure, with the ATSDR dependent upon the DOE's whims and politics for its funding of public health programs for exposed populations injured by DOE activities at federal facilities such as Hanford, serves only the interest of the DOE, inflicting yet more harm on already hurting populations. The ATSDR must have adequate funding to do its work, independent of any control or influence by DOE.

Environmental Epidemiology

The very nature of the HTDS as environmental epidemiology provides another reason for the inappropriateness of the conclusions that the HTDS investigators made. Environmental epidemiology is an observational study of the effect on human health of physical, biological, and chemical factors in the external environment [87]. The aim of the HTDS was to study the effect of I-131 on thyroid disease. The HTDS can be further characterized as "risk-factor epidemiology"

[88-90] because it focuses on factors associated with excess disease in groups, such as thyroid disease, but lacks the direct evidence to "specify the cause of any particular case of disease" [91]. Risk-factor epidemiology has the capacity to produce a generalized statement about the probability or risk that members of a population have developed or will develop a given disease due to this exposure, but it is not able to deliver a definitive answer for people like my family and our former Richland neighbors who now suffer with thyroid cancer and thyroid disease. For this reason, the HTDS should never have been portrayed as a source of "reassurance" to us that our health has not been harmed by radiation emissions from Hanford.

The Hanford Health Information Network published an article that expounds on this point:

> Regrettably, given the way in which the draft results of the study were communicated, the HTDS actually inflicted a good deal of harm on those whom the study was intended to serve.
>
> The cause of this harm is not the fact that the HTDS investigators found no link between Hanford radiation and thyroid disease. The fact is, it is rare for individual epidemiologic studies to provide strong evidence for connections between low-dose exposures and diseases like cancer. More often than not, the results are inconclusive.
>
> The problem with the January 1999 release of the HTDS is that the draft results of the study were presented as if they were conclusive. The message from the researchers was that if you are among those who suspected (or believed) that Hanford emissions are responsible for an increase in thyroid disease among downwinders, you should be "reassured" that there is no such connection.
>
> Such statements by scientists are practically unheard of in connection with environmental epidemiologic studies. The simple reason for this is that scientists understand that the results of any such study (whether it finds a link, or doesn't) have to be viewed as a piece in a larger puzzle. This is because environmental epidemiology is not laboratory science where researchers conduct carefully controlled experiments that can be repeated by other scientists. It is an observational science, where a given hypothesis must be tested via repeated observations and evaluated within the context of animal studies, cellular and molecular research, etc.
>
> In the case of the HTDS, there is considerable evidence from previous studies that exposure to radioactive iodine does cause increases in thyroid diseases. Why the HTDS team would offer "reassurance" in light of this other evidence is puzzling. The mildest criticism one can offer is that their statements do not reflect the circumspection and caution that is the hallmark of the science [92, p. 5].

THE PERSONAL IMPACT OF THYROID DISEASE

It is important while discussing the vastness of a "truth" attempted through environmental epidemiology to take a moment to see through the statistics and power calculations to the impact of disease on the individual. Thyroid disease may seem like a minor inconvenience to those who have not experienced this disease firsthand.

As a child, I hadn't yet passed through the "latency" period before exposure-caused disease manifested itself. My family and neighbors in Richland remember me as a healthy child. It wasn't until my teens that I began to experience the first uncomfortable symptoms of the failure of my thyroid.

My childhood was a happy one, playing in picket-fenced yards in back of our two story "F" house or in the front yard of our neighbor's "B." We boated on the Columbia River, played on its windswept islands, and made mud pies in the wet sands of the riverbanks. It wasn't until almost four decades later that we would learn that the milk we drank from the local dairy was laced with radioiodine, and that the muddy sands were infused with cobalt-60 released from the reactors into the Columbia. After my anger and shock at the fact that I had been involuntarily exposed to stuff that was very bad for children, and that there was nothing I could do about it, I, like many of my neighbors and friends from those days in Richland, trusted that the HTDS would finally answer our questions about why we had developed thyroid disease and thyroid cancer, diseases previously unknown within our families.

Thyroid disease is a mean disease. If you haven't been unlucky enough to experience thyroid disorder, it isn't a mere inconvenience. Many of us who developed thyroid disease after our time within Hanford's downwind region suffered for years with unexplained symptoms that we experienced as extreme, disabling discomfort. These symptoms included migraines, intense pressure in the head, dizziness, gastrointestinal problems, extreme fatigue, and severe muscle contractions, all without a correct diagnosis. In my own case, since there was no thyroid disease in my family, medical personnel were not looking in that direction. From testing, they knew it wasn't diabetes, and it didn't appear to be leukemia. These problems would worsen and remain mysterious for decades. And with its disabling effects came decreased hours on the job due to chronic fatigue, days of disabling pain, life's goals lost, not knowing the cause. So many of the women who grew up with me experienced miscarriage or infertility, some of the greatest losses a woman may experience. My father's death of thyroid cancer was one of extreme pain; his esophagus and trachea quickly closed off by the wildfire spread of tumorous growths that metastasized from his thyroid. Tracheotomy tube protruding from his neck, his airway suctioned every hour, he died a death of irony and of extreme pain. Irony because he believed in the safety of Hanford operations and the reassurances of his bosses, the Hanford site contractor at the time, General Electric. Even when it was finally revealed in 1986 that Hanford had covertly released an estimated 750,000 curies of I-131 in addition to other biologically harmful radioactive substances off-site, my father still clung to his trust that Hanford's contractors and the AEC had been upfront in their operations of the Hanford facility. Only when he was diagnosed with rapidly metastatic thyroid cancer did he begin to understand that it was too late.

The HTDS was the study that was intended to bring some closure, some answers to those of us who now deal with the debilitating health impacts of thyroid disease. My mother, who suffered from hyperparathyroidism and thyroid disease, had hoped that such answers would come from the HTDS. She died of a very aggressive form of malignant melanoma just after the January 28, 1999 public pronouncements of the Fred Hutchinson/CDC researchers that we should be reassured that our health had not been harmed from Hanford's releases.

For those of us who suffer now with thyroid disease, thyroid cancer, or who have lost those who are very important to our lives to thyroid or other cancers, the HTDS gives a very unclear picture of what really happened at Hanford. Perhaps all we can ask is public acknowledgment that HTDS is not consistent with the results of other studies on I-131 exposed populations, in which increased incidence of thyroid disease and thyroid cancer was found, and that the HTDS is inconclusive at best. A health survey conducted by the Northwest Radiation Health Alliance (NWRHA), an alliance of Hanford downwinders, physicians, scientists, and social activists, found an excess of illness, including thyroid disease and cancer, among Hanford exposed participants [93]. The R-11 Health Study, a study of the rate of prevalence of radiogenic illnesses in selected populations in the Hanford downwind areas, found that there was considerably more goiter (hyperthyroidism) and other diseases of the thyroid reported than in national survey data [94]. The burden should be upon those who *released* radioactive iodine onto our communities to show that our thyroid disease was *not* caused by their releases, not upon those of us with thyroid disease or who have lost family members to the cruelty of thyroid cancer to prove that our disease was more likely than not caused by our involuntary exposures. We already carry the burden of a lifetime of suffering.

This is not true closure for those of us dealing with the debilitating effects of thyroid disease or with loss of family members who we really need to be here, but it at least does not carry the distorted and insulting message that no harm came from Hanford's radioactive contamination of the air we breathed and the milk we drank day after day after day. If more than 750,000 curies of I-131 released onto the playgrounds and entered into the milk of babies does not cause harm, then why is the U.S. government currently distributing potassium iodide tablets to protect its citizens against terrorists using dirty bombs possibly containing radioiodine? If so much I-131 in my baby milk, air, and water didn't cause me harm, then it's time for the DOE, the successor agency to the Atomic Energy Commission which put me in harm's way, to bear the burden of showing where this debilitating disease, prevalent in so many of my neighbors from 1940s and 1950s in the Tri-Cities, *did* come from. Until that time, the HTDS is just an epidemiologic attempt to answer the question, inconclusive at best.

APPENDIX: Letter of 18 February 1999 to Dr. Richard Jackson, director, NCEH Signed by over 22 representatives of the Native American and Downwinder groups

The introductory portion of the letter to Dr. Jackson appears below:

February 18, 1999

Dear Dr. Jackson,

We are writing to express our profound dismay and objections to the manner and process by which the results of the Hanford Thyroid Disease Study were released last month. The way in which the report was realized showed a contemptible lack of sensitivity to the individuals whose personal well-being and family and community health have been, and continue to be, jeopardized by past exposures to Hanford radiation. Moreover, it is already clear that the substantive basis for the report's conclusions is dubious; that uncertainties about the accuracy of the doses assigned to study subjects should have [been] reconciled before such definitive conclusions were offered to the Congress, the press, and the public at large.

We would like to emphasize at the outset that we are not objecting to the news, per se, that an epidemiologic investigation could detect no correlation between exposures and health outcomes. Obviously, such findings are going to occur, more often than not, as scientists test environmental epidemiologic hypotheses with limited observational tools. That's not the issue here.

Our grievance with the Hanford Thyroid Disease Study is that the conclusiveness of the study's findings is not yet warranted by the quality of the science. Officials and scientists at the Centers for Disease Control and Prevention had advance knowledge of these shortcomings and limitations. It is inexplicable that they failed to publicly disclose them. Furthermore, it is inexcusable that they did not seek to explain how the conclusions drawn in the draft report are, at best, premature.

NOTES

1. Lt. Col. Matthias had been sent from the East Coast by Gen Leslie Groves, who took command of the US secret atomic weapons project in September of 1942. D'Antonio, M. 1993. *Atomic harvest: Hanford and the lethal toll of America's nuclear arsenal.* New York: Crown.
2. The Manhattan Project took its name from the fact that the first headquarters of the Corps of Engineers district in charge of bomb work was located in Manhattan. The Manhattan Project encompassed research and scientific projects in 37 facilities

throughout the U.S. and Canada, but the key to the project was the creation of three "top secret" atomic cities, Los Alamos (Site Y), the Clinton Engineer Works (later called Oak Ridge) (Site X), and Hanford (Site W). Sanger, S. L. 1995. *Working on the bomb: An oral history of WWII Hanford*. Portland, OR: Portland State University.

3. Except to the Pacific Northwest, New Mexico, and Tennessee.
4. There were 22 house plans available, mostly entitled with letters of the alphabet, in the later 1940s and 1950s. Many of these houses still stand in Richland, with minor modifications made by owners. See http://hanford.houses.tripod.com/
5. D'Antonio, M. 1993. *Atomic harvest: Hanford and the lethal toll of America's nuclear arsenal*. New York: Crown.
6. Groves, L. R. 1962, 1983. *Now it can be told: The story of the Manhattan Project*. New York: Da Capo.
7. Gallagher, C. 1993. *American ground zero: The secret nuclear war*, xxiii and 109ff. Cambridge, MA: MIT Press.
8. Sanger, S. L. 1995. *Working on the bomb: An oral history of WWII Hanford*. Portland, OR: Portland State University.
9. Chemical separation involves dissolving spent fuel rods and then isolating and concentrating the plutonium, uranium, and other radionuclides they contain.
10. When irradiated fuel rods from production reactors were immersed in an acid solution to dissolve the metal cladding, radiation was released into the atmosphere.
11. Aside from "normal" operations, Hanford conducted at least three experiments that released large amounts of radioiodine. The "Green Run" occurred December 2-3, 1949, releasing 7,800 curies of I-131.
12. Thomas, J. 1990. Hanford Education Action League. The human toll. *Perspective* (3):6.
13. A curie is the amount of a radioactive species which produces 37 billion radioactive decays per second.
14. It would eventually be revealed that Hanford's I-131 exposed large areas of eastern Washington State, Idaho, western Montana, northeastern Oregon, and traveled into parts of western Canada.
15. D'Antonio, M. 1993. *Atomic harvest: Hanford and the lethal toll of America's nuclear arsenal*. New York: Crown.
16. A micro-curie is one millionth of one curie. A curie is the amount of a radioactive species which produces 37 billion radioactive decays per second.
17. Thomas, J. 1992. Hanford Education Action League. Atomic deception: Oh, what a tangled web! *Perspective* (10-11):3.
18. Thomas, J. 1990. Hanford Education Action League. The human toll. *Perspective* (3):3-4.
19. Schneider, K. 1988. Seeking victims of radiation near weapon plant. *New York Times*, October 17.
20. Cantril, S. T., and Parker, H. M. 1945. Status of health protection at Hanford Engineer Works. HW-7-2136. (RL: HEW, August 24, 1945), p. 1. See also: *Diary of Colonel Franklin T. Matthias*. 24 August 1945, p. 104.
21. Leon and Juanita Andrewjeski, who lived on one of the farms closest to the Hanford reservation in Ringold had also kept track of the cancer and heart ailments in the area after Leon was first diagnosed with heart disease. By 1985, Juanita's map indicated

35 heart attacks among people of relatively young age—in their fifties—and 32 cases of cancer. D'Antonio, M. 1993. *Atomic harvest: Hanford and the lethal toll of America's nuclear arsenal*. New York: Crown.

22. See http://nuclearhistory.tripod.com/radiation.html
23. HEAL was formed in 1984 to raise questions about the past and present safety of Hanford.
24. The Freedom of Information Act established a procedure for citizens to receive government documents, but it also allowed agencies to hold documents deemed sensitive to national security. See 5 USC. § 552, As Amended By Public Law No. 104-231, 110 Stat. 3048.
25. Hanford Health Information Network. September 1996. A listing of radionuclides released from Hanford.
26. This estimate is associated with appreciable uncertainty because it depends on the use of mathematical models to substitute for direct measurements.
27. Heeb, C. M., Gydesen, S. P., Simpson, J. C., and Bates, D. J. 1966. Reconstruction of radionuclide releases from the Hanford Site, 1944-72. *Health Physics Journal* 71:545-555.
28. Napier, B. A. 2002. A re-evaluation of the I-131 atmospheric releases from the Hanford site. *Health Physics Journal* 83:204-226.
29. When the Three Mile Island reactor accident in Pennsylvania in 1979 released between 15 and 24 curies of I-131, people were evacuated and milk was impounded near the plant.
30. The average for the first half of 1955 was 5.1 curies per day, HW-55569 RD, p. 6.
31. Steele, K. D. 1987. Downwinders. *Spokesman Review* 2 Dec:A10.
32. Office of Environmental Management. January 1995. Closing the circle on the splitting of the atom. Washington, DC: USDOE.
33. Manning, M. 1995. Atomic vets battle time. *Bulletin of Atomic Scientists* 51:54-60.
34. Nussbaum, R. H., and Kohnlein, W. 1995. Health consequences of exposures to ionizing radiation from external and internal sources: Challenges to radiation protection standards and biomedical research. *Medicine and Global Survival* 2(4):195-213.
35. CDC established a second independent panel, the Hanford Historical Documents Review Committee (HHDRC), to continue analysis of DOE documents. See http://www.cdc.gov/nceh/radiation/hanford/htdsweb/guide/timeline.htm
36. Steele, K. D. 2005. Radiation study set up as defense records show. *Spokesman Review* 23 February.
37. This dose reconstruction study was to be conducted in a joint effort with the HHDRC.
38. The DOE completely de-funded the HHDRC by early 1988.
39. The Native American Working Group coordinated Hanford-related tribal research and recommended research activities to the TSP. Batelle altered its conflict of interest policies in 1992 to prohibit HEDR staff from also working for legal defense in the Hanford litigation, yet Batelle's chief records manager continued for work for both the study and for the government's defense litigation team in the Hanford litigation. These clear conflicts of interest raise major concerns over the independence, credibility, and integrity of HEDR. If HEDR source code or radiation estimates were inaccurate, this could greatly impact the outcome of the Hanford Thyroid

Disease Study, since it was the HEDR data used in the study to explore the link between Hanford's I-131 releases and thyroid disease in 3,440 study participants, exposed as children within the Hanford downwind region. Some of the Batelle staff in Richland who worked on HEDR also worked for the Justice Department and for Kirkland and Ellis, the Chicago law firm hired to defend Hanford contractors against radiation injury claims.

40. "Initial Hanford Radiation Dose Estimates," Technical Steering Panel, Hanford Environmental Dose Reconstruction Project, 1990.
41. Hanford Thyroid Disease Study. 1999. *Summary final report of the Hanford Thyroid Disease Study*, Seattle, WA: Fred Hutchinson Cancer Research Center. p. 56.
42. Public Law 100-607, directing CDC to conduct a study of thyroid morbidity among persons who lived near the Hanford Nuclear Site between 1944 and 1957.
43. The study used computer software developed under the HEDR project to estimate the radiation doses to the thyroid that HTDS participants received as children while living within the HEDR area, limited to the 246 by 306 mile area around the Hanford facility.
44. HTDS studied those exposed as children because exposure to radioactive iodine would most likely have affected children, who are more sensitive to the harmful effects of radiation than are adults.
45. There was an element of HTDS that looked at the feasibility of a similar design for the nine Native American tribes exposed to Hanford's I-131 releases. It was determined that a study with the same design as HTDS would not be capable of detecting radiation effects that existed. See transcript of Hanford Health Effects Subcommittee Meeting, 26-29 February 1999.
46. When possible, the participant's mother or another close family member was asked about dietary habits for the participant.
47. The evaluation included: residential and dietary history, past medical or occupational radiation exposures, and any history of thyroid disease, thyroid ultrasound evaluation, blood sample to test for thyroid function, the presence of antibody markers for autoimmune thyroiditis, and physical exam of the thyroid. Serum calcium levels were taken to check for hyperparathyroidism. See *A Guide to the Hanford Thyroid Disease Study Final Report.* CDC/FHCRC. 21 June 2002.
48. HTDS was conducted first as a pilot study, to test the feasibility of the methods proposed, and then as a full scale epidemiologic study. The full study fieldwork was completed in 1997.
49. Steele, K. D. 1999. Fallout from thyroid study: Critics fault CDC for early release of Hanford results, unreviewed research. *Spokesman Review.* 14 February.
50. Davis, S., and Kopecky, K. 1998. Executive summary. *HTDS draft final report*, 18. Seattle, WA: Fred Hutchinson Cancer Research Center.
51. Torvik, S. 1999. Study further muddies Hanford waters. *Seattle Times.* 28 February 1999.
52. Over much of the course of HTDS, I served as a long-term member of the Hanford Health Effects Subcommittee (HHES), a citizens' advisory committee to the Agency for Toxic Substances and Disease Registry and CDC, which had been following the development of HTDS. I had had great faith in science to reflect reality, and that the downwinders like me would hear the story of our lives and our damaged health confirmed within the results of HTDS.

53. Cary, A. 1999. Thyroid study to continue. *TriCity Herald.* 29 January 1999. See also: Hanford downwinders up against study results. *TriCity Herald.* 29 October 2004. http://www.hanfordnews.com
54. The NRC is the principal operating arm of the NAS (chartered in 1963) and the National Academy of Engineering. Its work is funded by the CDC. It is a private nonprofit organization that provides advice on science and technology under a congressional charter. As part of the extended NRC Subcommittee review of the HTDS draft report, the CDC included both communications questions and scientific questions within the charge to the NAS committee. The three communications questions asked were:
    1. Was the material accurate and appropriate in providing guidance to the public in understanding the study's findings?
    2. If these messages needed to be amended, how should the revised messages best be communicated to the public?
    3. How can the CDC improve the public communication process in the release of future study reports?
55. This is one of the first such extended reviews to be carried out by NAS, requested by people affected by Hanford's I-131 releases, reviewing not just the scientific components and qualities of a study typically involved in such a review, but concentrating as well upon the way the study's preliminary findings were communicated to the public, Congress, and the media.
56. The National Academy of Science's National Research Council (NRC) Subcommittee of the Board on Radiation Effects Research released the results of its extended review of the draft final HTDS report on 12 December 1999 in a public meeting in Spokane, Washington
57. NAS review report. 14 December 1999, p. 1.
58. The milk pathway is one of the primary means by which radioiodine is ingested, and is a particular concern with infants and children. The radioiodine deposits on pasture grass, the cows or goats eat the contaminated grass, and then the radioiodine is ingested by humans as the milk is consumed. A child's thyroid uptakes far more radioiodine than an adult's thyroid. This is because children often consume a greater quantity of milk than adults, because their thyroids are smaller and more vulnerable than those of adults, and because of a faster metabolism than that of adults.
59. See Ruttenber, A. J., et al. 30 March 2004. *A technical review of the final report of the Hanford Thyroid Disease Study.* p. 3, citing Hoffman 1991, Hoffman et al., 1993, Hoffman et al., 1996, Hoffman 1999. Prepared as an expert report for the Hanford litigation, to respond to suggestions and recommendations of the NRC Subcommittee's 2002 Hanford Thyroid Disease Study Draft Final Report. See also Hoffman, F. O., Ruttenber, A. J., Apostoaei, A. L., Carroll, R. J., and Greenland, S. 2007. The Hanford Thyroid Disease Study: An alternative view of the findings. *Health Physics Journal* 92(2):99-111.

    a. HTDS results do not show statistically significant elevations in risk but are not inconsistent with other published studies *supporting* risks for certain thyroid diseases from I-131 exposures, if the upper bounds of the calculated confidence intervals are considered (as pointed out for the situation of thyroid cancer and I-131 exposure from NTS fallout by the NRC). [emphasis added]

b. Applying a strict interpretation of the lack of statistical significance found in the results of HTDS, we find that the results of HTDS are consistent with the finding of thyroid risk in some but not all studies of I-131 exposures, but not consistent with those studies which show elevated thyroid risk, or;

c. If the results are subjected to strict interpretation based upon statistical significance, then HTDS is not inconsistent with other studies which show that chronic exposure to I-131 is not associated with thyroid disease.

60. NAS-BRER. 2000. Review of the Hanford Thyroid Disease Study draft final report. Washington, DC: National Academy Press, p. 7.
61. Ruttenber, A. J., et al. 30 March 2004. *A technical review of the final report of the Hanford Thyroid Disease Study*. p. 3 See also Hoffman, F. O., Ruttenber, A. J., Apostoaei, A. L., Carroll, R. J., and Greenland, S. Feb. 2007. The Hanford Thyroid Disease Study: An alternative view of the findings. *Health Physics Journal* 92(2): 99-111.
62. Instead, only NTS fallout was taken into account within HTDS. Doses were divided into two parts based on the median dose for all subjects (5.3 mGy) and then put through simple analysis as a confounder or effect modifier in dose-response models. These simple analyses caused HTDS authors to conclude that NTS fallout doses were not confounders or effect modifiers in any model, and so could be disregarded. The expert panel found that, for people who consumed fresh milk, the cut-off dose utilized for NTS fallout I-131 exposures within HTDS appeared to be very low and relevant only to people who did not consume fresh milk. Use of the National Cancer Institute's online I-131 NTS fallout dose calculator http://ntsi131.nci.nih.gov/ shows, for counties included in HTDS, that typical NTS doses from drinking fresh milk are much higher than 5.3 mGy. For those individuals who had not consumed any milk at all, other milk consumption scenarios reveal NTS I-131 doses which were substantially higher than the 5.3 mGy assigned within HTDS. 1,616 of the HTDS participants were assigned NTS I-131 doses of less than 5.3 mGy by HTDS researchers. Because only 8 percent of HTDS participants reported no consumption of raw or processed milk products, it was not reasonable that 1,616 participants would have NTS doses less than 5.3 mGy. "Therefore, it appears that the NTS doses calculated for members of the HTDS cohort have been underestimated." Ruttenber, A. J., et al. 30 March 2004. *A technical review of the final report of the Hanford Thyroid Disease Study*, p. 9.
63. See Commission on Life Sciences. 1998. Letter report-review of analysis plan for the Hanford Thyroid Disease Study (HTDS). National Academies of Science.
64. Fallout from thyroid study: Critics fault CDC for early, unreviewed results. *Spokesman Review*, 19 February 1999.
65. Letter of 18 February 1999 to Dr. Dick Jackson, then Director of NCEH, re: problems with HTDS, signed by more than 22 citizen groups.
66. Greenland, S. 1977. Response and follow-up bias in cohort studies. *American Journal of Epidemiology* 106(3):184-187.
67. Fred Hutchinson Cancer Research Center/CDC. 1998. Preliminary technical review of the Hanford Thyroid Disease Study draft final report, p. 6.
68. Greene, G. 1999. *The woman who knew too much: Alice Stewart and the secrets of radiation.* Ann Arbor, MI: University of Michigan Press, p. 216.

69. The incidence of thyroid cancer found within HTDS was very close to that which was predicted by the medical monitoring program plan. See Spengler, R. F. July 1997. Hanford medical monitoring program: Background consideration document and ATSDR decision. US DHHS, ATSDR.
70. HTDS Newsletter, February 1997.
71. Davis, S., Kopecky, K. J, and Hamilton, T. E. 1999. Hanford Thyroid Disease Study final report, p. 326, 370.
72. Davis, S., and Kopecky, K. 1998. HTDS final report, summary and conclusions, p. 5
73. Ruttenber, A. J., et al. 30 March 2004. *A technical review of the final report of the Hanford Thyroid Disease Study.* This technical report was written in support of Hanford plaintiffs in litigation. The report as such is not independent, but it has no relationship to the authors of HTDS nor CDC.
74. This was the most supportable interpretation, particularly because of the HTDS overestimates of statistical power and the incomplete characterization of the effects of dose uncertainty.
75. Considerably more goiter and other thyroid disease was reported in the R-11 Hanford Survey than in national survey data. See Report of R-11 survey results. 14 November 1995. JSI Center for Environmental Health Studies. See also Grossman, C. M., Morton, W. E., and Nussbaum, R. H. 1997. Malignancies among Hanford downwinders. Presented at the Health of the Hanford Site Conference, 3 December 1997.
76. Friedman, S. M. 2001. Risk communication, the Hanford Thyroid Disease Study and draft reports. 12 *Risk: Health, Safety & Environment.* 91(Spring):91-103. The initial seven members of the HTDS Advisory Committee were appointed in early 1991. The committee was disbanded 6 months before the release of the draft final HTDS, without communicating with committee members. CDC then did not renew the committee's charter, also without explanation to the Advisory Committee.
77. See David, S., Kopecky, K., and Hamilton, T. 1999. Letter to the Editor. Findings of study "clear and unequivocal." *Seattle Post-Intelligencer,* 14 March 1999.
78. See Centers for Disease Control and Prevention. 1999. Press release. Draft report: Results of the Hanford Thyroid Disease Study 28 January 1999. Quoting Scott Davis.
79. See Congressional Briefing. 27 January 1999. Document on Hanford Thyroid Disease Study. Centers for Disease Control and Prevention, Summary of the Study and the Primary Findings.
80. See Fred Hutchinson Cancer Research Center. January 1999. Questions and answers about the HTDS results. *HTDS Newsletter.*
81. *Hanford Medical Monitoring Program.* January 1998. A publication of the Agency for Toxic Substances and Disease Registry.
82. Downwinders program gets 5 million from DOE. *TriCity Herald.* 23 January 1998. http://www.hanfordnews.com
83. Galloway, A. 1999. Another look at radiation report urged. *Seattle Post-Intelligencer.* 15 December 1999.
84. Friedman, S. M. 2001. Risk communication, the Hanford Thyroid Disease Study and draft reports. 12 *Risk: Health, Safety & Environment* 91(Spring):101.

85. See *Trisha T. Pritikin v. United States Department of Energy et al.,* 47 F. Supp. 2d 1225 (E.D. Wash. 1999), affirmed at 254 F.3d 791 (9th Cir. 2001), cert. denied 19 February 2002 at 534 US 1133; 122 S.Ct. 1076; 151 L.Ed.2d 977.
86. See NAS/IOM. 1999. Exposure of the American people to iodine-131 from Nevada nuclear bomb tests: Review of the National Cancer Institute report and public health implications. Washington, DC: National Academy Press.
87. National Research Council's Committee on Environmental Epidemiology's definition. See Connor, T. 1997. *Burdens of proof.* Energy Research Foundation, p. 11.
88. Skrabanek P. 1992. The poverty of epidemiology. *Perspectives in Biology and Medicine* 35:182-185.
89. Skrabanek P. 1993. The epidemiology of errors (commentary). *Lancet* 342:1502.
90. Wing, S. 1994. Limits of epidemiology. *Medicine and Global Survival* 1:74-86.
91. Hanford Health Information Network. September 1994. Radiation health effects, A monograph study of the health effects of radiation and information concerning radioactive releases from the Hanford Site 1942-1972, p. 21, cited in Connor, T. 1997. *Burdens of proof.* Energy Research Foundation, p. 12.
92. Hanford Health Information Network. March 2000. Perspectives on the Hanford Thyroid Disease Study: The HTDS has done more harm than good for Hanford downwinders, p. 5.
93. See Nussbaum, R. H., Hoover, P. P., Grossman, C. M., and Nussbaum, F. D. 2004. Community-based participatory health survey of Hanford, WA, downwinders: A model for citizen empowerment. *Society and Natural Resources* 17:547-559.
94. R-11 study respondents reported goiter and other thyroid diseases approximately 6-10 times as frequently as respondents in the latest National Health Interview Survey. See Report of R-11 survey results. 14 November 1995. JSI Center for Environmental Health Studies.

http://dx.doi.org/10.2190/TORC3

CHAPTER 3

A Community's Experience with Environmental Health Research at the Fernald Feed Production Plant

Edwa Yocum

In 1951, the U.S. Department of Energy (DOE) built a nuclear feed processing plant, formerly known as the Fernald Feed Material Production Center (FMPC), in Crosby Township, Ohio, a semirural community 17 miles northwest of Cincinnati, Ohio.

The Fernald facility processed uranium ore, which was chemically converted into a series of uranium salts (orange oxide) and uranium tetra fluoride (green salt). Later, the focus shifted to processing other uranium feed material in the form of uranium metal extracted from the salt at high temperatures. Metal was then machined or extruded into tubular form and fabricated into reactor fuel cores and target elements that were shipped to other DOE sites in the nuclear weapons complex.

During the 34 years of plant operation, from 1954 to 1988, an estimated 310,000 kg of airborne uranium dust was released into the atmosphere. An additional 99,000 kg of radioactive liquid waste from water used for processing uranium was released in services and storm drains that emptied into the Great Miami River and Paddy's Run Creek. In addition to radioactive contaminants, other nonradiological toxic substances were released, including chlorinated and nonchlorinated solvents, metals, and metal salts. These releases were of great concern to families living within a five-mile radius of the Fernald site (Figure 1) because groundwater and the Great Miami aquifer were the main sources of water

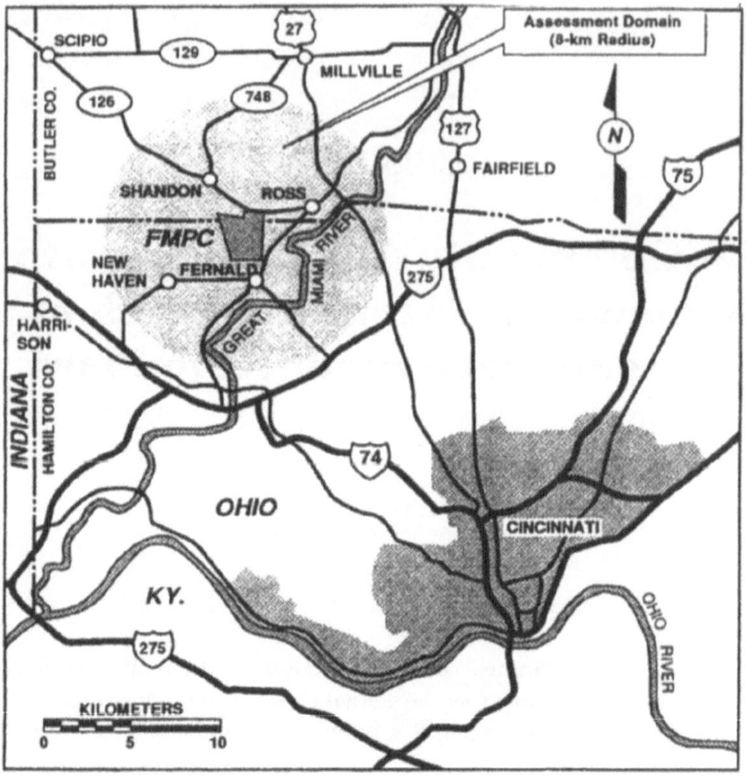

Figure 1. Location of the FMPC. The assessment domain is the region around the site with which this study is principally concerned. Doses will be calculated (Task 6) for people within the assessment domain.

that supplied their wells and cisterns. Community residents may have been exposed to both radiological and nonradiological contamination through groundwater pathways, soil contamination, and air dispersion of emissions from the plant [1]. This chapter describes how the community has felt a burden to prove the possible health risks of these contaminations.

THE NEED TO BUILD AND MAINTAIN TRUST

The following events are discussed here to provide an understanding of why residents of the communities surrounding the DOE Fernald site lost all trust in the credibility of the local, state, and federal health and environmental protection agencies—the very agencies formed to protect the public's health and the environment.

Between 1961 and 1984, academic researchers, the U.S. Geologic Survey, the Ohio Public Health Service (OPHS), and the Ohio Environmental Protection Agency (OEPA) discovered the first evidence that the DOE's lack of waste management at the Fernald site had led and would continue to lead to the contamination of surface water, groundwater, and soil. In 1981, the OEPA detected uranium contamination in groundwater south of the Fernald site and three residential wells across from the Fernald site. Neither the OEPA nor the OPHS notified the three residents that their wells were contaminated. In January 1982, the OEPA sampled fourteen residential wells in the Fernald area to determine the extent of uranium contamination off-site. When Congressman Thomas Luken became aware of the contaminated residential wells through newspaper articles, he notified residents Ken and Lisa Crawford that their well was one of the three wells contaminated by the Fernald plant operation. For seven years the Crawfords had been drinking, bathing, and cooking with uranium-contaminated well water measuring 190 micrograms per liter.

The Crawfords and other residents became enraged and frightened about the possible health impacts from the Fernald dust releases and contamination found in the groundwater. Residents contacted and requested the aid of their local and state public health services to test their wells and cisterns for uranium and toxic chemicals coming from the Fernald site. The OPHS (formerly known as the Ohio Department of Health) denied the request because the health agency did not have the adequate equipment for testing for uranium. Furthermore, they replied that the contamination came from a federal facility, therefore making it a federal issue. Both local and state health agencies were unable to offer information on what steps the community needed to take for their protection. During this period the city and state health departments refrained from communicating with residents living in the contaminated communities. Several years later, OEPA began to address the community's concerns.

In December 1984, Congressman Luken requested that the DOE hold a public meeting. The DOE staff held the public meeting and assured the community that there was no health risk from the uranium contamination. Residents who attended this public meeting demanded the DOE provide testing of all residential wells and cisterns in the contaminated area (South Plume). Due to the residents' demands, the DOE contracted with the OPHS to perform environmental sampling on residential wells and cisterns. The OPH staff collected water samples from the residents' kitchen faucets. Many of the residents with cisterns felt that the faucet samples were inadequate and should have been taken directly from the bottom of the cisterns. The DOE Fernald mailed letters of the sampling results to residents. The results were expressed in three different measurements: parts per billion of water (ppb), milligrams of uranium per liter of water (mg/l), and picocuries of uranium per liter of water (pCi/l). To a lay person, the three different measurements only added to the confusion of understanding the results.

The letters also informed residents of the background concentration of naturally occurring uranium in the Fernald area in picocuries (0.07 to 2.0 pCi/l.), and stated that the well samples were slightly higher than background. If a resident's well within a two-mile radius of the Fernald site showed above background levels, the Fernald contractor took monthly water samples. It was not until 1991 that the DOE supplied bottled water to residents living in the contaminated south plume whose wells were above background.

RESIDENTS BEAR THE BURDEN OF PROOF

Residents realized the burden of proof of a health risk would lie on their shoulders. In late 1984, the area residents formed a grassroots environmental group: The Fernald Residents for Environmental Safety and Health (FRESH) to educate themselves, the affected community, public officials (county, state, and federal), and local physicians on the possible contamination related to the Fernald site.

FRESH members needed to have their questions and concerns addressed, namely, "what is the health risk of being exposed to radionuclides and toxic chemicals released from the Nuclear Feed Material Production Center?"

FRESH recognized the need to get the attention of the National Center for Environmental Health (NCEH) or independent researchers to address their health concerns. In 1990, as the FRESH Health Chairperson, I was concerned about the health risks associated with exposures to radionuclides and toxic chemicals and designed a cancer incidence map to be used as an educational tool (Figure 2). To develop the map, I collected names of residents living in the Fernald communities who had health concerns that could be potentially related to living near the Fernald site. I placed pins on the map to represent the location of the residents with cancers and/or illnesses, such as multiple chromosomes, lung cancer, breast cancer, urinary system diseases, male and female reproductive problems, multiple miscarriages, multiple skin disorders, pituitary tumors, brain tumors, thyroid disease, and Hodgkin's disease. The first 100 pins depicted clusters of people possibly impacted by living near the Fernald site having certain cancers and other illnesses. Patterns formed in the northeast direction consistent with the prevailing wind and in the southeast direction consistent with the southern flow of the contaminated ground water. This was confirmed five years later by the CDC's Dosimetry Reconstruction Project [1].

FRESH planned to use this information from the map to attract the interest of the NCEH or an independent researcher to come to our community and further our study. We hoped that they would confirm the health effects caused by the releases from the Fernald site and use this data to correct the wrong done to residents and workers. Community members visited Senator John Glenn and requested an epidemiologic study. In 1988, Congress mandated that the NCEH

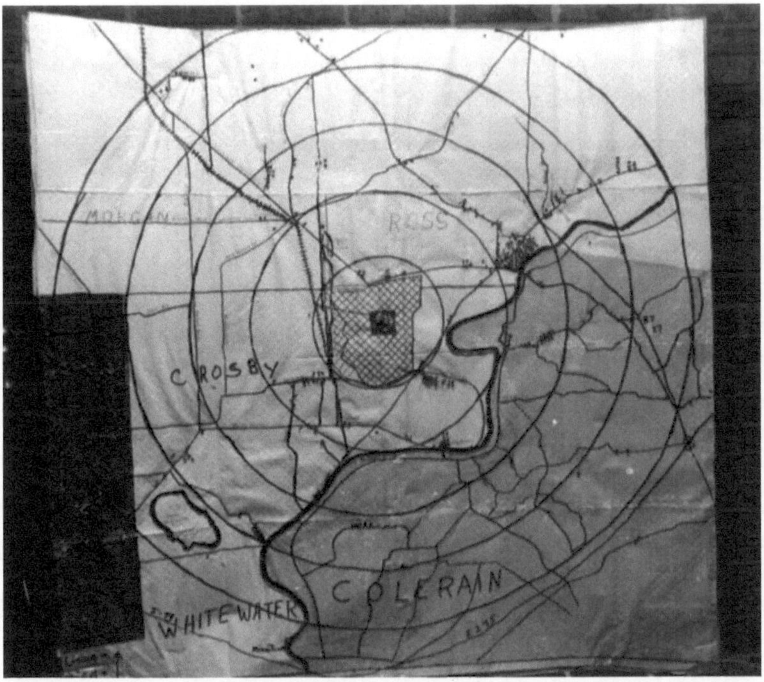

Figure 2. Cancer incidence map.

conduct an epidemiologic study in the Fernald community to evaluate health risks from possible radiation exposure.

DESCRIPTION AND FINDINGS OF THE NCEH INVESTIGATIONS

From 1990 to 2000, the NCEH Radiation Studies Branch determined that a dose reconstruction, a risk assessment, and a public health assessment needed to be undertaken to assess whether the health problems in the Fernald community could be related to exposure to radioactive material from the FMPC.

FINDINGS OF THE FERNALD DOSIMETRY RECONSTRUCTION PROJECT

Between 1990 and 1998, the CDC and the Radiological Assessments Corporation (RAC) conducted the Dosimetry Reconstruction Project (also known as the Dose Reconstruction Study) to estimate radiation doses and risks to people who lived near the FMPC during its years of operation. The project was divided into six tasks:

Task 1. Identify release points at the FMPC site.

Task 2. Determine the amounts of radioactive material released to the environment and the variability of release rates.

Task 3. Determine uncertainties associated with those historic releases.

Task 4. Develop methods to describe environmental transport of the released material and how people may have been exposed to those materials.

Task 5. Present monitoring data to be used for model validation in Task 6 and for source term reconstruction in Tasks 2 and 3.

Task 6. Calculate doses for people within the assessment domain (a five-mile radius around the Fernald facility).

The final results suggested that the primary radiation exposure to Fernald residents resulted from the inhalation of radon-decay products released into the atmosphere from the K-65 Silos used in processing uranium ores. The results also indicated a potential increased risk of lung cancer mortality and other fatal cancers, as well as a likelihood of toxic effects on the kidneys due to exposure to other radionuclides, such as thorium, radium, and uranium [2].

NCEH RISK ASSESSMENT PHASE 1 AND PHASE 2

The Dose Reconstruction Study was followed by the NCEH Risk Assessment Study conducted by the CDC to estimate the radiation-related health risk to people who lived near the FMPC and to assist in evaluating the feasibility of an epidemiologic study within the communities. The study, also known as the Fernald Risk Assessment Project, was conducted in two phases:

Phase 1: Assessed the potential lifetime risk for death from lung cancer that expanded beyond the risk projected in the Dose Reconstruction Study. The result was that an estimated number of lung cancer deaths among the assessment population may increase one to twelve percent over a lifetime.

Phase 2: Provided screening-level estimates of lifetime risk of developing kidney cancer, female breast cancer, bone cancer, and leukemia. The result of using worst-case estimates of the number of cancer cases that may result from exposure to radioactive material, including exposure to contaminated well water, among the population in the assessment domain is

4 or fewer additional cases of kidney cancer;
3 or fewer additional cases of female breast cancer;
4 or fewer additional cases of bone cancer; and
23 or fewer additional cases of leukemia [3].

NCEH recommended not doing a more detailed analysis of radiation-related risk for kidney, breast, bone cancers, and leukemia because the power of the study was too low to identify the effects, which included other risk factors, such as smoking [4].

Findings of a Feasibility Assessment for an Epidemiologic Study of Lung Cancer

The Fernald risk assessment was used in evaluating the feasibility of conducting an epidemiologic study of lung cancer within Fernald communities. The findings of the feasibility assessment are as follows:

- An epidemiologic study would take enormous resources to identify and locate past and present residents who lived in the assessment domain (a five-mile radius around the Fernald site) during 1952-1984.
- An epidemiologic study would take 10 years and possibly cost tens of millions of dollars.
- Information on smoking history and other potential risk factors may be poor because information would likely have to be provided by proxy respondents.
- The statistical power would be too low to estimate radiation dose.
- The study would be unlikely to detect an association between lung cancer and FMPC-related radiation exposure if it exists [4].

THE ATSDR'S FINAL REPORT OF THE FERNALD PUBLIC HEALTH ASSESSMENT

In May 2000, the Agency for Toxic Substances and Disease Registry (ATSDR) released for public comment a draft report of the Fernald Public Health Assessment (FPHA). The Fernald community made comments which are included in the final FPHA report. However, the report was not completed in a timely manner. After four years of peer review, the final FPHA report was released in August 2004. When Fernald area residents asked ATSDR why it took four years to complete the report, the ATSDR explained that there were two rewrites of the report, and that the ATSDR staff was occupied with another health study not related to Fernald.

The ATSDR presented the FPHA final report at a public meeting. The public attending the meeting was disappointed in the report because it was four years late. What was the purpose for discussion? The community felt betrayed and forgotten. Also upsetting to the community was the recommendation of the May 2000 FPHA draft report for an in-depth assessment of past exposure to chemical and radioactive contaminants in privately owned residential wells near the Fernald site because of the following past public health hazards: (1) ingestion of uranium in water from privately-owned wells in the South Plume area; and (2) inhalation of radon, radon decay products, and air-borne uranium. By contrast, the final 2004 report recommended the following: "If only additional pertinent information becomes available, an in-depth assessment of past exposure to air-borne, non-uranium chemical contaminants in privately-owned residential wells near the Fernald facility should be conducted" [2].

Furthermore, the researchers did not investigate cisterns as a possible pathway of exposure. This was a concern to residents because water stored in a cistern can come from potentially contaminated well water transported by truck from wells in the contaminated area and/or the filling of a cistern with rain from a roof that was covered with dust released from the Fernald site.

COMMUNITY PARTICIPATION IN NCEH HEALTH STUDIES

The Fernald Health Effects Subcommittee

In June 1996, the CDC's Radiation Studies Branch and the ATSDR sponsored the Fernald Health Effects Subcommittee (FHES). The FHES was formed as a formal Federal Advisory Committee for the community to provide advice and recommendations for research conducted by the CDC, ATSDR, and the NIOSH (National Institute for Occupational Safety and Health).

The FHES was the fourth Federal Advisory Committee formed under the Memorandum of Understanding with the DOE and the federal health agencies. The FHES members included regional and local residents, the Fernald contractor and former workers, labor representatives, scientists, local physicians, and four liaison members that included representatives from the Ohio Environmental Protection Agency (OEPA) and the Ohio Department of Health Services (ODHS). The meetings were open to the public and held approximately four times a year in the Fernald area. The CDC Executive Secretary was responsible for planning, organizing, and publicizing meetings. He prepared agendas and assisted the FHES chair with facilitating discussion. The NIOSH and ATSDR presented progress reports of their research activities. FHES members formed three work groups: (1) education for local physicians, (2) position papers and mission statement, and (3) strategies for community outreach.

The work groups met during each subcommittee meeting and held conference calls to accomplish certain tasks. Work groups reported back to the full subcommittee and presented recommendations. Some of the recommendations were to

- Conduct educational workshops for area physicians. Two workshops were implemented.
- Develop community outreach strategies, fliers, fact sheets, and meeting announcements. This was accomplished.
- Draft a mission statement and position paper. This was never implemented.

The subcommittee did not receive training to evaluate the risks and benefits of certain health research methods. At FHES meetings, the public and subcommittee would receive an explanation of the health agency's chosen health study, what research method would be used, and its benefits. Most area residents played a passive role as participants, believing the researcher knew what research projects would address their health concerns related to the Fernald site.

The FHES members and the researchers had a different interpretation of the subcommittee's role in the research advisory process. The subcommittee believed their purpose was to advise the researchers on what health studies should be conducted after the Dosimetry Reconstruction Project estimated radiation doses and possible health risks. By contrast, the subcommittee felt that the researchers believed the role of the subcommittee was to provide consensus on the researchers' chosen health study. Therefore, the researchers found meeting the request of the FHES for additional information on a proposed health study, which would be helpful to FHES in their advisory role, to be time-consuming and distracting from their health study.

Recommendations of Community and Subcommittee Members

1. During the Dosimetry Reconstruction Project, the community directed the Radiological Assessments Corporation (RAC) to:
   a. Hold evening meetings to accommodate working residents.
   b. Write and present reports in layman's terms.
   c. Consider community members' local knowledge, which is very useful in filling in gaps of Fernald historical data.

2. During the risk assessment, the FHES recommended that CDC delay assessing the feasibility of an epidemiologic study on lung cancer, and instead evaluate other risks of excess cancers (i.e., kidney cancer, female breast cancer, bone cancer, and leukemia) and medical conditions potentially caused by exposure to uranium.

3. The FHES recommended that the CDC should not do an epidemiologic study on lung cancers due to other confounders like smoking, as smoking was very prevalent during the production period at the Fernald site. Other reasons included the cost of the study, the projected length of time, and a potential lack of a benefit to the affected communities. The FHES believed the resources from the epidemiologic study could be better spent studying the health effects of low-level exposure to radiation and toxic chemicals and the possible cumulative effects of exposure to uranium and other chemicals. The resources could also be used to study the risk of illnesses and diseases of concern in the affected community, such as, but not limited to, birth defects, urinary system diseases, and colon and breast cancer.

4. The FHES recommended that researchers follow up on the Dose Reconstruction Study's recommendation for an in-depth look into the groundwater pathway relating to radionuclide exposure and possible toxic effects on the kidneys. CDC refused this recommendation.

5. The FHES recommended two educational workshops for Fernald area health professionals. The ATSDR educational program staff along with Mercy Health Partners from a local hospital and University of Cincinnati College of Medicine sponsored two workshops in 1998 and 2000. The workshops helped health professionals gain knowledge of historical exposures of former employees and residents and pathways of exposure. The workshops also taught health professionals to identify specific types and potential human health effects of radiological and toxicological exposure.

6. The FHES recommended a health study of non-cancer health outcomes. The ATSDR accepted this recommendation and contacted the UC College of Medicine to do the study using data from the Fernald Medical Monitoring database. The subcommittee did not participate in the research process.

Disbanding of the Fernald Health Effects Subcommittee

The researchers came into the Fernald community to do a congressionally-mandated epidemiologic study on radiation exposure to the area residents. At an FHES meeting in March 2000, CDC researchers announced they would not be doing an epidemiologic study, therefore their mission was complete. They then announced the discontinuation of the FHES, which came as a surprise to the subcommittee. When the FHES was established, no discussion or planning took place regarding how long the subcommittee should operate or criteria for discontinuation. Furthermore, the community had not been given the chance to express its support or to voice its concerns. The subcommittee was confused and stated their opposition to disbanding because they had just completed a successful membership drive under the direction of the FHES Executive Secretary. It was decided that the subcommittee would meet for further discussion.

Before the next FHES meeting, the subcommittee put together a public petition called, "In Support of the Continuation of Activities Conducted by the Fernald Health Effects Subcommittee." The meeting was attended by a large number of residents, members of the Fernald labor force, interested scientists, and members of the Greater Cincinnati medical community. Community members stated the need to address research on the groundwater pathway because groundwater is the main source that supplies residential wells and cisterns. After all, the ATSDR's Fernald Public Health Assessment draft report recommended an in-depth assessment of past exposures to chemical and radioactive contaminants in privately-owned residential wells using up-to-date modeling techniques because the contaminated South Plume area posed a public health hazard under *past* conditions at the Fernald site. Community members also stated that the Dosimetry Reconstruction Project data was not being used to its full potential.

The CDC indicated that they could not respond to the signed public petition and stated that their specific mission to investigate the health impact of radiation on the Fernald communities (through an epidemiological study) was complete. The Fernald Health Effects Subcommittee was disbanded in August 2001.

Obstacles to Community-Driven Research

Five obstacles to community-driven research are identified here. These obstacles provide an emphasis for how the NCEH and ATSDR response to community health concerns from the radiation releases of the Fernald plant became inadequate and incomplete.

1. Community members lacked sufficient scientific knowledge and background related to radionuclides, toxic chemicals, and the pathways of exposure. The lack of knowledge allowed the researchers to control the directions of the research. Community members need the assistance of an available independent researcher who can assist them through the process of a health study and help them determine what questions to ask so that they may make informed decisions and not remain passive participants.

2. Different interpretations of the advisory process led to different expectations. The subcommittee believed that the researchers saw the role of the subcommittee as that of providing consensus on the researchers' chosen health study, and the subcommittee believed their purpose was to advise the researchers on what health studies should be conducted in order to better address the community's health concerns.

3. The subcommittee made comments on the ATSDR's studies, but was not welcome to actively participate in the health studies (particularly in providing local knowledge to health investigations).

4. Health agencies had limited personnel and funding to address the needs of the affected community.

5. Scientists and researchers lacked adequate communication skills in relating with the affected community. Some scientists refuse to address the public. Scientists do not understand the frustration and the fear of the unknown that causes the community members to lash out when their questions related to low-level exposure cannot be answered directly or when a health study is never conclusive.

ATSDR Health Activities and Public Participation at Fernald

In 1999, the ATSDR came into the Fernald community and organized four public availability sessions where residents voiced their opinions, stated their health concerns, and asked questions about health issues related to the Fernald site and the contamination. These sessions were the only community participation in the ATSDR research activities.

Responding to community concerns, the ATSDR released results of four public health consultations [5] based on environmental data that ATSDR collected on the four following exposure issues:

- Ambient radon levels and radon emissions from the K65 Silos
- Consumption of milk products at local dairies near the Fernald site
- Consumption of produce grown on farms near the Fernald site
- Nonpotable use of uranium-contaminated groundwater

As a result of the four consultations, the ATSDR found that there was "no public health hazard to the community" [6-9]. The community was not satisfied with the process used to come to this conclusion for the following reasons: (1) The background measure used for radon was the background reading at the time of the consultations. The ATSDR should have used the background measure during the early years of no exposure when it would have been lower. (2) Researchers did not communicate with residents, and therefore they were not familiar with their lifestyle. (3) The sampling of food from local fruit stands had a mixture of local and out-of-town produce. (4) The findings of the groundwater sampling for nonpotable water did not suggest a health hazard from radionuclides. (5) The findings did not indicate that the groundwater used for potable water was safe. Some residents recommended changing the words describing "nonpotable" to "nondrinking purposes" and "potable" to "drinking purposes."

Also in 1999, the subcommittee had recommended a study of noncancer health outcomes. The ATSDR coordinated with the University of Cincinnati Medical Center to conduct a study on the prevalence of adverse health outcomes in persons living near the Fernald site. The University used data from the Fernald Medical Monitoring Program (FMMP). The FMMP is for off-site residents set up as part of the 1994 class-action settlement with the government. This allows volunteer residents to obtain free periodic examinations to detect possible adverse health outcomes. In 2001, the study findings were released. The findings suggested that the exposure domain (types and levels) in the past is related to health effects on urinary system function. The subcommittee did not participate in the research process.

Community and Academia Form a Partnership

In 2001, when the CDC and the ATSDR disbanded the Fernald Health Effects Subcommittee, the Fernald area residents formed a community-based health organization "The Fernald Community Health Effects Committee, Inc.

(FCHEC)." Area residents believed there was an ongoing need for continued research of potential health issues related to the Fernald site and the need for better communication of the results. The FCHEC formed a partnership with the University of Cincinnati Environmental Health Foundation (UEHF).

The FCHEC members and a UEHF technical advisory committee, referred to here as "The Research Team," used the Community-Based Participatory Research (CBPR) approach in the development and conduct of their research project. The CBPR methods afforded the FCHEC members opportunities to conduct numerous research tasks described below.

1. The research project was reviewed and approved by the Institutional Review Board (IRB). This is required to conduct research involving human participants.

2. The Research Team established the roles and responsibilities to support and promote the community and academic partnership. All parties meaningfully contributed to the design, data collection, data analysis, and communication of the findings. The specific research methods used include a self-administered survey, interviews, mapping wells in the five-mile area, and gathering information about Fernald water quality. Techniques for maintaining confidentiality and obtaining informed consent were also used.

3. The research team planned procedures for publicizing the survey, documenting outreach, contacts, and distributing and collecting surveys at distribution outlets. To announce the survey project, an article was placed in three local newspapers and local organizations' newsletters and the Research Team recorded a video to help in their presentations at local meetings. Two drop-off stations centrally located in the five-mile area of the exposure domain were set up for resident's to pick up and drop off surveys. In addition, the Research Team distributed surveys to gas stations, convenient stores, and banks. All presentations, drop-offs, and distributions were recorded in the outreach log.

4. The Research Team registered completed surveys by recording receipts in the logbook by an identification number and entered them into an electronic database. Surveys requiring additional information or clarification were flagged for Research Team members to follow up by phone.

5. The Research Team developed a work plan for creating a database of sources of water quality data for the Fernald area. The team also created an electronic inventory of the wells logged in the five-mile exposure domain.

The goal of the research project is to inform the public of possible exposure routes so that they could prevent or minimize exposure. The public is empowered with knowledge about potential exposure and the associated adverse health outcomes. When they share this information with their physician, it may help the physician manage the patient's care. This research project is an essential step in collecting information that can be used to further additional studies related to wells and cisterns.

CONCLUSION

Members of a community that believe there is a health risk from radiological, heavy metal, or toxic chemicals contamination must bear the burden of gathering information related to the health risk. This information is critical in convincing the appropriate people to help them address their health concerns.

The average affected community member will likely be a passive participant in ongoing health studies due to the lack of technical knowledge. To help community members be active participants, an independent scientist could assist them in having a better understanding of the scientific language and limitations of a study, and in asking the appropriate questions during the health study and research process. An independent scientific advisor would allow the study scientists and researchers to direct their time toward completing the health study in a timely manner. To extend the community's participation, the scientist should provide quarterly progress reports, communicate in layman's terms, and answer questions directly.

Community members may take an active role in their own research project that can address their health concerns by contacting a university that offers a Community-Based Participatory Research (CBPR) program. CBPR academic researchers can be of great help and guidance to the community in addressing their health concerns.

NOTES

1. Voilleque, P. G., Meyer, K. R., Schmidt, D. W., et al. 1995. *The Fernald Dosimetry Reconstruction Project, Tasks 2 and 3—Radiologic source terms and uncertainties.* Radiological Assessment Corporation (RAC) Report No. CDC-5. Neeses, SC.
2. Killough, G. G., Case, M. J., Meyer, K. R., et al. September 1998. The Fernald Dosimetry Reconstruction Project, Task 6—Radiation doses and risk to residents from FMPC Operations from 1951-1988. Volumes I and II (final report). Radiologic Assessment Corporation (RAC) Report No. CDC-1. Neeses, SC.
3. CDC. 1999. Screening level estimates of the lifetime risk of developing kidney cancer, female breast cancer, bone cancer, and leukemia resulting from the maximum estimated exposure to radioactive materials released from the Former Feed Materials Production Center (FMPC). Draft. Centers for Disease Control and Prevention (CDC). Atlanta, GA.
4. Garbe, P. 1999. Feasibility assessment for a community-based epidemiologic study of lung cancer and radiation exposures near the Former Feed Materials Production Center. Presentation to the Fernald Health Effects Subcommittee. September 22.
5. A public health consultation is a review of available information or collection of new data to respond to a specific health question or request for information about a potential environmental hazard. Health consultations are focused on a specific exposure issue. Health consultations are therefore more limited than a public health assessment, which reviews the exposure potential of each pathway and chemical. http://www.atsdr.cdc.gov/glossary.html

6. ATSDR. June 1995. Health consultation for milk produced near the Fernald Environmental Management Project. U.S. Public Health Service, Agency for Toxic Substances and Disease Registry (ATSDR).
7. ATSDR. May 1995. Health consultation for the K-65 silos. U.S. Public Health Service, Agency for Toxic Substances and Disease Registry (ATSDR).
8. ATSDR. February 1996. Health consultation for nonpotable use of uranium contaminated groundwater near the Fernald Environmental Management Project. U.S. Public Health Service, Agency for Toxic Substances and Disease Registry (ATSDR).
9. ATSDR. January 1996. Health consultation for consumption of produce grown near the Fernald Environmental Management Project. U.S. Public Health Service, Agency for Toxic Substances and Disease Registry (ATSDR).

http://dx.doi.org/10.2190/TORC4

CHAPTER 4

Democracy and Public Health at Rocky Flats: The Examples of Edward A. Martell and Carl J. Johnson

LeRoy Moore

A fundamental contradiction exists between democracy and the practice of building nuclear weapons. This truth is strikingly evident in the history of public health science as played out at the Rocky Flats nuclear bomb factory near Denver, Colorado, where over a period of nearly 40 years the fissionable plutonium "pit" for every nuclear weapon in the U.S. arsenal was manufactured.

This chapter, written to counter the art of denial, explores two versions of public health science: one oriented to the "nuclear establishment," the other to public service. The former includes personnel affiliated with the industry and with government agencies that at least implicitly give priority to the industry. The latter comes to focus here on two individuals, the late Edward A. Martell, a radiochemist with the National Center for Atmospheric Research (NCAR), a private nonprofit research body located in Boulder, Colorado, and the late Carl J. Johnson, MD, who for several years was the chief public health officer for Jefferson County, where Rocky Flats is located. Martell was the first to alert the public to dangers at Rocky Flats about which insider scientists remained silent. Johnson became a lightning rod for efforts to curb abuses resulting from operations at Rocky Flats.

I. EDWARD MARTELL: PUBLIC SERVICE FOR PUBLIC HEALTH

Martell's Revelation

On the afternoon of May 11, 1969, people throughout the Denver area saw smoke billowing from a building at the Rocky Flats nuclear bomb factory located at the base of the mountains 16 miles northwest of central Denver. The fire, soon labeled the most expensive industrial fire to date in U.S. history, caught the attention of NCAR radiochemist Ed Martell. He feared that the strong winds common at Rocky Flats had carried potentially lethal particles of plutonium toward unsuspecting people in the Denver area. So he asked Rocky Flats officials to sample off-site soil for plutonium. When they declined, he and colleague Stuart E. Poet took their own samples. At various locations east of the facility they found plutonium deposits in the top centimeter (0.39 inch) of soil up to 400 times average background concentrations from global fallout [1].

In February 1970, Martell and Poet met with officials from Rocky Flats and the Colorado Department of Health (CDH) [2] to discuss their findings. Plant officials insisted that what they found didn't come from the May 1969 fire. A more likely source was either a fire that occurred on September 11, 1957 [3], or leaks from thousands of drums of plutonium-laced waste stored outside in the plant's 903 area from 1954 until 1968. These two events were the sources of the largest plutonium releases from Rocky Flats since operations began at the plant in 1953. Thus did the state government and the public learn about the worst accidents ever at Rocky Flats [4].

In this meeting, a high-ranking Atomic Energy Commission (AEC) official, having learned that two of Martell's colleagues worked for the Commerce Department and that NCAR was a private research center supported by the National Science Foundation, let it be known that he would "bring this matter up with the appropriate officials of the Department of Commerce and the National Science Foundation." He said he had "a personal hang-up about one federal agency engaging in activities critical of another federal agency" [5]. This moment cast a dark shadow over Martell's future career.

Shortly after the meeting, Martell distributed a paper that included the following observations:

- Anyone who inhales particles of plutonium like those released from Rocky Flats would be "subject to radiation millions of times more intense than from an average naturally occurring radioactive dust particle of the same size. . . . Only minute amounts in the lung are sufficient to cause cancer."
- Neither Rocky Flats officials nor Colorado public health officers had provided any data on plutonium in the environment.

- Whether production should continue at Rocky Flats needs to be resolved based on a "thorough assessment" of health effects "by qualified medical researchers who are independent of the AEC" [6].

AEC Response to Martell: Krey

The AEC brought in P. W. Krey, a specialist of their own, to sample for plutonium in soil off the Rocky Flats site. He not only confirmed Martell's results but also showed that plutonium from Rocky Flats was very widely distributed throughout the metro area. When Krey reported his results in *Health Physics*, he mapped plutonium distribution in a series of amoeba-like isopleths graded to show concentrations ranging from higher levels near the facility to lower ones further out until deposits from Rocky Flats could not be distinguished from background [7] (see Figure 1).

Most of Krey's samples consisted of a composite of material from the top 20 centimeters (7.8 inches) of soil. This sampling method may have enabled Krey to estimate the total inventory in soil of plutonium released from Rocky Flats, but it could not show surface concentrations, since his method diluted surface deposits by mixing them with less contaminated soil from below the surface. Also, his isopleths only approximate reality, since they were based on samples taken at only twenty-five off-site locations over a very large area, with Rocky Flats plutonium found at only fifteen.

Colorado Sets a Standard for Plutonium in Soil

In response to revelations of major releases of radiation from Rocky Flats, Colorado established the first standard anywhere for plutonium in soil. In January 1973, it mandated that land where plutonium contamination exceeds 0.2 disintegrations per minute per gram of soil (dpm/g) is "unfit for residential use, subdivision development, or commercial and industrial uses" [8]. Less than two months later, the state increased by tenfold the amount of plutonium to which exposure was allowed, from 0.2 to 2.0 dpm/g. At the same time, the state lifted its prohibition against residential, commercial, or industrial uses in areas too contaminated to meet the standard; hereafter it would merely require "special techniques" for construction in such areas, such as plowing plutonium under [9]. Thus, the standard was completely gutted of its original provisions for public health. In 1975, Martell criticized the state standard for being at least twenty times too high and not protective of public health [10]. Nonetheless, the revised standard remains in effect today.

The State's Misleading Soil Sampling Practice

In February 1974, the Rocky Flats site more than tripled in size by the addition of 4,550 acres eleven months after the establishment of the state's 2.0 dpm/g

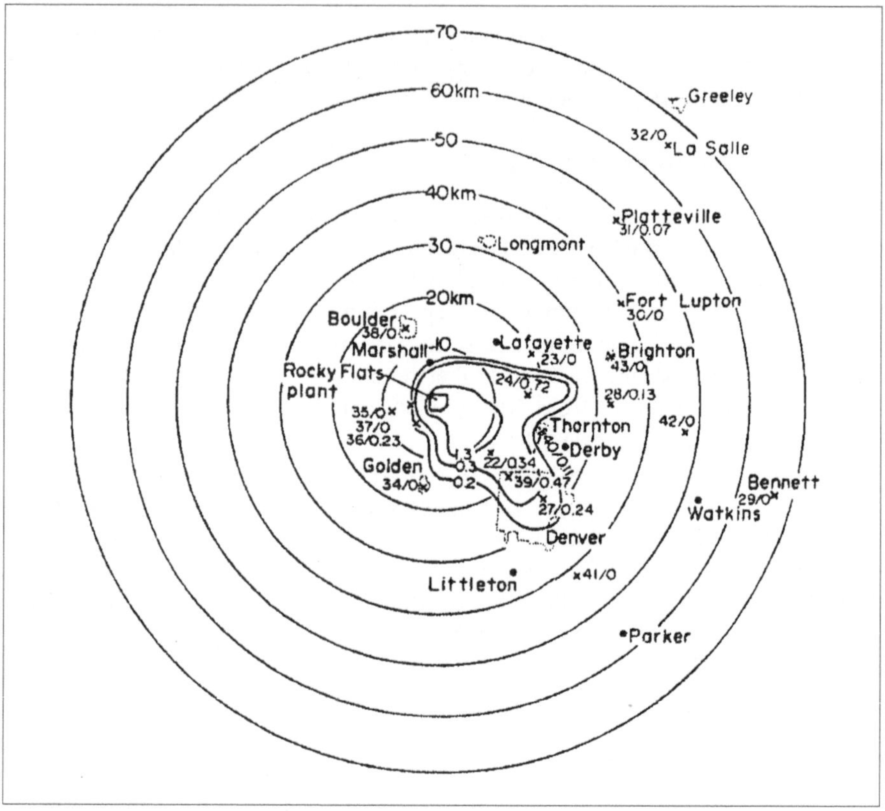

Figure 1. Soil sampling sites in north central Colorado are designated by X. The first of the adjacent pair of numbers to the site represents the site number. The second (following the slash) represents the Rocky Flats plutonium in millicuries per square kilometer (mCi/km^2) measured at the site (one millicurie is 1/1000th of a curie). The heavy irregular lines of the isopleths reflect the isoconcentration contours of Rocky Flats plutonium in the soil expressed as mCi/km^2. The concentric circles reflect the radial distances from the center of the Rocky Flats plant. From Krey, "Remote Plutonium Contamination and Total Inventories from Rocky Flats," *Health Physics,* 30, February 1976, p. 210, reprinted with permission.

standard for plutonium in off-site soil. The site's boundary on the predominantly downwind, down gradient east side was moved out to Indiana Street. In enforcing its new standard for areas east of the enlarged site, the CDH employed from the outset a sampling method that thwarted its ability to locate places where the plutonium concentration exceeded the standard. Rather than analyzing specific samples for their radiation content, the CDH divided the area to be sampled into large sectors, then calculated the average plutonium concentration in each sector by compositing all the soil collected from twenty-five samples taken from within that sector [11]. This approach may show average distribution in large areas, but it dilutes particular points with high readings by averaging them with lower ones, making identification of hot spots impossible.

The CDH's soil sampling also misrepresented reality in that over time it collected samples to increasingly greater depth, thereby diluting the material measured and giving the impression that the quantity of plutonium in the soil was steadily decreasing. An internal study criticized this practice and concluded that plutonium concentrations in soil around Rocky Flats had changed little from 1970 until 1991 [12]. For public health assessments, the CDH eventually adopted the practice of compositing samples taken from the top quarter-inch of soil within a given area. The words of German analyst Ulrich Beck are apt: "Whoever limits pollution has also concurred in it." Standards for "permissible" exposure "may indeed prevent the very worst from happening, but they are at the same time 'blank checks' to poison nature and humankind a bit" [13].

Martell and the Public

Martell's revelations after the 1969 fire sparked public awareness and action. "Nobody knew anything about Rocky Flats until his study," said Judy Danielson, a physical therapist recently returned from doing humanitarian work in Vietnam. She used Martell's work to organize people to go door-to-door in areas east of Rocky Flats asking residents if they could collect a scoop of dirt from their yards to test for radiation content. They labeled these samples with names and addresses and took them to public meetings of candidates for Congress in 1972, asking those running for office to get the samples analyzed and to explain what they'd do about Rocky Flats [14]. This attracted media attention and helped make Rocky Flats an issue that candidates for public office could not ignore.

In 1974, Danielson, a Quaker, and Pam Solo, a nun from the socially active Sisters of Loretto, were hired to share a staff position at the Denver office of the American Friends Service Committee (AFSC). Their focus: nuclear weapons production at Rocky Flats. Thus began what by the end of the decade had blossomed into a national and global movement of resistance to nuclear weapons. The Rocky Flats Action Group, an umbrella body that grew out of the AFSC activities, labeled Rocky Flats a "local hazard and a global threat." The "local hazard" was the public health and environmental danger Martell had exposed, the "global threat" the nuclear holocaust whose possibility haunted him. Observing bomb tests in the South Pacific as an Army radiation health specialist made him, he said, "quite a pacifist. If you appreciate the effects of thermonuclear explosions, you aren't going to be disposed toward the military and wars as the means of settling national affairs" [14, p. 162]. The Rocky Flats movement thus articulated and elaborated Martell's twin concerns.

Back in 1970, Martell had called for a "thorough assessment" of plutonium health effects at Rocky Flats. This never happened. But pressure from those he had energized led to the creation, in late 1974, of the Lamm-Wirth Task Force on Rocky Flats by newly elected Governor Dick Lamm and Congressman Tim Wirth, whose district included Rocky Flats. In 1975, the Task Force recommended that Rocky Flats be closed and its work be relocated [15].

The government's response was to form the Rocky Flats Monitoring Committee, probably the first citizen oversight group created for a nuclear weapons facility anywhere. Pam Solo, who says she was the only "adversary" appointed to this body, reported that they met on a regular basis, toured the Rocky Flats buildings, saw everything, were dazzled with technology, and were treated like VIPs. "The language and euphemisms that they used—a nuclear excursion, as though it was a trip up the Colorado River. You kind of kill off the language." She pressed them: "The Task Force says shut it down and convert it. How are we going to move on this? They would all look at me like I had pulled their pants down." Those meetings, she said, left her "totally numb and sick" [16].

Meanwhile, through the early and mid-1970s, Martell was in considerable demand as a speaker on radiation issues. Toward the end of the decade he cut back on this activity out of frustration "with the media and others whose claims exceeded the scientific evidence" [14, p. 182]. Science could be used, but it could also be abused. In 1986–87, when the DOE wanted to incinerate plutonium-laced waste at Rocky Flats, Martell supported a small group of scientists who worked directly with local people to defeat this plan.

Needless to say, the DOE was in no rush to shut down Rocky Flats. After the Lamm-Wirth recommendation fourteen contentious years would pass—years of repeated workshops, vigils, large demonstrations, and acts of civil disobedience—before production was halted in 1989 because it could not be done without violating federal environmental laws. The change of the Rocky Flats mission from production to cleanup was finally made in 1992 [17].

ALPHA RADIATION: NATURAL BACKGROUND AND GLOBAL FALLOUT

According to Martell, alpha particles released by plutonium taken into the body don't distribute uniformly in an organ as assumed by those "who persist in using the average whole organ dose as the measure of cancer risk" for setting exposure standards. Instead, within the body, alpha particles clump in "hotspots" where their energy is concentrated at levels 100 to 1000 times their average organ concentrations. Also, by means of alpha recoil, they subdivide into a cloud of smaller particles, thereby enhancing their microdistribution and intensifying the potential for harm to surrounding cells, possibly inducing cancer or creating conditions for other ailments [18]. Martell pointed out that "plutonium in fallout from nuclear tests is now present at measurable levels in all human organs." While the amount is very small, it "will certainly contribute to the initiation and progression of malignancy in the general population," particularly when radiation from other sources is added [18, ch.7, pp. 7-8]. He estimated that 80 percent of all cancers are radiation induced, most of them "attributable to lifetime exposures to natural background radiation" [19]. Those who ignore the adverse role of naturally occurring radiation, he noted, find it easy to allow additional exposure from human-made sources. Internal alpha emitters, from natural as well as unnatural sources, "may be the principal agent of radiation-induced cancer" as well as the major contributing factor in arteriosclerosis and resultant cardiovascular disease [20]. The record from Rocky Flats and other plutonium-processing sites suggests increased incidence of coronaries among plutonium workers [21].

Effects of Radiation on Plutonium Workers

In 1975, Karl Z. Morgan, for 29 years head of health physics at DOE's Oak Ridge Lab and a major figure in establishing radiation exposure standards, proposed reducing the maximum allowable lifetime plutonium body burden for nuclear workers 200-fold [22]. Martell noted that this "well justified recommendation" was ignored by standard-setting agencies, but said that he thought Morgan had nevertheless overlooked data that indicate that the worker standard should be reduced by a factor not of 200 but of 1000 or more [18, ch. 6, p. 38].

In early 1994, encouraged by the openness initiative of then-Energy Secretary Hazel O'Leary, Martell wrote to her specifically about plutonium workers:

> [A] complete, objective, independent follow-up of the medical histories and body burdens of plutonium . . . workers is long overdue and would shed considerable light on the full magnitude of plutonium cancer risks. . . . [It is] exceedingly important to have the best possible assessment of plutonium cancer risks *before* cleanup of plutonium contaminated sites at Rocky Flats and elsewhere. . . . For more than 40 years, assessment of the health risks of radionuclides has been controlled by a vested interest establishment that has contrived to minimize or ignore adverse effects of all sources of human exposure to ionizing radiation [23].

All such research, Martell's letter concluded, should be removed from the nuclear establishment. O'Leary made no reply. Now, two decades later, the plight of former workers at facilities like Rocky Flats whose health was destroyed by on-the-job exposures has become a national disgrace, mainly because many of them cannot get promised compensation [24].

Martell: A Whistleblower

When Martell died in 1995, chemist Niels Schonbeck of Denver's Metro State College called him a "whistleblower" who, despite three decades of original radiochemical research at NCAR, was never named a Senior Scientist [25]. In the early 1980s, perhaps because of the aforementioned intervention of an AEC official, his research group was broken up and he lost his lab; he kept his job only due to the support of colleagues [26]. Not long before his death, he said he didn't realize when he joined NCAR in 1962 that "the point was, if there's something disturbing going on, look the other way. . . . I worry about all future generations, because we're not studying radiation-induced health effects, not objectively, not thoroughly" [27].

II. CARL JOHNSON: AGAINST THE TIDE

Innovative Dust Sampling Stops Residential Development

In September 1973, Carl Johnson became Director of the Health Department of Jefferson County, which, with a population of about 250,000, was then the second-most populous county in Colorado. His involvement with Rocky Flats began in December 1974 when Jefferson County Commissioner Joanne Paterson sought his opinion on whether the commissioners should permit a new housing development on land just east of Rocky Flats. The CDH had already approved the project, despite their having found plutonium in surface soil there up to seven times the state standard (they would require plowing prior to construction). "If she had not called me," Johnson later said, "the land would have been developed and there'd be about 10,000 people living there" [28]. He was not deterred by the CDH's prior approval, having already seen "gross errors" in other CDH work [29]. The county commissioners gave Johnson the go-ahead to do a "validation survey of plutonium around the plant" with two soil-science specialists from the U.S. Geological Survey. Johnson and his USGS colleagues developed a protocol for the study and got concurrence from scientists with CDH and the Colorado School of Mines. The samples would be split and analyzed by two labs, one at the CDH, the other at Rocky Flats [30].

This project began in the spring of 1975, using Johnson's innovative method of sampling respirable dust. Dust samples taken at 25 locations showed plutonium concentrations, on average, 44 times greater than what had been measured at the same locations in previous surveys using whole-soil samples collected to a variety of depths. Several of the readings exceeded previous ones by 100 times or more, one by 285 times [31]. Readings were 10 to 40 times greater than what Martell and Poet had found in the top centimeter of soil [32]. When the County Commissioners saw Johnson's results in September 1975, they vetoed residential development on the land in question. Later that year, Marcus Church, owner of the land, sued the Energy Research and Development Administration (ERDA, predecessor to the DOE) and its Rocky Flats contractors, Dow Chemical and Rockwell International, for damages.

Meanwhile, Johnson, having stopped a housing development on contaminated land, suddenly met resistance. Though the principal parties had been consulted beforehand and had accepted the dust-sampling protocol Johnson and his USGS colleagues had developed, as soon as their results became known, officials at the ERDA, EPA, CDH, and Rockwell began to criticize their sampling method, and the CDH and Rocky Flats labs announced they would no longer analyze samples taken by Johnson's group. The negativity would affect all Johnson's future work related to Rocky Flats. Martell, to the contrary, saw Johnson's sampling method as a stroke of genius "that shouldn't be overlooked in any discussion of off-site risk and health studies" [33].

When Johnson and his colleagues reported their work in *SCIENCE*, they faulted the Colorado plutonium-in-soil standard for making no provision for what to do if additional plutonium gets deposited atop what is already present, and for allowing those who build where plutonium contamination exceeds the standard to plow it under; in their view, future activity like gardening or construction could bring it back to the surface. A "more realistic" standard for plutonium in surface soil, they said, would be based "on the respirable-dust fraction because the very small particles in this fraction have the greatest potential for suspension and inhalation" [34].

Johnson Proposes a New Standard for Plutonium in Soil

In October 1975 Johnson formally proposed that for purposes of assessing health risk, the state set a new standard based on plutonium in respirable dust on the surface of the soil [35]. "The coarser materials which are not inhaled and retained," he pointed out, "have no bearing on the actual hazard to health and serve only to dilute the amount of radioactivity found by analysis, and may yield a spurious low concentration of plutonium that is misleading" [36].

The CDH did not welcome Johnson's proposal. To resolve the issue, the Colorado Land Use Commission brought in Karl Z. Morgan, former chair of the internal dose committee of both the National Council on Radiation Protection and Measurements and the International Commission on Radiological Protection and recently retired from the DOE's Oak Ridge Lab. Morgan was asked whether for assessing the public health risk from plutonium in surface soil it was better to follow Johnson in using dust samples or the CDH in collecting whole-soil samples. Morgan sided with Johnson, in favor of using samples limited to "the respirable portion, less than 5 microns dust particles." Employing Johnson's method, he realized, would make the state's 2.0 dpm/g plutonium standard far more protective, since, for samples taken at the same location, Johnson's method shows concentrations 40 or more times greater than the CDH whole-soil approach. He added a cautionary note that it would be best to apply the 2.0 dpm/g standard as a limit not for plutonium alone but for the sum of all radionuclides in the environment [37]. Colorado officials, having gotten from Morgan the advice they sought, chose to ignore it.

Shortly after his visit, Morgan wrote Johnson: "The situation is much worse than I had suspected. . . . I am amazed that the State of Colorado . . . has not been out front from the beginning, collecting this type of data, pointing out the environmental hazard and doing all it could to ameliorate the problem" [38].

Enlarged Survey of Plutonium in Surface Respirable Dust

Johnson's group soon followed up their plutonium sampling done on land near Rocky Flats with a much larger survey in which they collected dust samples from 72 locations along the compass coordinates and in areas of known or suspected contamination out as far as 32 kilometers, or about 18 miles, from Rocky Flats. Krey had said that at about this distance out, Rocky Flats plutonium could not readily be distinguished from background; Johnson's group, however, found plutonium at this extremity in varying amounts up to as high as 17 times background. Their highest reading was 3,390 times background, at a point just east of the site boundary. Values generally decreased with samples taken further to the east and southeast, displaying a nonuniform pattern of distribution [39].

Cesium, Strontium, and the Criticality Question

In doing this larger survey, Johnson's group found cesium-137 at four offsite locations with concentrations considerably higher than plutonium sampled at the same places. The presence of cesium suggested the likelihood of "a significant fission reaction," or "criticality," of plutonium at the plant. If so, other fission products, such as strontium-90 and iodine-131, should also be found. Johnson wanted off-site soil sampled for these radionuclides and "a review of incidents" on site "to determine the source of the cesium" [39].

When Johnson learned that an explosion had accompanied the 1957 fire, he suspected it was a fission reaction. He thus countered the Rocky Flats orthodoxy that there had never been a criticality at the site. He soon had results from eight more samples that also showed cesium, with two from widely separated locations east of the site giving readings of 30 and 31 times background respectively [40]. The CDH, ignoring Johnson's findings, declared that there was no proof that cesium found locally had come from Rocky Flats [41]. Johnson later saw reports uncovered in the discovery proceedings of the Church case that referred to elevated levels of both cesium and strontium in soil at the site [42]. The issue of strontium remains contentious at Rocky Flats [43].

Another Innovation: Isopleths and Census Tracts

To assess adverse health effects among residents of off-site areas shown by Krey to be contaminated with plutonium from Rocky Flats, Johnson introduced into the field of epidemiology an important innovation. Rather than determine his area of study by drawing concentric circles around the point-source of the contaminant (i.e., Rocky Flats), he defined his study area by the pattern of wind-blown distribution of plutonium from the source as indicated by Krey's isopleths [44]. Comparing 1975 leukemia and lung cancer death certificates for residents of contaminated census tracts near Rocky Flats and in Golden with death certificates from noncontaminated tracts elsewhere, he found a significantly higher incidence of death from these two causes in the former areas by comparison with the latter [45]. Again employing the isopleth approach but focusing on different census tracts, he found an excess of birth defects in the City of Arvada [46]. The method of combining isopleths with census tracts he would soon use for a cancer incidence study for the Denver metro area, his best known but also most controversial project.

Interlude: The 1957 Fire

Based on previously secret documents uncovered by discovery proceedings in the Church landowner lawsuit filed in 1975, Johnson concluded that adverse health effects he had documented probably resulted from exposure to plutonium released during the 1957 fire. He learned the following:

- The fire and explosion totally destroyed the bank of 620 large (2′ × 2′) filters that existed to protect the public, allowing plutonium particles to escape unimpeded.
- These filters had not been changed since operations began four-and-a-half years earlier, so they were caked with plutonium.
- The smokestack radiation monitors were not operational from the time the fire began until seven days later.
- Production resumed before either filters or monitors were restored.
- When stack monitors were turned back on eight days after the fire, the guidelines for stack emissions were exceeded by 16,000 times for that day.
- Soil samples were collected after the fire at only three off-site locations. High levels of "possible enriched uranium" were found at two widely

separated schools. The only sample analyzed for plutonium (taken on Church property) registered 225 times background.

- The amount of plutonium released, while unknown, was large.
- No effort was made to survey the extent of contamination in off-site downwind areas [47].

Is It Safe to Live Near Rocky Flats?

In 1978, Johnson began a study that raised quite forcefully the question whether residing near Rocky Flats was more dangerous than living further away from the site. Funded by a grant from the National Cancer Institute, Johnson adapted Krey's isopleths for an epidemiological investigation of cancer incidence (not death rates) in Denver-area census tracts known to be contaminated with Rocky Flats plutonium compared with those contaminated only from global fallout. He made no attempt to estimate dose. It was the first attempt anywhere at a comprehensive analysis of the effect on an off-site population of carcinogens released from a nuclear weapons production facility [48].

Johnson framed his study with a review of plutonium's toxicity and the history of its releases from Rocky Flats, especially from the 1957 fire. He modified Krey's isopleths to reflect his own more extensive sampling (he had collected three times as many samples within a much smaller area), producing "three study areas with populations in the same order of size" [49]. His resultant "approximate but useful" figures divided the Denver Standard Metropolitan Statistical Area (1970 population: 1,019,131) into four areas [50].

For each of these areas, he determined the cancer incidence among Anglos for 1969 through 1971, corrected for age, race, sex, and ethnicity [51]. Comparing the cancer data with the contamination data, he found a correspondence between zones of increased cancer and zones of increased contamination. Cancer incidence in Area IV, his noncontaminated control area, was essentially identical to the rest of the state. Area I, nearest Rocky Flats, showed 16 percent more cancer incidence than Area IV and 8.5 percent more than Area II, the urban center [52]. The incidence for Area II was 10 percent above Area IV; Area III was 6 percent greater than Area IV. Incidence of cancers of "radiosensitive organs" (those found in excess among Hiroshima and Nagasaki survivors) was higher near Rocky Flats. Overall, he "found a higher incidence of all cancer in areas contaminated with plutonium, compared to the unexposed area" [53] (see Figure 2).

Johnson first presented his findings in a paper dated February 9, 1979. What he had to say was big news in the Denver area. The CDH, DOE, NRC, and EPA produced critiques, all answered point by point by Johnson. The essence of the CDH critique showed up in a May 11, 1979, *Denver Post* editorial. A decade later a *Post* reporter revealed that the DOE had given its contractor, Rockwell, a

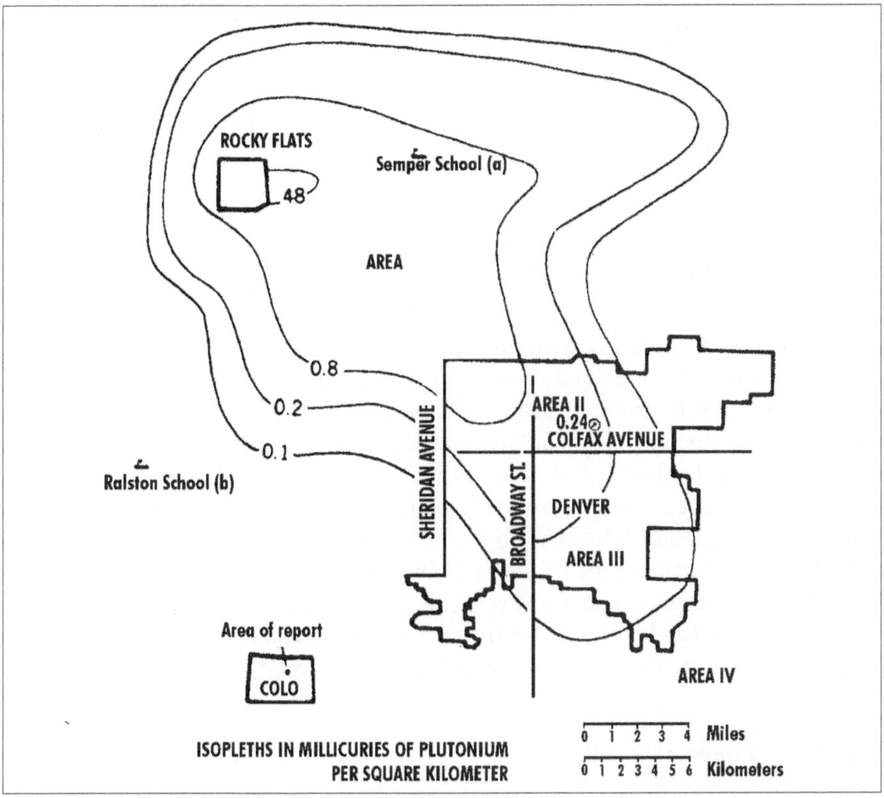

Figure 2. Carl Johnson studied cancer incidence for 1969-1971 among Anglos in three areas downwind of Rocky Flats defined by levels of plutonium contamination in millicuries per square kilometer (mCi/km^2) as compared to the uncontaminated control area. See the text above for cancer incidence rate for each area. From Johnson, "Cancer Incidence in an Area Contaminated with Radionuclides Near a Nuclear Installation," *Ambio*, 10, 4, October 1981, p. 177 and Table 3 (copyright Royal Swedish Academy of Sciences, reprinted by permission of Allen Press Publishing Services).

bonus for persuading the *Post* to publish the editorial questioning Johnson [54]. Through 1979 and 1980 Johnson used criticisms of his study to continue revising his paper, even as he presented it at several national and international scientific gatherings. In October 1981, after extensive peer review, the finished study was published in *Ambio*, the journal of the Royal Swedish Academy of Sciences [55]. Subsequently, reports of the study and replies to critics appeared in other publications [56].

In 1982, Rockwell gave a citizen review group its report listing eight negative reviews of Johnson's study. It fell to Johnson to inform the group that all the critics cited by Rockwell were linked to nuclear agencies, that he had already responded in detail to their criticisms, and that Rockwell had failed to cite any of the numerous positive reviews his study had received from other specialists [57].

The Rocky Flats Advisory Notice

Johnson's study clearly disturbed people associated with the nuclear establishment. But it also troubled those who wanted unimpeded development in the burgeoning suburbs moving closer and closer to the Rocky Flats site. Perhaps the biggest threat to real estate interests came in March 1979 when the federal Department of Housing and Urban Development required anyone seeking federal mortgage insurance on property being bought within 10 miles of Rocky Flats to sign the "Rocky Flats Advisory Notice." The notice referred to "varying amounts of plutonium contamination of the soil" and said an "Emergency Response Plan" would be implemented in the event of "an accidental release of radioactive materials" from Rocky Flats. Shortly after Ronald Reagan took office in January 1981 the Advisory Notice requirement was abandoned.

Johnson Loses His Job

In May 1981, five months prior to publication of his cancer incidence study in a prestigious journal, Johnson lost his position as Director of the Jefferson County Health Department. He had worked for two bodies, the County Commissioners and the County Board of Health, the latter appointed by the former. Though his Rocky Flats work had often been opposed by the President of the Board of Health (a wealthy individual who owned 20 acres of land within a mile of the Rocky Flats site), he always had the support of a majority of both the Board of Health and the Commissioners. The makeup of the Board of Health began to change, however, after the election in 1980 of a realtor as a County Commissioner. In April 1981 a reconstituted Board of Health held a secret meeting at which they voted to ask Johnson to resign. He requested a hearing, which occurred on May 15, 1981. The Board's attorney advised them that they did not need to state a reason for discharging a health officer who served "at the pleasure of the Board." When the Board, by a vote of three to two, gave Johnson the choice of being fired (and losing all accrued benefits) or of resigning immediately, he resigned [58]. Martell, on hearing this news, called Johnson the "only man in the Denver public health community who is concerned about public health" [59].

Johnson Goes to Court to Save His Job

Within days of his termination, an ad hoc Citizens Health Committee persuaded Johnson to file suit in the Jefferson County Court to seek reinstatement to the position from which he had been terminated. This group thought the Health Board had violated Johnson's rights and flouted due process by failing to reveal their own conflicts of interest. When the case went to trial, one of the three Health Board members who had voted against Johnson said that, in his view, a health officer "could be fired for the color of his tie" if the Board didn't like it [60]. The judge ruled that since Johnson served at the pleasure of the Board, he could not be reinstated.

The case was appealed to the State Supreme Court, which on April 18, 1983, in a unanimous decision, annulled the County Court verdict and remanded the case for retrial. The Supreme Court also disqualified the original judge for saying that "it would be a disaster if Johnson gets his position back."

Meanwhile, in December 1984, before Johnson's case could be retried, the Church lawsuit was settled. The owners of the land near Rocky Flats on which Johnson had prevented residential development were paid $9 million, and it was mandated that the contested land could be used only for open space or an industrial park. One week after announcement of this settlement, the Jefferson County Commissioners offered to settle with Johnson for $150,000. He accepted [61]. By this time he had become the chief public health officer for the State of South Dakota.

Crump and Johnson

Johnson was gone from Colorado, but not forgotten. The DOE paid Kenneth S. Crump and colleagues $70,000 (a hefty sum at the time) to refute Johnson's cancer-incidence study. Using the same data that Johnson had used, Crump and colleagues replicated his findings. When they examined data from a decade later (1979 through 1981), they found a reduced cancer incidence in Area I nearest Rocky Flats (the opposite, they said, of what one would expect), with the highest incidence now in Area II, the urban core. They advanced the thesis that the cancer incidence levels in both 1969–71 and 1979–81 had nothing to do with Rocky Flats but were due to the "urban effect" measured by distance from the state capitol building in Denver. They found no evidence of "a relation between environmental exposure to plutonium from Rocky Flats and cancer incidence" [62].

Johnson, in a published response, pointed out that Crump and colleagues were able to claim less cancer for areas near Rocky Flats only by setting aside his isopleth approach in favor of dividing the Denver region into six sectors radiating out from the state capitol building in downtown Denver. The sector on their map containing the Rocky Flats area also includes the sizeable unexposed

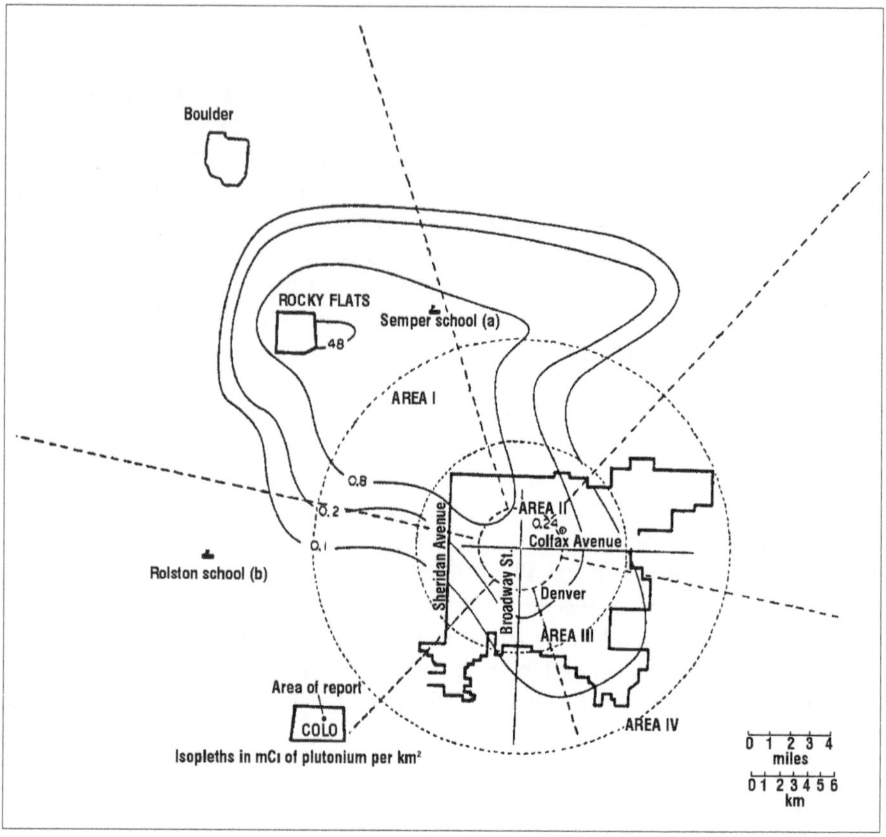

Figure 3. Crump divided the Denver area into six sectors radiating outward from the state capitol building, then analyzed data from these sectors to demonstrate the "urban effect" on cancer incidence patterns. The figure above superimposes Crump's sectors on Johnson's map, showing that the city of Boulder is included in the sector that contains Rocky Flats; this results in gross undercounting of cancer incidence attributed to Rocky Flats. For Crump's sectors, see Crump et al., "Statistical analyses of cancer incidence patterns in the Denver metropolitan area in relation to the Rocky Flats plant," Report of research done under DOE contract #DE AC04-76EV01013, Subcontract 8115006 from the Lovelace Inhalation Toxicology Research Institute, Albuquerque, NM, August 20, 1984, p. 80. The image above is from an unpublished paper by Johnson, "Rocky Flats Revisited: Follow-up Studies," April 1988, p. 15.

upwind city of Boulder (1970 population 66,870). This results in greatly undercounting cancer incidence related to Rocky Flats per se (see Figure 3).

When, on the other hand, Crump et al. used Johnson's isopleth approach they got the same results he had for 1969–71, while for 1979–81 they found, as noted, a decline of cancer incidence in the area nearest Rocky Flats. Johnson attributed this reduction to the very large in-migration into Area I through the 1970s, significantly diluting the contaminated population he had counted in his earlier study [63]. Despite Johnson's careful rebuttal, government agencies ignored what he wrote and continued to tout the Crump study as a definitive refutation of Johnson.

The Staging of the Church Case: The CDH Shows Its Hand

Though the 1984 settlement of the Church lawsuit had confirmed Johnson's original position that housing should not be allowed on the contaminated land, in other respects the case played out in ways not favorable to Johnson. First, in his words, according to the settlement, the plaintiffs (landowners) were paid $9 million "in exchange for a court hearing staged for the judge and the press by the attorneys and witnesses for the defendants. Nothing was to be heard from the experts for the plaintiffs [including Johnson], and there was to be no cross examination of defendants' witnesses" [64].

With Johnson effectively gagged, Stanley W. Ferguson of the CDH, citing Crump, pointedly dismissed Johnson's cancer incidence study, then stated the position of CDH: "There is no scientifically valid evidence of the creation or intensification of any health effects as the result of the existence and operations of the Rocky Flats Plant, or by the existence of any materials from the Rocky Flats Plant on soils outside of the plant" [65]. Also, reversing their earlier statement that plutonium on Church land exceeded the state's 2 dpm/g standard by up to seven times, the CDH now gave the landowners a certificate stating that plutonium contamination on their land did not exceed the standard.

From Johnson's unheard testimony:

> Based on my education, training, and experience as a medical doctor, and my understanding of how the body works, and of the effects of ionizing radiation on the human body, and based on my studies of the radioactive emissions of the Rocky Flats Plant and the area-wide contamination of the Denver area from those releases, and my studies of cancer mortality and cancer incidence in contaminated areas, and having considered other possible causes, it is my opinion, within a reasonable degree of medical probability, that the radioactive emissions from the Rocky Flats Plant have caused an excess of cancer in the exposed areas [66].

Johnson called for a standard for plutonium in surface respirable dust of 0.4 dpm/g, evacuation of all residential areas within four miles of the plant site and no new housing within ten miles—due to contamination already present or likely to be added later [66].

The Public Betrayed: Secrecy Prevails

In settling the Church case, the DOE and the contractors gained control of all internal documents reviewed in the case and had them sealed, thereby depriving the public of access to crucial information regarding contaminants released from Rocky Flats [14, pp. 200-201]. This was repeated with a vengeance after the June 1989 FBI raid of Rocky Flats; federal authorities used the subsequent grand jury investigation to gather evidence of wrongdoing and then sealed the record [67]. In both instances, the court allowed the Rocky Flats operators to withhold from the public data about the nature and extent of contamination on and off the site. In October 2006, the DOE announced completion of the Rocky Flats "cleanup" without this information being available. There seems a conspiracy of silence, whether unconscious or otherwise, between those who contaminated the land and those who prefer not to know that it's contaminated. Neither is interested in the truth. Johnson, at least, stood against this collective denial, as well as and as long as he could.

Context: Risk Assessment and Cost-Benefit Analysis

In the 1970s and 80s, at just the time Martell and Johnson were most active in efforts to protect public health, others were developing the tools of risk assessment and cost-benefit analysis. These tools enable U.S. decision-makers to deal with threats to public health and environmental integrity without unduly impeding enterprises like the nuclear industry. Incorporation of these tools into the decision-making process is based on the assumption that scientists can understand the impact of human activities on ecological and human systems well enough to predict harm and to estimate risk. The resultant risk-based regulatory regime that now prevails in the United States puts a price on human health and ecological well-being without really knowing what that price is. It presupposes that some level of harm is acceptable without asking those affected whether it is acceptable to them. Abstract and abstruse formulations of risk are employed to consign some to disease, deformity, and premature death, whether soon or in the wholly unknown long term.

Persistence of Johnson's Question: Varied Answers

Dose-Reconstruction Project

In response to the June 1989 FBI raid on Rocky Flats to collect evidence of alleged lawbreaking, DOE funded the CDH to manage a dose-reconstruction study for Rocky Flats. The goal was to determine the history of contaminant releases and to estimate doses that people off-site may have received in order to decide whether further study was warranted. Colorado Governor Roy Romer appointed a 12-member oversight Health Advisory Panel that included, besides prominent scientists and local people, two officials from CDH (one would chair the panel) and one each from DOE and CDC. Such a panel would not stray far from the risk assessment orthodoxy that typically informs studies of this sort.

The nine-year study (1990–1999) estimated that total offsite plutonium releases for the production years, 1952–1989, ranged from 4.8 to 51.3 curies [68]. One curie is the quantity of any radioactive material that undergoes 37 billion disintegrations or releases of radiation per second. Thus, according to the foregoing estimate, plutonium released from Rocky Flats to the off-site environment emits between 176.6 billion and 1.9 trillion bursts of alpha radiation each second. After 24,110 years (the half-life of plutonium-239), the number of alpha bursts per second will be reduced by half. The material remains in the environment in the form of particles too small to see, but not too small to be inhaled or ingested.

Periodic meetings to involve the public in the study were fairly well attended, though often held when most working people could not attend. The meetings could be informative, tedious, and contentious. Technical specialists and the engaged public interacted intensely in efforts to reconstruct major accidents and contaminant releases. But when it came to estimating risk, the abstractions of the "experts" left me, and I suspect others, with the sense of being reduced to a spectator. The study's final report session had something of the feel of a triumphal celebration, as if those affected were expected to rejoice at learning that, though as much as 51.3 curies of plutonium may have been released off-site, risks were inconsequential and further studies were not warranted. It was a bit unnerving.

The CDH calls the dose-reconstruction study a "health study," but it was no such thing. Indeed, it concluded that an actual health study was not warranted. The only situation in which a dose-reconstruction study would point to the need for direct health study would be where there is an indisputable correspondence between known large releases of a particular contaminant and its known physical effects. An example is large releases of radioactive iodine from the DOE's Hanford facility matched by the high incidence in the area of childhood thyroid cancer, a cancer attributed solely to the presence of iodine in a single organ [69]. Plutonium released from Rocky Flats can certainly cause cancer in exposed people, but any cancer caused by plutonium can also have other causes.

The CDH has generally interpreted the study as providing scientific confirmation of the absence of adverse health effects. Unknown to outsiders, some members of the Health Advisory Panel wanted additional research on plutonium in water as it affects downstream communities, a proposal vetoed by the panel's CDH chair. Others thought the final report should emphasize in the strongest manner possible that the Denver-area population had been subject to the risk of a major cataclysm due to careless operation of the plant. Specifically, had the 1969 fire breached the roof of the building where it raged, Denver almost certainly would have faced evacuation [14, ch. 8]. Because the final report downplayed this matter, David Albright, a prestigious independent scientist who had been a very active member of the panel, refused to sign on to it [70].

The study concluded that the largest single plutonium release was from the 1957 fire and that the person likely to have received the highest exposure was a laborer working outdoors in the direct path of the plume of plutonium-laden smoke from that fire (see Figure 4). The researchers produced a dose calculator that could be used by persons present in the Denver area at the time of the fire to estimate their dose according to their location. By the time the calculator was finished, however, the CDH had in effect dissolved the oversight panel by the simple expedient of convening no more meetings. The calculator thus was never made available, and affected people were denied the chance to learn of the dose they may have received back in 1957. Might they have learned of dangers like those to which Johnson and Martell had pointed but that the CDH had denied?

Calls for Further Studies

Despite the conclusion that there is no need for further health studies, several have disagreed. In 1982, Martell said that the plutonium in the soil east of Rocky Flats "involves risks that are sufficiently serious that only epidemiological studies of the next several generations of people living in that area can really find out what is going on" [71]. In 1996, nurses at the University of Colorado conducted a community needs assessment and concluded that community-based epidemiological studies should occur in areas affected by Rocky Flats [72].

Also in 1996, Boston University epidemiologist Richard W. Clapp found excessive incidence of lung and bone cancers in areas near Rocky Flats and concluded that "the most recent data are indicative of an ongoing health effect and support the need for surveillance of the incidence of cancer and other diseases on a continuing basis in the exposed communities" [73].

The programs that Clapp and others proposed have never taken place. Indeed, there has never been any direct health study or medical monitoring of people who live in areas contaminated with plutonium released from Rocky Flats [74]. Hence, no one really knows the actual health effects of living in such areas.

Alternate Assessments of Risk in Off-Site Areas

In 1998, the Colorado Central Cancer Registry of the CDH issued a report that purports to show that people who live near Rocky Flats have no higher incidence of cancer than those who live elsewhere in the Denver area [75]. German radiation specialist Bernd Franke criticized this report as seriously flawed: "It appears that the study design was chosen to calm people down, for public relations purposes, rather than for any real scientific reason" [76].

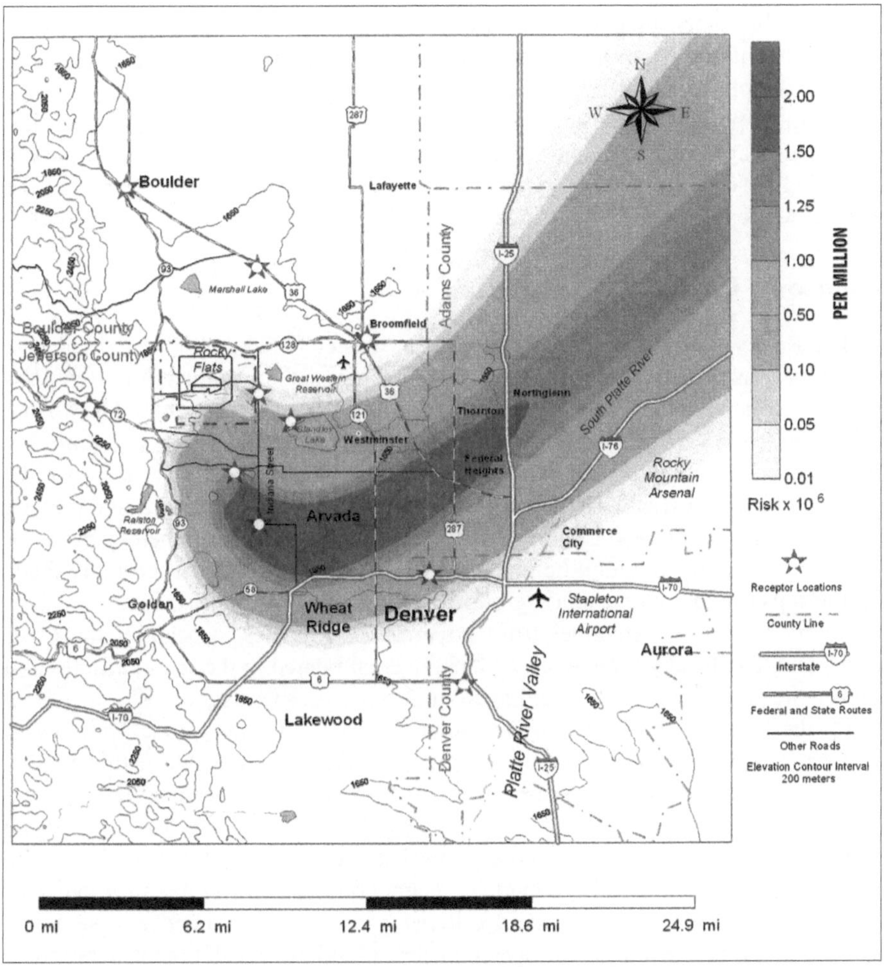

Figure 4. Trajectory of the plume of plutonium-laden smoke from the September 11, 1957, fire at Rocky Flats as calculated in the dose reconstruction study. Note that the map covers only the area defined for this study and thus presents no estimate for how far the plume traveled. From *Historical Public Exposure Studies on Rocky Flats,* Colorado Department of Public Health and Environment, August 1999, p. 19.

On February 14, 2006, the jury in a class action case heard in the federal court in Denver found Dow and Rockwell, the former operators of Rocky Flats, liable for harming the property of people who lived in areas shown by Krey to be contaminated with plutonium released from Rocky Flats and by implication endangering their health [77]. The jury assessed penalties of $554 million. This suggests that when essentially uninformed people are presented evidence of a kind with which Johnson was very familiar, along with countervailing arguments, they are likely to reach conclusions approximating Johnson's views regarding the dangers posed by Rocky Flats. The huge sum of money, a record-breaking amount, awarded as compensation by the jury to the property holders in the specified off-site contaminated area may never reach those affected, since the verdict was overturned by the Appeals Court in March 2010.

Johnson's Legacy

The Rocky Flats work for which Johnson was celebrated and vilified and for which he was forced from office was done in the final six years and five months of his seven years and eight months term as Director of Public Health for Jefferson County. Since the termination of his very brief tenure, no one remotely like him has occupied an official position related to public health vis-à-vis Rocky Flats—no county official, no state official, no federal official. Johnson stands alone as an untiring advocate for people with public health concerns, whether inside or outside the facility. Though he made himself available to concerned individuals and groups (he met with a study group I organized in 1979), the primary arena of his work was with personnel from government agencies, especially the DOE and CDH. His Rocky Flats work is densely documented in the many articles and reports he prepared as well as in his voluminous correspondence [78].

By the time Johnson died on December 29, 1988, he was a much-published, internationally respected practitioner and specialist on radiation health effects. At the urging of former Interior Secretary Stewart Udall, he did the first-ever study of downwinders from the Nevada Test Site [79]. He was in considerable demand abroad as well as elsewhere in the United States. But in Colorado he was in eclipse, dismissed by nuclear technocrats as well as by promoters of urban sprawl. Indeed, the constant criticisms of his cancer incidence study by nuclear establishment figures gave boosters of urban development a rationale for ignoring his warnings.

On December 18, 1988, less than two weeks before he died, Johnson published in the *New York Times* an op-ed called "Rocky Flats: Death, Inc." He recounted his years with Jefferson County, explaining various studies he had done and how, "as a result of the buildup of enormous political pressures by vested interests," he was forced from office. He concluded that if people are "to be properly protected, all studies of nuclear contamination and associated health effects should be conducted primarily by independent scientists who are insulated from cynical retaliation."

The *Denver Post* published a tribute to the deceased Johnson headlined "Doctor warned of Rocky Flats danger" six days after the FBI raided Rocky Flats on June 6, 1989, to collect evidence of environmental crimes allegedly committed at the facility. The article came close to saying that Carl Johnson was right all along. An anonymous Rocky Flats insider said Johnson "wasn't as off-base as we used to say he was," while a CDH official praised him as a "workhorse," but said he presented some of his results in ways that "overstated reality." For many, the fact that the FBI was investigating Rocky Flats confirmed that Johnson knew what he was talking about.

III. CONCLUSION: PROPER HEALTH PROTECTION

Johnson and Martell blew the whistle on Rocky Flats. They delved into the details of radiation health effects to understand in the most thorough way possible what "proper" protection of public health would entail. They remind us that any purportedly "safe" dose of radiation may be the one that will tip the scales against us. They warn that our fate may be sealed 20 or 30 years before symptoms appear. They were exemplars of caution on behalf of the unassuming public. But the rules by which they worked were not the rules by which others played the game. There is a striking difference between public health as service to the public and public health as obeisance to the nuclear industry and the economy of denial.

The tale told here is one of systemic failure of the U.S. system of representative democracy, by means of which, purportedly, the well-being of the public is served by elected representatives and the bureaucrats and technocrats up and down the governmental chain of command who are charged with implementing the will of the people. The system fails because of the fundamental conflict between the democracy professed on the one hand and denied on the other. Nuclear weapons that supposedly protect our democracy destroy it, because, to exist, they require secrecy and centralized decision-making which in turn allow deceit, damage, and denial.

Martell, in discovering that plutonium had been released from Rocky Flats to the off-site environment, exposed damage that led to the unraveling of some of the deceit. He and the public learned for the first time about previously unknown major accidents. But an AEC official, practiced perhaps in the art of denial, made sure that Martell would pay for what he'd done. Martell kept his job because of the support of colleagues, but the loss of his lab and of funding for research hobbled his career in ways that are beyond measure.

Johnson, who did lose his job, seems clearly to have fallen victim not to the lords of the nuclear priesthood but merely to the greed and corruption of local government. But this is only half the story. The Colorado Department of Health had already tried to marginalize him by rejecting his innovative dust sampling method that, as Karl Morgan pointed out, was up to 40 times more protective than the method they employed. Undeterred, Johnson proceeded with a series of reports culminating in his major study that showed a correspondence between zones of cancer incidence and zones of contamination from Rocky Flats. The DOE, in a fit of denial, hired Crump to refute Johnson and then buried Johnson's own rebuttal in a repetitious tide of deceit that can only lead to more of the very kind of damage Johnson was exposing. The CDH, not to be outdone, after Johnson was gagged in a federal courtroom, cited Crump to dismiss Johnson, only later to have him in mind when they produced their PR piece asserting that living near Rocky Flats is no riskier than living anywhere else in the metro area. Some within the CDH undoubtedly viewed Johnson as an impediment to economic development, like the realtor who became a Jefferson County Commissioner so he could ax Johnson. This sort of distorted cost-benefit calculation is not simply an instance of corrupt local or regional politics; it's a characteristic blindness of the culture, essential to the economy of denial.

In the dead end of this failed system, one has two responsibilities: first, to create a public record for those who will come after and, second, to articulate as clearly as possible a positive alternative to the failed system. The present narrative contributes to the essential public record. It can be supplemented by my account of the inadequate "cleanup" at Rocky Flats [80]. The second responsibility, pointing to an alternative, can here be alluded to only in outline. To deal with radiation health effects in and around facilities like Rocky Flats, we need to begin anew and to implement what can most appropriately be called "ecological democracy." By this term I mean direct democracy informed by the awareness that we are inseparable from the ecology in which we live and move and have our being. For any human action likely to affect public health or environmental integrity, insofar as possible, affected parties must participate directly in decisions about the action. Otherwise, they are forced to endure the results of decisions made by others, which is what has happened at Rocky Flats, where the range of public participation has been limited at best to spectator activities and at worst to disdainful dismissal. In the practice of ecological democracy, the only role for representative democracy is to ensure that voice is given to parties who cannot be present—that is, to the very young, the very old, the infirm, the unborn, plus the whole spectrum of nonhuman creatures that inhabited the land long before we arrived and will be there long after we have passed.

Public health science deserves to align itself with ecological democracy because its primary intent is to sustain ecological well-being and to work with and for people rather than against them and without them. The problems for Johnson and Martell were not that they lacked independence but, as Johnson made clear, that they were vulnerable to "cynical retaliation" from those who deny harmful effects even as they foster harmful ends. All science serves some interest. Ecological democracy entails a shift in decision-making power that puts science irrevocably in the service of people and planet.

NOTES

1. Martell, E. A. 1995. Interviewed by Niels Schonbeck for the Health Advisory Panel as part of the Rocky Flats Dose Reconstruction Study, 21 February 1995, p. 25.

In this same interview Martell pointed out that P. W. Krey (see note 7 below) measured plutonium at the east boundary of the Rocky Flats site at 1,500 times background.

2. On July 1, 1994, CDH changed its name to Colorado Department of Public Health and Environment. Throughout this article this agency is referred to as CDH.
3. Within one month in 1957 a major disaster occurred at a production facility in each of the only three countries then known to be making nuclear bombs, the U.S., Britain and the USSR. http://www.rockyflatsnuclearguardianship.org/leroy-moore/papers-by-leroy-more-phd-2/
4. After the 1957 fire, AEC officials told the *Denver Post* that it "resulted in no spread of radioactive contamination of any consequence." Atomic Plant Fire Causes $50,000 Loss, *Denver Post*, 12 September, p. 1, 1957. Avaiable online at www.rockyflatsnuclearguardenship.org/site-map.html
5. Metzger, P. 1972. *The Atomic Establishment.* New York: Simon and Schuster, p. 259.
6. Martell, E. A. 24 February 1970. *Plutonium contamination in the Denver area.* Press release of the Colorado Committee for Environmental Information, Boulder, Colorado. See also Poet, S. E., and Martell, E. A. 1972. Plutonium 239 and Americium 241 contamination in the Denver area. *Health Physics* 23:537.
7. Krey, P. W. February 1976. Remote plutonium contamination and total inventories from Rocky Flats, *Health Physics* 30. See also Krey, P. W., and Hardy, E. P. 1 August 1970. *Plutonium in soil around the Rocky Flats plant,* HASL-235. New York: U.S. Atomic Energy Commission, Health and Safety Laboratory.
8. Cleere, R. L. 24 January 1973. Public notice of plutonium contamination in the area of the Dow Chemical Rocky Flats Plant, signed R. L. Cleere, Executive Director, CDH.
9. Amendment to the State of Colorado Rules and Regulations Pertaining to Radiation Control, Subpart RH 4.21.1, adopted Colorado State Board of Health, 21 March 1973.
10. Martell, E. A. January 1975. *Basic considerations in the assessment of the cancer risks and standards for internal alpha emitters.* Statement presented at the public hearings on plutonium standards, US EPA, Denver, pp. 17, 20.
11. Love, J. June 1994. *Rocky Flats Soil Plutonium 239+240 Survey from 1970 to 1991.* Denver: CDH.
12. Jones, R. H., and Zhang, Y. 19 September 1994. *Spatial and temporal analysis of the Rocky Flats soil plutonium data*. Denver: CDH.
13. Beck, U. 1992. *Risk Society: Towards a new modernity*, trans. Mark Ritter. London: Sage. p. 64.
14. Ackland, L. 1999. *Making a Real Killing: Rocky Flats and the Nuclear West.* Albuquerque: University of New Mexico Press, p. 169.
15. Lamm-Wirth Task Force on Rocky Flats. October 1975. *Final Report.*
16. Solo, Pam. Interviewed by L. Moore. Newton, MA. 23 September 1996.
17. For more on local activism, see Moore, L. et al. 1992. *Citizen's Guide to Rocky Flats.* Boulder: Rocky Mountain Peace Center, pp. 52-54; and Ackland, L. *Making a Real Killing*, chaps. 9, 10, and 13.
18. Martell, Edward A. *Natural radionuclides and life* (unpublished manuscript), chap. 4.

19. Martell, Edward A. Chap. 7, p. 11. Martell viewed naturally occurring radiation as the likely source of the energy necessary for the evolution of life. See Martell, E. A. 1992. Radionuclide-induced evolution of DNA and the origin of life. *Journal of Molecular Evolution* 35:346-355.
20. Martell, E. A. 1975. Tobacco radioactivity and cancer in smokers. *American Scientist* 63:409-410.
21. Martell, E. A. Interviewed by Robert Del Tredici, 22 July 1982.
22. Morgan, K. Z. 1975. Suggested reduction of permissible exposure to plutonium and other transuranium elements. *American Industrial Hygiene Association Journal* 567-575.
23. Martell, E. A. to Energy Secretary H. O'Leary, 9 February 1994.
24. Denver journalist Laura Frank has covered this issue extensively for former Rocky Flats workers but also for workers at other DOE facilities. http://www.zoominfo.com/people/Frank_Laura_393007209.aspx
25. Schonbeck, N. Obituary for Martell. Delivered 19 July 1995.
26. Medrud, N. (Martell's NCAR colleague). Interviewed by Moore. 3 June 2005.
27. Martell, E. A. Interviewed by Niels Schonbeck for the Health Advisory Panel as part of the Rocky Flats Dose Reconstruction Study. 21 February 1995. On an explicit threat to Martell and colleagues by an AEC official, see note 5.
28. Johnson, C. Interviewed by Robert Del Tredici, 20 July 1982.
29. Some errors are cited in Johnson, C., and Holland, J. R. 1985. Politicization of Public Health. Presented at the U.S. Conference of Local Health Officers, and the American Public Health Association, Washington, DC, 18 November 1985, p. 8.
30. Johnson, C. (no date). The public health impact of the Rocky Flats nuclear weapons plant in the Denver Area: A case history with recommendations.
31. Johnson, C. 12 September 1975. Survey of land proposed for residential development east of Rocky Flats, for plutonium 239 contamination of respirable dust on the surface of the soil and proposal of a new standard to define the potential airborne-plutonium-particle hazard in terms of concentration of plutonium in respirable dust. Report to the Jefferson County Commissioners and the Colorado State Health Department.
32. Martell, E. A. Interviewed by Robert Del Tredici, 22 July 1982.
33. Martell, E. A. Interviewed by Niels Schonbeck, 21 February 1995.
34. Johnson, C., Tidball, R. R., and Severson, R. C. 6 August 1976. Plutonium hazard in respirable dust on the surface soil. *Science* 193:488-490. Johnson et al. answered criticisms regarding dust particle size made by John A. Hayden of Rockwell in *SCIENCE* 196 (June 3, 1977):1126.
35. Johnson, C., to Colorado Board of Health, "Proposal of a new interim standard to define the potential airborne-plutonium particle hazard in terms of concentration of plutonium in respirable dust on the surface of the land," 14 October 1975. For Johnson's detailed response to EPA on sampling methods and related matters, see his "Critique of the EPA's 'Proposed Federal Radiation Protection Guidance on Dose Limits For Persons Exposed to Transuranium Elements In The Environment,'" 14 October 1975.
36. Johnson, C. 21 January 1976. "Remarks to the State Board of Health concerning a proposed new interim standard for contamination of soil with plutonium." See Hazle, A. J., and Johnson, C. 20 January 1976. "Joint statement of some alternatives to

the State Board of Health concerning the proposal for a new interim standard for plutonium based on the respirable dust on the surface of the ground."

37. Morgan, K. Z. 21 January 1976. Transcript of Presentation, Colorado Land Use Commission Meeting, pp. 12-13.
38. Morgan, K. Z. to C. Johnson. 30 January 1976.
39. Report to the Jefferson County Board of Health, 31 March 1977.
40. Johnson, C., to A. Robbins, Executive Director of CDH, 17 May 1977.
41. Johnson, C. to A. Robbins. 5 October 1977. Refers to a 27 September 1977 CDH report on this matter.
42. Johnson, C. (no date). The public health impact of the Rocky Flats nuclear weapons plant in the Denver Area, p. 10. Refers to Murray, R. L., "Gamma analysis of plutonium-contaminated soil at Rocky Flats." Unpublished report. E.S. 376-77-197. Rocky Flats Plant. 10 January 1977; and Anon., Rocky Flats Environmental Monitoring Results, Dow Chemical Corp., Rocky Flats Plant, Golden, May 1970.
43. Strontium as a contested issue reappeared in January 2005 when former FBI agent Jon Lipsky, who had led the June 1989 FBI raid of Rocky Flats, announced at a news conference in Denver that he had seen documentation of high levels of strontium contamination at the site. For more on the strontium issue, see McKinley, W., and Balkany, C. 2004. *The ambushed grand jury: How the Justice Department covered up government nuclear crimes and how we caught them red handed.* New York: Apex, pp. 122, 187, 194-196.
44. Johnson, C. interviewed by Del Tredici, R. 20 July 1982.
45. Johnson, C. 1977. Leukemia death rates of residents of areas contaminated with plutonium. Proceedings of the 105th Annual Meeting of the American Public Health Association, Washington, DC, 1 November 1977; Johnson, C. 1977. Evaluation of the hazard to residents of areas contaminated with plutonium. *Proceedings of the IVth International Congress of the International Radiation Protection Association,* Paris, 24-30 April 1977. 1: 243-246; and Johnson, C., to Jefferson County Board of Health. 20 November 1977. "Report on death rates from lung cancer in the eight census tracts near Rocky Flats and in Golden, and in nineteen census tracts at the south end of Jefferson County.
46. Johnson, C., to Jefferson County Board of Health. 31 March 1978. "Report on rates of congenital malformations in an area contaminated with plutonium."
47. Johnson, C. 26 September 1980. Comments on the 1957 fire at the Rocky Flats Plant, Jefferson County, Colorado. Johnson, C. 17 September 1980. A case history of a disaster at the plant which could serve as a model for a future disaster emergency response plan exercise.
48. Johnson, C. 1982. Environmental and health effects of the nuclear industry and nuclear weapons: a current evaluation. *Ecology of Disease* I(2/3):135-152.
49. Johnson, C., to S. Ferguson of CDH, 2 May 1979.
50. Johnson, C. October 1981. Cancer incidence in an area contaminated with radionuclides near a nuclear installation. *Ambio* 10(4):178.
51. Johnson restricted his study to Anglos because the population of suburban areas nearest Rocky Flats was at the time predominantly Anglo.
52. In a 2 May 1979, letter to S. Ferguson of CDH, Johnson explained that the Area I census tracts closest to Rocky Flats had a very small population when operations

began at the plant but later grew rapidly from in-migration. Many residents of this area thus had not lived there long enough to develop Rocky Flats-induced cancers by 1969-71. Including these newcomers in his calculations meant that he understated actual cancer incidence for Area I compared to Area IV.

53. Johnson, C. 1981. Cancer incidence. *Ambio* 10(4):181.
54. Obmascik, M. Rockwell won bonuses despite errors. *Denver Post,* 7 January 1990.
55. Johnson, C. 1981. Cancer incidence. *Ambio* 10(4):176-182; see also Johnson, C. 1982. Rocky Flats revisited. *Ambio* 11(6):377-378.
56. Places of presentation and/or publication are referenced in Johnson, C., and Holland, J. R. "Politicization of Public Health," notes 13-22.
57. Johnson, C., to J. W. Spensley, Executive Director, Rocky Flats Blue Ribbon Citizens' Committee. 21 January 1983. Comment on the *Safety Analyses and Risk Assessment Report* for the Rocky Flats nuclear weapons plant, prepared by Rockwell International. November 1982.
58. Johnson, C., and Holland, J. R. *Politicization of Public Health.* This document provides details regarding Johnson's termination. I personally was present when the Board of Health forced him to resign.
59. Lange, T. They fired Dr. Johnson. *Westword* 28 May 1981.
60. Citizens Health Committee. January-March 1982. *Citizens Healthwatch.*
61. Johnson, C., and Holland, J. R. *Politicization of Public Health,* p. 44.
62. Crump, K. S. et al. 1987. Cancer incidence patterns in the Denver Metropolitan Area in relation to the Rocky Flats Plant. *American Journal of Epidemiology* 126(1): 127-135. See also Crump K. S. et al. 20 August 1984. Statistical analyses of cancer incidence patterns in the Denver metropolitan area in relation to the Rocky Flats plant. Report of research done under DOE contract #DE AC04-76EV01013, Subcontract 8115006 from the Lovelace Inhalation Toxicology Research Institute. Albuquerque, NM.
63. Johnson, C. 1987. Cancer incidence patterns in the Denver Metropolitan Area in relation to the Rocky Flats Plant. *American Journal of Epidemiology* 126(1):153.
64. Johnson, C. Two Landmark Radiation Cases, p. 14.
65. Affidavit of S. W. Ferguson in the U.S. District Court for the District of Colorado, Civil Action No. 75-1162. 15 February 1985. See Johnson, C., to Colorado State Board of Health. 21 August 1985. The role of CDH in the decision of Judge Matsch in the Rocky Flats case.
66. Johnson, C. (no date). The public health impact of the Rocky Flats nuclear weapons plant in the Denver Area: A case history with recommendations.
67. See Moore, L. [80] January-February 2005. Rocky Flats: The bait-and-switch cleanup. *Bulletin of the Atomic Scientists,* p. 55. http://bos.sagepub.com/content61/1/50full and McKinley, W., and Balkany, C. *The Ambushed Grand Jury*, chap. 13.
68. Summary of Findings, Historical Public Exposures Studies on Rocky Flats. August 1999. Health Advisory Panel and CDPHE.
69. Connor, T. 1997. *Burdens of proof: Science and public accountability in the field of environmental epidemiology, with a focus on low dose radiation community health studies.* Columbia, SC: Energy Research Foundation.
70. Personal communication with D. Albright, Washington, DC, 30 March 2004.

71. Martell, E. A. Interviewed by Robert Del Tredici, 1982.
72. Brown, N. J. et al. 1996. *Rocky Flats community needs assessment final report.* Denver: UCHSC School of Nursing, p. 46.
73. Clapp, R. W. Report submitted 13 November 1996 for plaintiff's counsel in *Cook vs. Dow Chemical and Rockwell International,* United States District Court, District of Colorado.
74. An example of what is needed but has never been available for Rocky Flats is the Fernald Medical Monitoring Program established at DOE's Fernald uranium processing facility near Cincinnati, Ohio. Created as a result of a class action lawsuit, this program, which ended in 2007, provided comprehensive monitoring of the health of about 9,500 individuals over a period of 18 years. The monitoring relieved some individuals of worry while for others it provided an early warning of problems in need of attention. http://www.genmed.uc.edu/fmmp/ A program of this sort should have been set up by the federal government for all DOE nuclear weapons facilities.
76. Colorado Central Cancer Registry. 1998. *Ratios of cancer incidence in ten areas around Rocky Flats, Colorado compared to the remainder of Metropolitan Denver, 1980-89 with update for selected areas, 1990-95.* CDPHE.
76. Franke, B. of Institut fur Energie-und Umweltforschung, Heidelberg, to C. Balkany, Esq. 2 December 2002. A copy of this letter is in my possession.
77. Civil Action No. 90-cv-00181(JLK), *Cook vs. Dow Chemical & Rockwell International*, U.S. District Court, District of Colorado, 14 February 2006.
78. The papers of both C. Johnson and E. Martell are archived at the University of Colorado, Boulder.
79. Johnson, C. 1984. Cancer incidence in an area of radioactive fallout downwind from the Nevada Test Site. *Journal of the American Medical Association* 251:230-236.
80. Moore, L. January/February 2005. Rocky Flats: The bait and switch cleanup. *Bulletin of the Atomic Scientists*. http://bos.sagepub.com/content/61/1/50.full See also Moore, L. 28 March 2010. People and plutonium don't mix. http://www.rockyflatsnuclearguardianship.org/ leroy-moore/papers-by-leroy-more-phd-2/

http://dx.doi.org/10.2190/TORC5

CHAPTER 5

A Collaborative Effort to Address the Distribution of Plutonium-Contaminated Sludge in Livermore, California

Patrice Sutton, Jacqueline Cabasso, Tracy Barreau, and Marylia Kelley

For over a half-century, the U.S. Department of Energy nuclear weapons laboratory in Livermore, California, has worked with plutonium in the course of its mission to research and develop nuclear weapons. Plutonium releases via the laboratory's sewer system resulted in the contamination of sewage sludge that was distributed and used widely as soil conditioner in parks, landscaping around public buildings, and in home lawns and gardens. The amount of sludge distributed and the concentration of the radioactivity in the sludge are uncertain.

In 1999, research was undertaken to investigate the historic distribution of sewage sludge (1958–1976) in Livermore. Navigating the uncertainties surrounding the sludge distribution more than forty years after it began presented an enormous ethical challenge. Community members who received the sludge at no cost were not told that the sludge they received may have been contaminated with plutonium, and the logbook that had recorded the names and addresses of sludge recipients had disappeared. The half-life of weapons-grade plutonium is about 24,000 years. Therefore, former, current, and future Livermore residents are at potential increased risk of cancer and other health impacts from their largely unrecognized and therefore unavoidable exposure to radioactive sludge.

Two research models to address the potential public health impacts of plutonium-contaminated sludge distribution were undertaken. One model was a collaborative approach that emphasized gathering and incorporating local knowledge into the scientific analysis and fostering the growth of mutually respectful relationships between scientists, and governmental, and nongovernmental collaborators. This model sought an ethical research framework that would maximize the benefits to community health while minimizing the potential for unwarranted fears, or stigmatization of individuals, households, or the entire community. Principles of community right-to-know and the precautionary principle were incorporated into the science. This investigation concluded that the distribution of sewage sludge posed an indeterminate health hazard due to a lack of data and recommended a process be implemented to inform and solicit further information from residents who may have obtained sludge, sample known areas of sludge disposition in order to gain a better understanding of the potential health risk, establish criteria for sampling residences and interpreting results, and provide a mechanism for sampling and, if necessary, removing plutonium-contaminated sludge. An outcome of the research was the convening of the Alameda County Plutonium Action Taskforce (ACPAT), a transparent, locally-based participatory process for scientific decision-making to address the large uncertainties surrounding the distribution of sludge. Since 2003, ACPAT members have conducted educational and other activities to carry out a work plan that they developed to implement the research recommendations.

The second research model undertaken was a dose-assessment approach that utilized existing data to estimate radiological doses from exposure to plutonium-contaminated sewage sludge and compared the estimated doses with those that have caused sickness or death. The investigation acknowledged the population-based implications of the sludge exposure, finding that many Livermore residents could have been exposed to plutonium-contaminated soil and that exposure may still be occurring. However, it did not make a quantitative estimate of the number of people potentially exposed to contaminated sludge over the lifetime of the plutonium and translate those doses to risk. The investigators received many public comments strongly objecting to specific assumptions and methods it incorporated into its dose assessment. This research concluded that there was no public health hazard stemming from the distribution of contaminated sewage sludge.

Identifying and implementing a collaborative model to address the large scientific uncertainties associated with the sludge distribution involved many hurdles, including: (1) lack of trust, unequal power, and different perspectives among collaborators; (2) lack of data; (3) opposition to the ACPAT process by Lawrence Livermore National Laboratory; (4) inconsistent Alameda County leadership in the ACPAT process; and (5) lack of funding to carry out the ACPAT process. Key limitations are that neither of the two investigations nor the ACPAT process address issues of intergenerational equity and primary prevention of exposure. In November 2005 the U.S. Department of Energy decided to double the plutonium storage limit at Livermore National Laboratory to more than 3,000 pounds—enough plutonium for about 300 nuclear bombs. Worldwide, there are 3.7 million pounds of this man-made substance. The wide dispersal of a radioactive substance having a lifetime of virtually forever, guarantees that the majority of Livermore's plutonium will still be waiting for the generations that follow. Therefore, prevention efforts undertaken today must also speak to the health of future generations. This will involve looking upstream of the plutonium and working toward sustainable solutions to security that do not involve the public health threats embedded in the global embrace of nuclear weapons.

PART I: PLUTONIUM, SEWERS, AND SLUDGE: A HALF-CENTURY OF LIVERMORE'S HISTORY

> When they had dried this speck of matter God had not welcomed at the Creation they simply snipped off the sides of the platinum dish, covered the sample with a layer of protective Duco Cement, glued the dish to a piece of cardboard labeled Sample A and set is aside until it decayed completely to 94^{239}. . . . Not until 1942 would they officially propose a name for the new element that fissioned like U235 but could be chemically separated from Uranium. But Seaborg already knew what he would call it . . . Seaborg would name the element 94 for Pluto, the ninth planet outward from the sun, discovered in 1930 and named for the Greek god of the underworld, a god of earth's fertility but also the god of the dead: *plutonium* [1].

The aftermath of World War II brought indelible change to Livermore, California. In 1952, Edward Teller won a second nuclear weapons laboratory in the southeast corner of the Livermore Valley, about 50 miles east of San Francisco, in Alameda County [2]. From its beginning, Teller's Livermore Radiation Laboratory was operated for the Atomic Energy Commission and later for the U.S. Department of Energy (DOE) by the University of California. For more than half a century, Livermore's National Laboratory has worked with plutonium in the course of its mission to research and develop nuclear weapons. The essential ingredients of every nuclear weapon are fissile materials compressed into a "supercritical mass" so that the number of fissions will escalate very rapidly and create a nuclear explosion [3]. Plutonium is one of the two principle fissile materials used to make nuclear weapons explode.

Plutonium both routinely and unintentionally left Livermore Laboratory via the sewer system. The laboratory's sewage effluent and the plutonium it carried were destined for the Livermore Water Reclamation Plant (LWRP). The end result of waste treatment at the LWRP is "sludge." Between 1958 and 1975, the LWRP's four sludge drying beds covered an area approximately the size of five football fields. The drying beds were filled yearly, up to four inches high, with sludge. Liquids flowed out of the sludge into an underlying layer of sand,

and were carried off into tile drains. Workers hammer milled and ground the dry sludge, while treated liquid effluents were placed in oxidation ponds, which covered approximately 37 acres, and then discharged to the Arroyo Seco and Arroyo Las Positas [4]. In 1958 the Livermore Radiation Laboratory was renamed the E. O. Lawrence Radiation Laboratory, to honor the nuclear physicist Ernest O. Lawrence [5], and the LWRP began to offer its sludge to Livermore's 13,000 residents, for free, for use as a soil amendment.

In 1960, two years after the LWRP began distributing sludge to the public, the State of California, Department of Public Health, Bureau of Radiologic Health, began conducting monthly monitoring of radiation in LWRP's effluent and digester sludge. Plutonium gives off radiation in the form of alpha particles. In 1964, routine monitoring by the state at the LWRP revealed relatively higher alpha activity in dried digester sludge, signaling a large release of plutonium to the sewer [4]. The State Health Department did not monitor radiation levels in the "end-of-the-pipe" sludge given to the public.

By the mid-1960s Livermore was growing, and so grew the LWRP. Between 1965 and 1967, in order to meet the needs of Livermore's 30,000 residents, "Phase II" expansion was underway at the LWRP. Two sludge lagoons were added. The LWRP now had a capacity to hold five to seven years of Livermore's waste. The oxidation ponds were shortened and liquid effluents were disposed of at the airport and discharged into the arroyos. The construction activities at the LWRP brought the distribution of sludge to the public to a temporary halt. The sludge remained in the drying beds for about one year before it was mixed and given out again.

In the spring of 1967 the laboratory inadvertently released a larger-than-usual quantity of plutonium to the city's sanitary sewer. Since "low-level" radioactivity was routinely released to the sewer from the laboratory, the source of these "extra" releases was never definitively established [6]. The 21-day-long discharge of plutonium left the sewage sludge at the LWRP contaminated, but no one knew by how much.

At the time of the incident, laboratory employees tried to estimate the amount of plutonium released into the sewer. But they faced a dilemma: the laboratory's radiation monitor was inoperative for five of the 21 days, so release data were available for only 16 days. Laboratory workers inferred the data for the missing five days, and estimated that the laboratory discharged approximately 32 millicuries of Plutonium-239-Americium-241 to the sewer [6]. During this time, high levels of alpha activity were also detected in dried digester sludge by the State Department of Health [4].

A year after the 1967 non-routine plutonium release, and after Phase II construction activities had been completed, the LWRP resumed giving sludge to the public and local agencies. Residents who picked up sludge were asked to sign their names and addresses in a log book. Sludge was also hauled by LWRP workers to the Altamont/Vasco Road landfill, stockpiled at the airport, and disposed of at a 200 acre ranch adjacent to the LWRP. Golf courses and arroyos began receiving liquid effluents from the LWRP.

In June 1968, Janis Turner and her husband moved into their newly built Livermore home. Janis was starting her teaching career in the Livermore School District and her husband was employed in the Computations Division at LLNL. Beginning in July 1968, Janis and her husband began the year-long effort to landscape their recently purchased Livermore home. They were delighted to read an announcement in a local newspaper about free processed sludge, and ferried truckloads of sludge from the LWRP to their new home in her dad's old yellow pickup truck. "Our LWRP sludge-fertilized garden has been growing for thirty-five years, feeding family, neighbors and friends organic produce harvested from my twelve fruit trees and vegetable garden," Janis relates today with pride.

Sometime between 1968 and 1971, a young Livermore father came home from work with news that free sludge was available at the LWRP. Martha Priebat recalls that her husband liked the idea of getting free sludge to use in several planting beds in their large backyard in Livermore. At least one LWRP worker recalls putting the sludge to use in his garden at the time.

And so the cycle continued: plutonium from Livermore Radiation Laboratory, through the sewer system, to the LWRP, to the sludge, to the public. The population of Livermore was now 41,000. No one had yet measured the amount of plutonium in the sludge given to the ever-growing public. About this time, the University of California removed the word "radiation" from the Livermore laboratory's name, and re-named it Lawrence Livermore National Laboratory (LLNL) [5].

In 1973, Livermore Laboratory monitored plutonium in processed LWRP sewer sludge for the first time, fifteen years after sludge was first distributed to the public. LWRP employees read about the presence of detectable levels of plutonium in the sludge drying beds in the laboratory's annual report. LWRP employees stopped giving the sludge away to the public. Sludge was still given out to local agencies and also to a half-acre worm farm on Buena Vista Avenue, an LWRP employee's yard, and to the rose garden at Great Livermore Junction/Portola Road.

In 1975, in view of what the laboratory described as the "widespread use of the sludge as a soil conditioner in parks, landscaping around public buildings, and in home lawns and gardens," Livermore Laboratory planted a garden to study how much plutonium a person would inhale and ingest if they used LWRP sludge to grow their food [7]. The LLNL study reported plutonium levels in processed sewage sludge as high as 4.4 picocuries per gram (piC/g). Notably, this concentration exceeds the 2.59 piC/g level used by the U.S. Environmental Protection Agency (USEPA) in setting goals for plutonium clean-up activities for residential areas [8]. The laboratory's 1975 garden study concluded that the radiation dose associated with use of the sludge would be 0.04 percent of the annual permissible dose. A year later, the LWRP stopped distributing sewage sludge to local agencies.

Although all sludge distribution by the LWRP had stopped by 1976, plutonium discharges from LLNL to the Livermore sanitary sewer system had not. On May 12, 1988, in a meeting between LLNL and LWRP personnel, Laboratory employees disclosed that elevated levels of plutonium were released to the city's sanitary system beginning in May 1987. The Assistant Director of Public Works at the time, John C. Hines, was apparently not pleased by this news, writing that LLNL's treatment of the release as a "non-incident" does not give consideration to the public's health concerns [9]. He was particularly concerned that LWRP workers were unprotected for possible radiation exposures, and were totally dependent on LLNL to advise them of potential health risks in a timely manner. Hines proposed that the LWRP conduct their own monitoring to insure the protection of the health of LWRP workers and the public, and that the cost be charged to LLNL. More than a decade later, community members would seek the same remedy—independent monitoring paid for by LLNL—when they found out about the possibility of plutonium in their sludge.

PART II: RESEARCH ETHICS IN ASSESSING THE PUBLIC HEALTH IMPACTS OF PLUTONIUM-CONTAMINATED SLUDGE

Setting the Research Agenda

In 1987 LLNL was listed as a Superfund site. Ten years later, and almost 40 years after the sludge was first distributed, the Agency for Toxic Substances and Disease Registry (ATSDR) initiated a scientific investigation of the potential human health impacts of LLNL activities. The health assessment was undertaken because ATSDR is required by law to conduct a Public Health Assessment at Superfund clean-up sites. Community members and advocates did not initiate, and some did not welcome, ATSDR's research. On the basis of reports from other communities living near DOE nuclear weapons facilities [10, 11], some community-health advocates feared that the ATSDR public health assessment process would involve a superficial look at limited data, yet lead to sweeping conclusions that exposures are "below levels of health concern."

The ATSDR conducted part of its LLNL research under a cooperative agreement with the California Department of Health Services' Environmental Health Investigations Branch (CDHS). CDHS researchers initiated a public participation process, called the "Site Team," to help guide the state and federal agencies' research efforts. The Site Team consisted of approximately 25 members, including representatives of the DOE, LLNL, city, county, and state government, environmental, peace, and antinuclear organizations, a small-business owner, a school nurse, and a Bay Area community member who had previously grown up in another nuclear weapons-impacted community, the Hanford Reservation in Washington State, home to what the DOE describes as the "world's largest environmental cleanup project" [12].

CDHS researchers attempted to incorporate meaningful public participation into their health investigation. One way CDHS researchers translated this ethic into the scientific process was by creating the opportunity for the public to suggest topics to be investigated. As Executive Director of Western States Legal Foundation, Jacqueline Cabasso had been closely tracking the environmental record of LLNL for over 15 years, along with Marylia Kelley, her counterpart at Tri-Valley Communities Against a Radioactive Environment. Together, these organizations had decades of experience uncovering and disclosing the environmental impacts of LLNL. During an early Site Team meeting, Jackie held up a newspaper article discussing the results of LLNL's "plutonium garden" [13], and asked, "This has always troubled me, why did LLNL plant a plutonium garden to assure us growing food in plutonium is safe? What happened to the sludge? How much plutonium was in the sludge?" Jackie suggested that CDHS researchers "look into the sludge issue," and they did. By 1999, the health agencies' preliminary investigation established that historic releases of plutonium from LLNL resulted in radioactive contamination of sludge at the LWRP. In May 1999, state and federal health agencies jointly recommended that the historic distribution of sewage sludge be investigated [14].

Research into the distribution of plutonium laden sludge was sparked by a single question posed in a public meeting almost four decades after the sludge was first distributed. However, the kindling had long been in place, as the investigation was just one thread in an interconnected web of events related to the release of radioactive materials from LLNL (see Table 1). For example, the sludge investigation took place in the context of community concerns about more widespread community contamination stemming from recent disclosure of plutonium contamination of three Livermore parks. The parks that had been sampled to obtain "background" levels of plutonium in community soil, as part of on-site LLNL plutonium remediation activities. All three parks showed elevated levels of plutonium, with the highest concentration found in Big Trees Park, about one-half mile west of LLNL. Moreover, inseparable from the scientific uncertainty as to the potential health risks associated with the releases illustrated in Table 1 was the longstanding and vast public relations effort by LLNL to minimize public concerns.

Research Methods

Although the recommendation to investigate the sludge distribution was made jointly by CDHS and ATSDR, the federal and state researchers completely diverged in their methods of inquiry. Two research models to address the potential public health impacts of plutonium-contaminated sludge distribution

Table 1. Timeline of Plutonium Sludge (1952 to 2005) and Some of the Known Unintentional Releases of Radioactive Material from Lawrence Livermore National Laboratory (1960-2005)

1952	Livermore Radiation Laboratory established.
1958	Livermore Water Reclamation Plant (LWRP) begins to distribute sludge to the public, for free.
1960	State of California, Department of Public Health begins monthly monitoring of radiation in LWRP effluent and digester sludge.
November 8, 1960	Curium fire in Building 251, may also involve plutonium-238.
March 26, 1963	Criticality accident in Building 261 triggers explosion, followed by 15 kilograms of weapons grade uranium burning uncontrollably.
1964	Routine monitoring by the State of California at LWRP reveals relatively higher alpha activity in dried digester sludge, signaling a large release of plutonium to the sewer.
January 20, 1965	350,000 curies of tritium goes up the stacks in Building 331.
September 13, 1965	Plutonium fire in Building 332 involves about 100 grams of plutonium.
April 20, 1967	Plutonium spill outside Building 332 spreads due to rain.
May 25 to June 15, 1967	Plutonium is released to sewer system.
August 6, 1970	Tritium accident in Building 331 releases 300,000 curies, elevated levels of tritium related to accident found by LLNL 150 miles away, in Fresno.
1973	Unknown quantities of plutonium released to soil during transfer of solid materials from "solar evaporators."
1973	Livermore Laboratory monitors plutonium in processed sewer sludge for the first time.
1973	LWRP stops distributing sludge to the public.
1975	Livermore Laboratory plants a garden to study how much plutonium a person would inhale and ingest if using LWRP sludge to grow food.
June 16, 1975	Contaminated liquids sprayed throughout a room in Building 332.
1976	LWRP stops distributing sludge to local agencies.
April 8, 1980	Burst plutonium "glove box" outside Building 332.
April 16, 1980	Flash fire in plutonium "glove box" causes pressure to blow the window out, Building 332.
March 1983	Plutonium, curium and americium spilled from waste drums in Building 612.
June 8, 1984	5,000 curies of tritium released from Building 331.
January 25, 1985	1,000 curies of tritium released from Building 331.
February 1986	Plutonium "glove box" leak due to degradation of the gloves.

Table 1. (Cont'd.)

December 15, 1986	Failed pump and cryogenic vessel releases 125 curies of tritium.
May 1987	Plutonium released to sewer system.
April 14, 1987	Equipment failure releases 198 curies of tritium.
1987	Lawrence Livermore National Laboratory declared a Superfund site. The USEPA places LLNL on the National Priorities List of hazardous waste sites due to groundwater contamination.
May 15, 1988	Unexpected presence of tritium in gases being vented, 653 curies released.
August 22, 1989	Container pressure relief fails, 329 curies of tritium released.
1989	Livermore Valley wines sampled by LLNL are found to contain four times the tritium of other CA wines.
1990	U.S. Department of Energy investigative team finds elevated levels of plutonium in off-site air monitor east of LLNL.
April 2, 1991	Improper preparation of reservoir releases 144 curies of tritium.
July 9, 1991	Increase in plutonium discharge found in sewer.
October 24, 1991	Torn bag results in plutonium powder spread on floor.
1994	USEPA soil samples find elevated levels of plutonium in three city parks; highest levels are found in Big Trees Park west of LLNL.
March 1994	Rainwater at LLNL is found to contain tritium at concentrations 7 times higher than state and federal maximum limits; equipment from Building 331 "off-gassing" is thought to be the cause.
1995	Additional soil sampling in Big Tree Park undertaken jointly by USEPA, LLNL, and the State of California reveals concentrations of plutonium up to 1.02 pCi/g in the top two inches of dirt.
February 7, 1996	Inventory reveals 12 pounds of plutonium at LLNL unaccounted for.
February 7, 1997	HEPA filter failure in Building 321 releases uranium-238.
February 1997	Plutonium-contaminated tissue cut out of worker's body.
March 1997	Uranium filings catch fire.
July 2, 1997	Curium contamination during filter shredding operation.
1997	The Agency for Toxic Substances and Disease Registry (ATSDR) initiates a Public Health Assessment of the potential human health impacts of Livermore Laboratory's activities.
1998	LLNL conducts a third round of sampling to investigate plutonium in Big Trees Park. Elevated levels of plutonium found at numerous sites in the Park, near (but no in) the nearby creek, along the baseball field that borders the elementary school and by a little grassy hill between the park and the sidewalk. Slightly elevated levels of plutonium also found behind an apartment complex between LLNL and Big Trees Park.

Table 1. (Cont'd.)

May 1999	The California Department of Health Services (CDHS) and ATSDR jointly recommend the historic distribution of sewage sludge be investigated.
November 2002	CDHS concludes, "sludge at LWRP was contaminated by routine and unintentional releases of plutonium from LLNL . . . [and] the historic distribution (1958-1976) of sewage sludge from the LWRP poses an indeterminate health hazard due to a lack of data." CDHS recommends that "LLNL/DOE [should] provide funding to Alameda County Department of Health Services to implement a process to address the historic distribution of sludge from LWRP."
August 2003	ATSDR concludes, "the historic distribution of Pu-contaminated sewage sludge is determined to be no apparent public health hazard."
October 2003	Plutonium "glove box" leaks due to missing seal, emergency generator, alarm system, and negative air flow system fail simultaneously.
May to August 2004	LLNL cited for "chronic airborne radiation levels" of plutonium over a 4-month period due to continual use of faulty equipment in waste packaging operations.
March 2005	LLNL cited for storing plutonium in paint cans and food tins.
April 22, 2005	Radioactive spill at LLNL tracked off-site; spill area left unsecured for several days.
November 2005	U.S. Department of Energy issues decision to double the amount of plutonium that can be kept at Livermore National Laboratory having determined its review showed no adverse environmental impacts associated with the weapons research even if more plutonium is made available.

emerged: (1) A collaborative approach, undertaken by CDHS; and (2) a dose-assessment approach pursued by ATSDR.

A Collaborative Approach

Key characteristics of the CDHS research method were: (1) gathering and incorporating of local knowledge into the scientific analysis; and (2) fostering the growth of mutually respectful relationships between scientists and governmental and nongovernmental collaborators by including them in all aspects of the research.

Absent a complete and accurate written record about the sludge, and by virtue of their commitment to a transparent, collaborative process, CDHS researchers recognized that input from workers and community members would be essential to their investigation. However, in 1999, over the protests of community-based members of the Site Team, the ATSDR unexpectedly withdrew its funding to the CDHS to convene the Site Team—leaving CDHS without a functional mechanism to gather the historical knowledge about the sludge. In May 2000, the CDHS convened an informal group, called the "Sludge Working Group," as a way to ensure the necessary collaboration. The ATSDR continued to convene the Site Team intermittently as a mechanism to complete other components of its Public Health Assessment.

The CDHS invited all members of the Site Team to participate in the Sludge Working Group. Site Team members who self-selected to join the Sludge Working Group included community members, representatives of three nongovernmental organizations (San Francisco-Bay Area Physicians for Social Responsibility, Tri-Valley Communities Against a Radioactive Environment and Western States Legal Foundation), state and local health officials, and a representative of the City of Livermore. Neither DOE nor LLNL representatives chose to participate in the Sludge Working Group.

Working together, the Sludge Working Group identified and interviewed retired LWRP workers who provided researchers with invaluable, and otherwise undocumented, data. The working group members also tried to locate the logbook that had the names and addresses of the households that received the sludge. Despite making Freedom of Information Act requests to LLNL, and searching the files at the LWRP, the location of logbook remains a mystery to this day.

For Sludge Working Group members, navigating the uncertainties surrounding the sludge distribution presented an enormous ethical challenge. Historically, the ethical implications of distributing plutonium-contaminated sludge had been virtually ignored or obfuscated. Community members who received the sludge at no cost were not told that the sludge they received may have been contaminated with plutonium. During the years that the sludge was distributed to the public, over 11,000 homes had been built in Livermore. As the century that ushered in the nuclear age came to a close, the population of Livermore had grown to over 76,000, and it continues to rise. This translates into ever larger numbers of people at risk of exposure to the plutonium.

Sludge Working Group members grappled with how to engage the community about the potential health hazard without knowing who took the sludge, where it went, and how much plutonium it contained. What was known was that the half-life of weapons-grade plutonium is about 24,000 years. Therefore, former, current, and future Livermore residents are at potential increased risk of cancer and other health impacts from their largely unrecognized and therefore unavoidable exposure to radioactive sludge. Sludge Working Group members tried to find an ethical research framework that would maximize the benefits to community health while minimizing the potential for unwarranted fears, or stigmatization of individuals, households, or the entire community.

Community members had differing experiences with the sludge and expressed their feelings about how to proceed in the face of uncertainties about the sludge in many ways. For example, some knew they had obtained and used LWRP sludge and were concerned about the implications for their family:

> It is frustrating to remember the hundreds of hours my son and I worked our soil with shovel, hoe, and rototiller. My son is now ready to start his own family. I will NOT allow my future grandchildren to play in my soil as long as I suspect plutonium is present. I am requesting a thorough soil test.
> *Janis Turner*

Others didn't know for sure they had contaminated their property, but were concerned that they may have transferred the risk to others:

> We sold the house in 1972. I do not know for sure that we used any sludge and, of course, do not know if it contained plutonium. However, I am concerned that the grounds at my old house may be contaminated with plutonium. The present owner would have no way of knowing about the possible radioactivity in their yard. Taking action about my concerns is the only way I have of remediating my unwitting contamination of that home.
> *Martha Priebat*

And some have gardened extensively in Livermore soil and have no way of knowing if plutonium was part of their exposure:

> As a person who works with the soil, I have been angry and disappointed that, despite the passage of years, location and removal of radioactive sludge once distributed to Livermore's gardeners, has not been completed. The health implications of contact with even small amounts of affected soil are severe and many of us may have been affected. It's time to address this problem.
> *Mary Perner*

However, the extent to which these feelings are representative of Livermore's residents is not known. LLNL is by far the largest employer in Livermore (see Figure 1). Other residents have expressed concerns about jobs; others support the laboratory and its mission; and others have expressed fear of social or work-related retaliation if they were to publicly express their questions about the plutonium.

It became clear that none of the people at the table could decide for the community what to do about the sludge. A shared understanding of the problem as one of science *and* ethics developed over time. The Sludge Working Group members felt that more information was needed and that members of the community should be provided information ("community right-to-know") [15] about historic sludge contamination. The right-to-know approach is based on the fact that community members were not made aware of the potential for plutonium

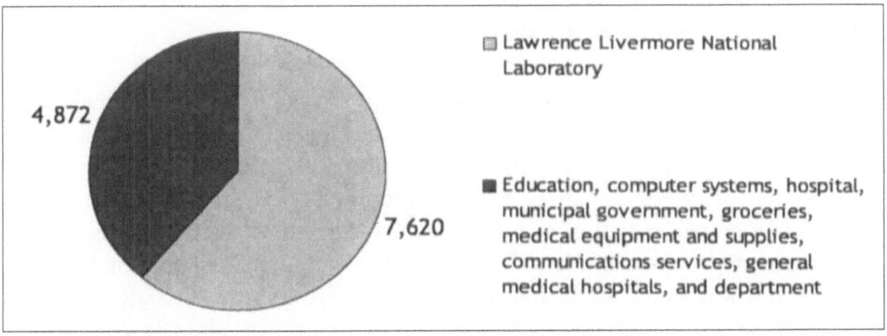

Figure 1. Top ten non-manufacturing employers in Livermore (*N* = 12,492 jobs).
Source: Economic Development Alliance for Business, City of Livermore,
http://edab.org/index.html?BODY=cities/livermore.html
Accessed February 29, 2005.

contamination when, or after, they received the sludge. Since the nature and extent of the potential health hazard remains uncertain, members also supported a process that approached these issues in a proactive manner and would be based on the "precautionary principle" [16]. A key component of the precautionary principle is to take precaution in the face of scientific uncertainty. By integrating community right-to-know and the precautionary principle into the science, the research led to the process proposed in the CDHS report.

The CDHS collaborative approach led to the November 2002 release of the CDHS report titled, *Proposed Process to Address the Historic Distribution of Sewage Sludge Containing Plutonium Released from the Lawrence Livermore National Laboratory* [4]. The CDHS report compiled what was currently known about the sludge and concluded that "sludge at LWRP was contaminated by routine and unintentional releases of plutonium from LLNL . . . [and] the historic distribution (1958–1976) of sewage sludge from the LWRP poses an indeterminate health hazard due to a lack of data." CDHS recommended that "LLNL/DOE [should] provide funding to Alameda County Department of Health Services to implement a process to address the historic distribution of sludge from LWRP."

The objectives of the proposed process were to inform and solicit further information from residents who may have obtained sludge, sample known areas of sludge disposition in order to gain a better understanding of the potential health risk, establish criteria for sampling residences and interpreting results, and provide a mechanism for sampling and, if necessary, removing plutonium-contaminated sludge. The ATSDR refused to sign off on the CDHS report, and CDHS released the report independent of the federal agency.

A Dose-Assessment Approach

ATSDR's approach utilized "existing data to estimate radiological doses from exposure to plutonium contaminated sewage sludge and compared the estimated doses with those that have caused sickness or death" [17]. The ATSDR was explicit in its development and incorporation of a "chronic minimal risk level" for ionizing radiation that the ATSDR considered to be "protective for both cancer and non-cancer health effects." The National Academy of Sciences, Nuclear and Radiation Studies Board has observed that the ATSDR's use of a threshold for evaluating the potential health impacts of chronic exposure to ionizing radiation is inconsistent with its claim to be incorporating health protective assumptions in its Public Health Assessments [18].

The ATSDR was also explicit that its method "was not designed to evaluate the *risks* associated with radiological releases, . . . but does address the radiological *doses* created by exposures to the Pu [plutonium]-contaminated sludge and whether those doses are at levels likely to create any adverse health effects" (emphasis added).

The ATSDR dose assessment made assumptions about the sufficiency of the available data and about exposure conditions or scenarios that would lead to the highest doses or worst-case exposure conditions for an exposed individual. Based on this methodology, ATSDR concluded that "the historic distribution of Pu-contaminated sewage sludge is determined to be no apparent public health hazard."

The ATSDR acknowledged the population-based implications of the sludge exposure, stating that "many Livermore residents could have been exposed to Pu 239-contaminated soil," and "exposure may have occurred, or may still be occurring." However, the ATSDR did not make a quantitative estimate of the number of people potentially exposed to contaminated sludge over the lifetime of the plutonium, and translate those doses to risk. As undertaken by the ATSDR, its dose-assessment methodology discounted a basic epidemiological principle of preventive medicine that large numbers of people exposed to "small" risks can lead to a large public health impact [19].

When its report was released in 2003, the ATSDR received many public comments strongly objecting to specific assumptions and methods it incorporated into its dose assessment [20]. However, even assuming that a scientifically competent dose assessment had been performed by the ATSDR, the divergent methods underlying the CDHS and ATSDR approaches are likely to account for much of the difference between the agencies' conclusions.

On August 11, 2004, the three community-based organizations and the individual community members of the ATSDR Site Team resigned *en masse* from the ATSDR Site Team. In their five-page letter, the community representatives stated in part:

> We have participated in good faith in the process for eight years, attempting always to mend the flaws in the ATSDR's public health assessment process. We have used our individual and organizational in-house scientific expertise and have also hired independent scientists to offer needed comment and criticism on the individual "health consults" and studies undertaken by ATSDR [of which the plutonium-contaminated sludge was but one]. . . . For eight years, ATSDR has disregarded our individual and collective scientific and community expertise. . . . [T]he site team process is being used by ATSDR to imply community participation and acceptance. . . . Therefore, we take the only ethical action available to us—to tender our resignations. . . .

PART III: FORMALIZATION AND EXPANSION OF THE COMMUNITY-GOVERNMENT PARTNERSHIP AS AN ETHICAL MODEL FOR PARTICIPATORY AND EQUITABLE DECISION MAKING

Alameda County Plutonium Action Taskforce (ACPAT)

The outcome of the CDHS collaborative research process was a report that proposed a transparent, locally-based, participatory process for scientific decision making to address the large uncertainties surrounding the distribution of sludge. The Alameda County Environmental Health Department convened an expanded working group in July 2003, named the Alameda County Plutonium Action Taskforce (ACPAT), to address the historical distribution of plutonium-contaminated sewage sludge.

The ACPAT began with approximately 25 members, including an expanded community member contingent along with Sludge Working Group members. The ACPAT process was designed to inform the public of plutonium contamination to sewage sludge from historical releases from LLNL to the LWRP, to increase public participation in environmental decision making, to provide environmental sampling and analysis to affected and interested residents, and to provide a mechanism for implementing appropriate follow-up action. Alameda County actively solicited community members' involvement in the process at public meetings, followed-up by letters and phone calls.

Under the leadership of Pamela Evans of the Alameda County Environmental Health Department, the ACPAT set up a regular, local meeting schedule with agendas that aimed to carry out a work plan that they developed to implement the CDHS report recommendations and to accommodate the interests and concerns of community members. For example, newer members wanted information about property owners' contamination disclosure responsibilities, health effects of plutonium, construction activities at contaminated sites, and appropriate sampling protocols for contaminated residential gardens.

Sludge Working Group and later ACPAT members collaborated on grant proposals, trainings for community members and scientists, and educational materials. To date, the results of this collaborative model have been:

- 1998–99 Submitted USEPA grant proposals for funding to conduct independent monitoring for radiation; conducted community and government "Radiation and Risk" workshops to strengthen the capacity of community members impacted by the historic distribution of sludge to make informed decisions about their health, and for state and local officials to respond to community concerns.
- 2002 Conducted government and community organization workshop on evaluating and communicating radiation risk; released CDHS Report and held community meeting.
- 2003 Developed work plan and grant proposal to Syracuse University to fund *Short Courses for Environmental Research Ethics, Case Study and Trainings for the Ethical Decision-Making for Widespread Distribution of Plutonium-Contaminated Sewage Sludge;* initiated ACPAT meetings which are on-going.
- 2004 Conducted government and community workshops on health risks.
- 2006 Developed and posted plutonium-sludge related fact sheets on the Alameda County Environmental Health Web-site [21].

Hurdles: Some Overcome, Some Persistent

Lack of Trust, Unequal Power, Different Perspectives, Lack of Data

What began in 1997 as what could be viewed as "unwilling but cooperative" participation on the part of the community organizations when ATSDR initiated the public health assessment process, developed over ten years into a truly collaborative process to address an uncertain environmental exposure. Although many factors may have contributed to this outcome, the participatory research framework nurtured by CDHS scientists was essential. The CDHS-led investigation served to equalize power among the scientists and community members and valued the contribution of all points of view, including a CDHS health physicist, city, county, and state government representatives, and community-based environmental and peace activists.

Members of the Sludge Working Group came to the table with very different perspectives, but all shared a commitment to protecting the public health. All participants were experienced at, and committed to, providing their respective constituencies with only the most scientifically-accurate information. All participants appeared familiar and comfortable with not having the answer and therefore with grappling with scientific uncertainty.

Although ATSDR and LLNL took the position that no public health risk exists due to the contaminated sludge, CDHS and county health officials gave more weight to the evidence that there were substantial data gaps. This led state and local agencies to determine that risk to residents living at properties where sludge may have come to rest is not established (and cannot be based) on the available information.

Opposition to the ACPAT Process by Lawrence Livermore National Laboratory

LLNL refused the county's request to provide funding for a process to address the sludge issue and sent a letter to the USEPA, essentially opposing the county's and other stakeholders' USEPA grant application. As previously noted, LLNL's extensive public relations efforts promote its message that the plutonium-sludge distribution and other LLNL releases carry no health risk to the community.

Inconsistent Alameda County Leadership in the ACPAT Process

Although representatives of Alameda County attended meetings of the Site Team convened by CDHS in 1997 to guide the public health assessment process, the county's commitment to interact with nongovernmental organizations in a collaborative process to address radioactive exposures in the county was actually prompted by the 1998 and 1999 findings of the Alameda Grand Jury recommendations to the Alameda County Board of Supervisors [22]. The Grand Jury recommended that the county collaborate with governmental and nongovernmental organizations to assure public safety from radioactive and other hazardous contaminants from LLNL and other sites in the county, mandate monitoring of radioactive contaminants, seek and allocate funding for independent monitoring, and disseminate information regarding radioactive contaminants [23, 24].

In January 2004, the county suddenly reversed itself when it refused to accept its first successful grant to support the ACPAT process, and it abandoned project leadership. Some of the grant funds (from Syracuse University) were redirected to Tri-Valley Communities Against a Radioactive Environment and the Western States Legal Foundation. This enabled the nonprofit groups to move forward with the work. However, the loss of the funding to the county did impede ACPAT's efforts to implement the work plan and caused the county's credibility to suffer among its community-based partners. Despite this setback, the ACPAT has continued to meet, to address community members' questions and issues, to plan for workshops, to develop fact sheets, and to strategize alternative approaches to implement the work plan.

Lack of Funding to Carry Out the ACPAT Process

As described above, LLNL/DOE have refused to fund the sludge follow-up process, and the county was not successful in its two grant requests to the USEPA. The process has moved forward through the in-kind contributions of all the collaborators, and limited funding from Syracuse University for trainings and case-study development. In 2005, ACPAT members met with elected officials at both the county and federal levels to present their concerns and to identify other funding sources to implement the work plan. In March 2005, the County Board of Supervisors voted to request a federal appropriation for this purpose.

Limitations: Intergeneration Equity and Primary Prevention

This case study has described the development of a process to address the issue of plutonium-contaminated sludge distribution in the Livermore Valley. At best, if implemented, the process developed will permit community members who may have received the sludge to get the necessary information, training, and environmental testing to make informed decisions about the health of themselves and their families. Key limitations are that the process does not address issues of intergenerational equity and primary prevention of exposure. The ACPAT process is happening against a backdrop of the DOE's November 2005 decision to double the plutonium storage limit at LLNL to more than 3,000 pounds [26], enough plutonium for about 300 nuclear bombs. Worldwide, there are 3.7 million pounds of this man-made substance [26]. The wide dispersal of a radioactive substance having a lifetime of virtually forever, guarantees that the majority of Livermore's plutonium will still be waiting for the generations who follow. Therefore, prevention efforts undertaken today must also speak to the health of future generations. This will involve looking upstream of the plutonium and working towards sustainable solutions to security that do not involve the public health threats embedded in the global embrace of nuclear weapons [27].

ACKNOWLEDGMENT

The authors acknowledge the valuable contribution of Pamela Evans of Alameda County Environmental Health to the development of this case study and thank her for her tireless efforts on behalf of public health.

NOTES

1. Rhodes, R. 1986. *The making of the atomic bomb.* New York: Simon and Schuster, pp. 354-355, 777.
2. U.S. Department of Energy, Office of Environmental Management. January 1997. Linking legacies. Connecting the Cold War nuclear weapons processes to their environmental consequences. DOE/EM-0319:12.
3. Mahkijani, A., and Saleska, S. 1995. The production of nuclear weapons and environmental hazards. In *Nuclear wastelands. A global guide to nuclear weapons and its health and environmental effects,* eds. A. Mahkijani, H. Hu, and K. Yih, 23-63. Cambridge, MA: MIT Press.
4. California Department of Health Services. November 2002. Proposed Process to Address the Historic Distribution of Sewage Sludge Containing Plutonium Released from the Lawrence Livermore National Laboratory. http://www. ehib.org/cma/papers/LLNL_Sludge_Health_Consultation.pdf
5. Schwartz, S. I. 1998. *Atomic audit: The costs and consequences of US nuclear weapons since 1940.* Washington, DC: Brookings Institute Press, p. 593.
6. Lawrence Radiation Laboratory (LRL). 22 August 1967. Letter to E. C. Shute, U.S. Atomic Energy Commission from D. C. Sewell, Associate Director, LRL re: Summary Hazards Analysis: Pu Am Release to Sanitary Sewer.
7. Myers, D. S. et al. 1975. Lawrence Livermore National Laboratory. Evaluation of the Use of Sludge Containing Plutonium as a Soil Conditioner for Food Crops. Livermore, CA: Prepared for presentation at the International Symposium on Transuranium Nuclides in the Environment, San Francisco, November 17-21, 1975, sponsored by the IAEA, USERDA, and LLL. 17 September 1975. Report No: UCRL-77318.
8. U.S. Environmental Protection Agency. *Waste cleanup and risk assessment. Preliminary cleanup goals for superfund.* http://epa-prgs.ornl.gov/
9. Lawrence Livermore National Laboratory. 17 May 1988. Letter to Robert O. Godwin, Associate Director Plant and Technical Services, from John C. Hines, Assistant Director of Public Works.
10. Agency For Toxic Substances and Disease Registry. Public Health Assessment, US DOE Facility Mound, Miamisburg, Montgomery County, Ohio, EPA Facity ID: OH6890008984. March 30, 1998. http://www.atsdr.cdc.gov/HAC/PHA/doemound/dmf_p2.html#conc
11. Agency For Toxic Substances and Disease Registry. Public Health Assessment, Pantex Plant, Amarillo, Carson County, Texas. CERCLIS NO. TX4890110527. September 30, 1998. http://www.atsdr.cdc.gov/HAC/pha/pantex/pan_ toc.html
12. U.S. Department of Energy, Richland Operations Office. http://www.hanford.gov/communication/reporter/rl/
13. Valley Times. September 10, 1989. *Lab downplays effect on plants in spiked gardens.*
14. California Department of Health Services, Environmental Health Investigations Branch. May 1999. *Health consultation plutonium in Big Trees Park, Lawrence Livermore National Laboratory.* Prepared for the Agency for Toxic Substances and Disease Registry, U.S. Department of Health and Human Services. http://www.ehib.org/cma/papers/LLNL_Sludge_Health_Consultation.pdf

15. Community Right-to-Know: Title III of Superfund law: In 1986 Superfund law was amended with a provision added to help increase the public's knowledge and access to information on the presence of hazardous chemicals in their communities and releases of chemicals into the environment. USEPA Superfund. www.epa.gov/oerrpage/superfund/programs/er/comunity/rt2know.htm
16. Precautionary Principle: When information about potential risks is incomplete, basing decisions about the best ways to manage or reduce risks on a preference for avoiding unnecessary health risks instead of on unnecessary economic expenditures. USEPA Terms of the Environment: Available from http://www.epa.gov/OCEPA terms/pterms.html Precautionary Principle: When an activity raises threats of harm to human health or the environment, precautionary measures should be taken even if some cause-and-effect relationships are not fully established scientifically. Science and Environmental Health Network. Fact Sheet: The Precautionary Principle: A Common Sense Way to Protect Public Health and the Environment: http://www.sehn.org/precaution.html
17. U.S. Agency for Toxic Substances and Disease Registry. 26 August 2003. Public Health Assessment: Plutonium-239 in sewage sludge used as a soil amendment in the Livermore community. Lawrence Livermore National Laboratory, Main Site (USDOE.) Livermore, Alameda County, California. http://www.atsdr.cdc.gov/HAC/PHA/livermore5/lll_p1.html#sect1c1
18. National Academy of Sciences. National Research Council. Nuclear and Radiation Studies Board. Review of Worker and Public Health Activities Program Administered by the Department of Energy and the Department of Health and Human Services. National Academies Press, WA DC, 2006, p. 104. http://books.nap.edu/openbook.php?chapselect=yo&page=104&record_id=11805
19. Rose G. 1992. *The strategy of preventive medicine*. New York: Oxford University Press, pp. 22-28.
20. San Francisco-Bay Area Physicians for Social Responsibility. 28 April 2003. Letter to Max M. Howie, Jr. Agency for Toxic Substances and Disease Registry, Division of Health Assessment and Consultation Program Evaluation, Records and Information Services Branch, from Robert Gould, San Francisco-Bay Area Physicians for Social Responsibility, Marylia Kelley, Tri-Valley Communities Against a Radioactive Environment, and Patrice Sutton, Western States Legal Foundation. Re: Public Health Assessment Plutonium 239 Sewage Sludge Used as a Soil or Soil Amendment in the Livermore Community Lawrence Livermore National Laboratory, Main Site (USDOE) Livermore, Alameda County, California EPA Facility ID: CA2890012584, 10 February 2003.
21. Alameda County Public Health Department Web-Site. Data and Reports. http://www.acphd.org/user/data/DataRep_ListbyCat.asp?DataRepdivId=2&DataRepdiv catid=44
22. On April 14, 1998, the grand jury issued a report that found, "Contaminants such as plutonium, tritium, and volatile organic compounds (VOCs) are present in several Alameda County facilities. The largest of these facilities is Lawrence Livermore National Laboratory (LLNL) where there have been releases of plutonium which have appeared on a nearby City of Livermore park and on citizens' lawns."

23. Alameda County Grand Jury. 14 April 1998. Letter from N. B. Goodhue, Foreman, 1997-1998, Alameda County Grand Jury to Supervisor Scott Haggerty.
24. Alameda County Grand Jury. 26 July 1999. Letter from L. M. Poe, Foreman, 1998-1999, Alameda County Grand Jury to Ms. S. Muranishi, County Administrator.
25. U.S. Department of Energy. National Nuclear Security Administration. Record of Decision. Final Site-wide Environmental Impact Statement for Continued Operation of Lawrence Livermore National Laboratory and Supplemental Stockpile Stewardship and Management Programmatic Environmental Impact Statement. November 29, 2005. Available from http://www-envirinfo.llnl.gov/SWEIS_ROD.pdf
26. Albright, D., and Kramer, K. June 2004. Plutonium watch: Tracking plutonium inventories. http://www.isis-online.org/global_stocks/plutonium_ watch2004.html
27. Sutton, P. M., and Gould, R. M. 2008. Nuclear weapons. In *War and public health* (2nd ed.), ed. B. S. Levy and V. W. Sidel, 152-176. New York: Oxford University Press.

http://dx.doi.org/10.2190/TORC6

CHAPTER 6

Institutional Preferences for Justice, Avoiding Harm, and Expertise in Public Health Policy Making about the Health Consequences of Iodine-131 Nuclear Weapons Testing Fallout

Seth Tuler

A total of one hundred and twenty-five atmospheric, surface, near-surface, and underground tests were conducted at the Nevada Test Site (NTS) between 1951 and 1963.These tests resulted in fallout of many different kinds of radioactive isotopes, including cesium, strontium, and iodine, exposing millions of Americans to radioactive contamination [1, 2]. The most extensive analysis of radioactive fallout from U.S. nuclear weapons testing concentrated on radioiodine, or I-131, which has a half-life of eight days [1]. An analysis performed by the National Cancer Institute (NCI) found that nuclear weapons tests released about 150 million curies of I-131 [1]. Virtually every county in the United States received some I-131 fallout. The highest levels of I-131 fallout were deposited immediately downwind from the NTS. The main pathway of exposure to humans was from consumption of fresh milk. Although in some groups (e.g., Native Americans), exposures may also have resulted from eating wild game and fish [3]. While the NCI study estimated doses of I-131 fallout, subsequent estimates were made of the risks of I-131 exposure, with particular emphasis on thyroid cancer. Estimates of thyroid cancer risk are questionable because of the many uncertainties associated with the actual levels of fallout deposited, individual exposures and doses (including the relative biological effectiveness of I-131), and the dose-response function. The possible excess thyroid cancers from the I-131 fallout have been estimated to range from 11,300 to 212,000, with a central estimate of 49,000.

Any effort to study the public health consequences of nuclear weapons testing or to determine appropriate public health responses raises a host of ethical issues. For example, does the government have an ethical responsibility to inform residents of the United States that they may have been exposed and have elevated risks of thyroid cancer or nonmalignant thyroid diseases? Should policy decisions about health responses be based on a concern for the most vulnerable or the average population risks? What are reasonable kinds of responses to choose from—screening of special populations, general public education efforts, outreach to medical professionals, or compensation? Are these risks significant enough to even warrant a public health response? And who should be involved in deciding what is an appropriate response to the study about I-131 fallout?

There are different ways to resolve complex risk issues that are permeated by ethical considerations. An oft-used approach is to separate questions of science from considerations of values or ethics [4]. Others argue that questions of fact and values—science and ethics—cannot be cleanly separated because values influence the assumptions and judgments that are inherent in technical and scientific analyses [5]. In this view, decisions should be made through an approach that integrates both scientific analysis and broad deliberation among interested and affected parties. New frameworks have been proposed to integrate science and values [6].

In this chapter, I highlight how considerations about public health responses to nuclear fallout are informed by different approaches to resolving ethical issues. I begin by providing a brief overview of the NCI study on I-131 fallout. Next, I explore the way that two different efforts responded to the news that millions of Americans were exposed to I-131 fallout from nuclear weapons testing by their own government. Finally, I argue that that the results of these efforts were largely a result of different ways of thinking about and integrating science and ethics.

THE NATIONAL CANCER INSTITUTE REPORT: THE FIRST ASSESSMENT OF I-131 FALLOUT EXPOSURES

In 1983, Congress directed the Department of Health and Human Services (DHHS) to assess the public health consequences of I-131 fallout from nuclear weapons testing (Section 7 of Public Law 97-414). More specifically, the DHHS was required to assess risks of thyroid cancer and estimate individual thyroid doses from the fallout. In addition, Congress directed DHHS to address the full range of radiogenic cancers and their individual probability of causation based on exposure to all the radionuclides from atomic bomb tests. The Secretary of the DHHS designated the National Cancer Institute to carry out the required studies. The study's reconstruction of I-131 doses was essentially complete in 1992. However, no report was finalized or released and the results were not conveyed either to Congress or the public. Information about the study was only available within a narrow community of researchers interested in radiological dose reconstructions.

By 1996, the DHHS Advisory Committee on Energy-Related Epidemiologic Research (ACERER) and others began asking questions about the status of the study. No information was forthcoming until *USA Today* published a series of articles in 1997, including maps illustrating I-131 fallout distributions across the United States based on the leaked executive summary of a draft report. Soon afterward, the NCI published a two volume report [1] addressing the second and third elements of the legislation [7], and voluminous amounts of supporting data and maps on the Internet. http://www.cancer.gov/i131 The reaction was swift. Members of the U.S. Senate voiced strong concern about their constituencies who were identified as receiving relatively high levels of exposure to the I-131 fallout. Others expressed their concern in the press around the country.

At the same time, the first requirement of the legislation—to estimate risks from thyroid cancer—was not addressed in the report. However, after the study was released, NCI staff person Dr. Charles Land wrote a memo to the NCI director estimating that 7,500-75,000 excess thyroid cancers would result during the lifetime of those exposed before the age of 20. He later revised his initial estimates, increasing the range to 11,300-212,000 with a central estimate of 49,000 excess thyroid cancers.

Several issues quickly became apparent. First, credible individual risk estimates were not possible because of the paucity of data and high uncertainties about fallout distribution and individual exposures. Second, while the average thyroid dose from I-131 to the approximately 160 million people in the United States during the period of weapons testing was 2 rads [8], some individuals—possibly numbering in the tens of thousands—could have received very high doses. For example, the dose to some children possibly reached as high as 160 rads. Third, high exposures were distributed across the United States, and not isolated to an area around the test site because of meteorological factors affecting fallout. East of Nevada and Utah, where most of the I-131 was deposited via rain, there were isolated "hotspots" in, for example, Iowa, Maine, New York, and Tennessee. Some of the highest recorded estimates were in Idaho. Fourth, factors that would be associated with elevated risk were identifiable. These included drinking fresh milk (particularly goats milk), age at time of exposure (the young were more vulnerable), and sex (women were more vulnerable). Location of residence was, of course, associated with exposure levels (e.g., proximity to the test site), but individual-specific factors played a significant role.

THE IOM/NRC REVIEW

In August 1997, the DHHS asked the National Research Council (NRC) and the Institute of Medicine (IOM) to conduct an independent assessment of the public health and medical implications of the estimated exposures to I-131 and to advise the Secretary of DHHS on future actions. This assessment, completed in 1999 [9], was conducted by two existing committees working together:

- The Committee on Thyroid Screening Related to I-131 Exposure, established by the IOM Board on Health Care Services, and
- The Committee on Exposure of the American People to I-131 from the Nevada Atomic Bomb Tests, established by the NRC Board on Radiation Effects Research.

It is important to note that the charge to the IOM/NRC committees did not focus only on thyroid cancer and recommendations for cancer screening. The charge was much broader, asking for an assessment and recommendations related to the effects of I-131 on public health [9]. Yet, the IOM/NRC committees chose to focus on thyroid cancer risk and thyroid cancer screening [10]. The primary conclusions were that (a) the dose reconstruction was valid, even though the uncertainties were large and (b) no type of thyroid cancer screening program associated with I-131 exposures from U.S. nuclear weapons testing was warranted. In the committees' words:

> [We reached] a somewhat unsettling combination of conclusions, first, that some people (who cannot be easily identified) were likely exposed to sufficient iodine-131 to raise their risk of thyroid cancer and, second, that there is no evidence that programs to screen for thyroid cancer are beneficial in detecting disease at a stage that would allow more effective treatment. To serve the public interest, the major contribution that the government can make is not to launch an ineffective but politically appealing screening program but rather, to develop effective ways to communicate with the public about iodine-131 exposure and health risks and to involve the public in determining what communication strategies people will find understandable, useful, and trustworthy [9, p. x].

In short, the IOM/NRC labeled any suggestion of screening as politically motivated and not grounded in good science. The committees believed that evidence-based criteria for national screening policy (e.g., an effective treatment for disease exists; an accurate, practical screening test is available; and early detection of disease improves survivability) could not be met. They concluded that it would be inappropriate to initiate a national screening program for asymptomatic people who may be at elevated risk of thyroid cancer because of exposures from the nuclear weapons tests. Thus, they suggested that the only reasonable response was to inform people, carefully, about possible risks, but not to provide any formal programs to ensure that clinical follow-up would be available. They also recommended that it would be important to promote health care provider education about I-131 health effects and thyroid cancer diagnosis.

THE ACERER'S RESPONSE TO THE NCI REPORT

The ACERER also deliberated about the public health and medical implications of the estimated exposures to I-131. When ACERER was established in 1992, its primary role was to review analytic epidemiologic research conducted by the Centers for Disease Control and Prevention (CDC) and the National Institute for Occupational Safety and Health (NIOSH) and to provide advice to the Secretary of the DHHS in setting the research agenda and conducting the research program. From its inception, however, the committee served a broader purpose: to ensure that the study of radiation health effects from the nuclear weapons program was both scientifically sound and publicly credible [11]. Many of the ACERER's members had long histories of conducting and assessing research on the risks from radiation exposure arising from DOE activities. Others had experience in public and occupational health programs, and one was a community activist.

In 1997, the ACERER established a Community Working Group that was transformed into the Subcommittee for Community Affairs (SCA) within a year. The purpose of the SCA was to improve the representation of community and worker perspectives in ACERER, including to help identify issues of concern in communities around DOE nuclear weapons facilities and to help ACERER prioritize its consideration of issues. Twenty-one individuals representing communities and workers within the DOE nuclear weapons complex were formally designated as consultants to the Subcommittee for Community Affairs and began meeting with ACERER. Many of the consultants had long experience with the DOE, NCEH, and ATSDR health-related studies at DOE nuclear weapons sites. Some were nurses or worked in the public health arena, and all were advocates within their communities or for national nongovernmental organizations. Community consultants identified public health consequences of fallout from nuclear weapons testing as a priority issue during their first meeting in 1997.

In July 1998, the SCA held a two-day meeting in Boise, Idaho. Three questions guided the discussions:

1. What additional research, if any, was needed to reduce the uncertainties of the NCI report?
2. What public and physician notification and education actions were necessary, given the current state of knowledge about fallout exposures?
3. What medical screening and medical monitoring programs should be considered in light of the NCI fallout study, and how should they be implemented?

It is clear from this meeting that a combined focus on ethics and scientific understandings would become foundational issues in the way that the ACERER approached this issue. For example, ACERER and SCA members talked about:

- A ban on nuclear weapons as a "primary prevention" approach to reducing public health risks from fallout.
- People need a range of options when responding to new information about health risks.
- Special risk populations can and should be identified (e.g., via the milk consumption pathway) for particular kinds of programs (e.g., medical screening).
- Attention should be given to the special character of the exposures, e.g., they were involuntary, the government was responsible, and the government failed to notify exposed populations even when it was known that they might be harmful—in some cases the government plainly lied.
- The ethical and practical aspects of a possible thyroid cancer screening program, including the relevance of U.S. Task Force for Preventative Medicine guidelines on screening, screening for the "general population" versus subgroups that may have received higher doses, the issues of false positives, unnecessary surgeries (or other invasive procedures), rates of increased survival from such a screening program, and physician diagnostic skills (e.g., conducting neck exams for thyroid nodules).
- The importance of acting immediately with some form of notification program, rather than waiting for further studies and reviews.

A few months and several drafts after the Boise meeting, ACERER member Tim Connor proposed recommendations for ACERER's action during a meeting in September 1998. This was also a meeting at which the chairs of the NRC and IOM Committees presented their findings and recommendations to ACERER.

ACERER's six recommendations [12] were that the Secretary of DHHS should:

1. Fulfill the legislative intent of Public Law 97-414.
2. Complete a comprehensive dose-reconstruction project for Nevada Test Site fallout.
3. Notify Americans of the factors that might help them to determine whether they received significant radiation doses from Nevada Test Site fallout.
4. Create a public and health care provider information service on Nevada Test Site exposures and resulting public health concerns.
5. Support archival projects to document experiences of exposed peoples.
6. Further evaluate screening opportunities for thyroid cancer. It is urgent, in the meantime, to evaluate the advisability and feasibility of screening for other (noncancerous) thyroid and parathyroid diseases, with a priority to evaluate this service for those at highest risk due to their exposures.

SIMILARITIES AND DIFFERENCES BETWEEN THE IOM/NRC AND THE ACERER

The recommendations of the IOM/NRC and the ACERER reveal two important areas of agreement. First, each effort resulted in a statement about a moral and ethical responsibility for the federal government to provide a public health response to the exposures of the American people to I-131 fallout from U.S. nuclear weapons tests. Both groups believed that the government should notify and educate residents of the United States and medical professionals about increased risks due to I-131 fallout. Second, each effort resulted in a recommendation about the inappropriateness of a thyroid cancer screening program for the general population. Both groups felt there was a good chance that there could be serious negative consequences associated with a general, nationwide public screening program for thyroid cancer. The IOM/NRC was quite forceful in recommending that no screening programs for thyroid cancer should be considered. The ACERER respected "the reasoning that discourages moving forward quickly with a general thyroid cancer screening program" because "there are legitimate and unresolved questions as to whether early detection of thyroid cancers can measurably improve the survival rate in the screened population" (Recommendation #6).

However, beyond these basic agreements there were serious and deep disagreements, even within the context of these two issues. Important differences between the IOM/NRC committees and the ACERER were:

- The IOM/NRC did not consider dose reconstruction of the NTS (and fulfilling the intent of Public Law 97-414) to be a national public health priority. The ACERER felt that understanding the effects of the full range of biologically significant radionuclides—hence, the public health emphasis—in fallout from the Nevada Test Site to be an important.
- The ACERER sought to overcome possible public distrust of further efforts to evaluate public health consequences of fallout from the NTS by recommending that special attention be given to creating a public oversight committee under the general supervision of the ACERER; the NRC/IOM viewed the role of public involvement as limited to the development of public notification and education programs, and they felt that public distrust was something that needed to be addressed in a public notification and education program.
- The IOM/NRC recommended against *any* program of thyroid cancer screening in response to concerns about NTS I-131 fallout. The ACERER was in agreement with this recommendation when applied to the entire U.S. population, but it also felt that screening might be warranted for certain exposed subpopulations and suggested further evaluation of such an effort.

- The IOM/NRC committees downplayed the importance of screening for noncancer thyroid disease outcomes by using blood tests. In contrast, the ACERER recommended a more proactive approach to screening for such diseases because it believed that the danger of false positives were far less than in a cancer-screening program.
- The ACERER recommended that the DHHS support archival projects with the intent of documenting the experiences and histories of people's exposures to NTS fallout. The IOM/NRC did not mention the role or need for such efforts.

The approaches, deliberations, and written documents of the two groups suggest that they adopted different normative frameworks for integrating considerations of science and ethics in the context of significant uncertainties [13]. In particular, social justice was at the center of the ACERER's framing of the findings and recommendations; justice-related issues were a secondary concern in the IOM/NRC report and presentations.

The IOM/NRC committees were driven primarily by their own expertise and interpretation of the state of scientific information available, and they attempted to stick to what they viewed as valid scientific knowledge and keep ethical considerations out. Institutionally, the IOM/NRC are geared toward consideration of the science and view themselves as free from "political" influences. They assemble experts in relevant fields from outside of the government to ensure independent advice on matters of science, technology and medicine. Their approach is intended to preserve the independence, objectivity, and scientific integrity of the advice provided by committees. There is a strong emphasis on acknowledged experts learning about and deliberating about the scientific aspects of an issue. The structure and process of committees are set up so that, presumably, they are free from the pressure of outside influences.

Concerns about independence, objectivity, and scientific integrity were also shared by the DHHS and ACERER. However, the ACERER's institutional history and context ensured that issues of justice, morality, and ethics were at the forefront of its concerns, as expressed in its recommendations and in its members' deliberations (as well as the criteria used to evaluate the research agenda, see Footnote 11). As one member stated, the issue of credibility was the central purpose of the ACERER: "Public credibility. I mean, to me that's the whole reason we're here" [14]. In its recommendations to the Secretary of DHHS, the ACERER wrote:

> The difficulties in identifying individuals whose injuries are caused by fallout exposures do not absolve the federal government of its civil and moral responsibility to aid the injured. The general obligation of the Government to attend to the well-being of its citizens is, in this instance, profoundly enhanced by the facts that the Government is responsible for the exposures

> and for failing to give people the information necessary to avoid or minimize the risks imposed upon them (Finding #2).

In contrast, the IOM/NRC were much more restrained in how they articulated these ethical and moral dimensions:

> Governmental decisions related to safety both on and off the Nevada Test Site were undoubtedly influenced by a sense of urgency about national security. One apparent consequence is a history of misleading government statements about the Nevada tests [9, p. ix].

> Since the tests have ended, governments and residents of areas adjacent to the test sites have engaged in intermittent, often acrimonious debate about possible health effects and about the release of information. The legacy is a government with a record of poor credibility as an information provider and a subset of the population convinced that the health consequences of the tests are significant and severe [9, p. 125].

In the following sections, I will discuss three ways that the IOM/NRC and ACERER committees balanced ethical concerns and integrated them with scientific considerations and how they ultimately affected their proposals for addressing issues associated with I-131 fallout.

Who Should Be Considered: Most Americans or Vulnerable Subpopulations?

The IOM/NRC focused on the general population and recommended against *any* thyroid cancer screening program because the harms would likely outweigh the benefits to the *general* population; they did not consider in detail the possible appropriateness of a targeted screening program for higher-risk subpopulations. According to the chair of the IOM committee, the two committees concluded that "there was no direct evidence that early detection of thyroid cancer through systematic screening rather than through *routine clinical care* improved survival or other health outcomes" [14, p. 18]. In fact they went further: "A program of systematic screening for thyroid cancer therefore is not recommended generally or *even among regional populations* believed to have been exposed to I-131 from the Nevada test [sic]" [14, p. 19, emphasis added].

On the other hand, the ACERER framed the issue of thyroid cancer screening risks and benefits around those with the highest risk, rather than "most" Americans with lower average exposures. While it is not possible to reliably identify specific individuals in high-risk subpopulations, there are factors that characterize them. It was widely noted that the individuals with the greatest chance of significant exposures were "young children at the time and who routinely drank milk from backyard cows and in particular goats" [15]. The

ACERER recommended "that DHHS move with deliberate speed to evaluate the opportunities for, and feasibility of, identifying and locating high dose subpopulations for whom thyroid cancer screening would merit further consideration" (Recommendation #6).

The NRC/IOM made its recommendation on thyroid cancer screening using an "evidence-based" approach that requires an assessment of relative risks and benefits. However, the committees used the lack of clear evidence for the benefits of early detection of thyroid cancer screening as justification for its inappropriateness, rather than using it to raise questions and suggest opportunities for further investigation of the need for a targeted program (e.g., pilot program for high-risk subpopulation). Regarding further research their main concern was the need to provide a better understanding of "people's perceptions of the benefits and risks of screening for thyroid and other cancers and the factors affecting such perceptions including the way quantitative information is presented" [9, p. 9]. How to weigh the evidence was a judgment in the face of uncertainty.

In the face of this uncertainty, the ACERER gave more weight to what it understood as the ethical and moral obligations of the government to provide a public health response, especially to more vulnerable subpopulations [16]. Furthermore, the ACERER noted the apparent tension between informing people they might be at risk and providing no way for them to follow up with their concerns:

> Although notification is not the same as offering enrollment in a thyroid cancer screening program, it inescapably invites many of the same ethical concerns [17].

> We are not talking about your standard asymptomatic population because we've energized that population with information. We've told them that they're more at risk . . . aren't we in fact creating a *de facto* screening experience when people get this information, which we all agree we should be giving to them, and in a sense herding them to their doctors for neck exams, aren't we in a sense doing what you [IOM/NRC] don't want them to do? [19, pp. 58-61].

The IOM/NRC noted this tension too:

> Given popular fears of cancer and concern about radiation, the often modest reach of public information programs, and conflicting recommendations from other groups, clinicians will likely see some patients who express concern about possible exposure to radioactive fallout and who request screening for thyroid cancer. Although the committee recommends against policies that encourage or promote routine screening, it is essential that clinicians respond sensitively and constructively to concerned patients" [9, pp. 7-8].

But it does not appear to have influenced their understanding of who a screening program should apply to (i.e., the anxious). The IOM/NRC adopted a widely used definition of screening which applies to the testing of *asymptomatic* people or as committee member Dr. Mazzaferri put it:

> Screening is testing someone who feels well, who their own perception of their health is, is that it's fine, there's nothing wrong. And I say no, you need a mammogram, or you need a PSA, or you need a thyroid test because I think you might be sick, versus the patient who is fatigued or losing weight or anxious, or has a host of symptoms, that's not screening [19, p. 50].

During a discussion of this tension, Bob Lawrence, Chair of the IOM committee stated: "There's some that would argue that an anxious, concerned patient is no longer asymptomatic. I think that's a little semantic dodge" [19, p. 56]. But, in fact it was the IOM/NRC that engaged in a semantic dodge in its report by excluding serious consideration of vulnerable subpopulations and maintaining a focus on the appropriateness of screening for "most" Americans. Furthermore, in its report, the IOM/NRC's response to this tension was to deflect responsibility for resolving it to individuals and their doctors. They implicitly dismissed the appropriateness of addressing it on a broader social scale when they wrote that "to serve the public interest, the major contribution that the government can make is not to launch an ineffective but politically appealing screening program but rather, to develop effective ways to communicate with the public" [19, p. x].

What Diseases Should Be Addressed?

The different approaches to identifying who should be the target of public health follow-up activities is also apparent in the way that each group handled the question of nonmalignant thyroid disease (e.g., hypothyroidism). In this case the IOM/NRC committee also attended to the risks of "most" Americans from I-131 exposures rather than those with the highest risk:

> The review in Chapter 3 cites considerable evidence of links at moderate and high exposures but little evidence suggesting a link between hypothyroidism or hyperthyroidism and I-131 doses in the range experienced by *most* of those exposed to fallout from the Nevada nuclear tests [19, p. 93, emphasis added].

> The data on nonmalignant disease induction rate is inconclusive in the dose range to which *most* people were exposed from fallout. As a result the IOM/NRC panel did not further consider the implications of nonmalignant disease [19, p. 71, emphasis added].

The scientific evidence available at the time suggests that such diseases may result from exposures within the range of the most highly exposed individuals

(100+ rem [20]), which, as they note in their report, might number in the tens of thousands of individuals. There was no discussion in the IOM/NRC report of special follow-up activities for people who may have received higher exposures, except insofar as notification programs might identify those who could be at higher risk.

On the other hand, the ACERER recommended a proactive approach to screening for nonmalignant thyroid disease (hypothyroidism) and that the "DHHS develop strategies to help ensure that those at highest risk for hypothyroidism have the earliest access to screening" (Recommendation #6). The ACERER and its SCA consultants were very concerned about individuals who might be at higher risk because of exposures within the range of what the scientific evidence suggests might be associated with nonmalignant thyroid disease and thyroid cancer. Hypothyroidism or hyperthyroidism are easily testable via a blood test and do not require the more complex diagnostic testing required for thyroid cancer that can lead to an unacceptably high rate of false positives.

A clue to the rationale for these divergent recommendations is found in the justice-related concerns that the ACERER raised in its recommendation on screening:

> Notwithstanding the uncertainties about individual doses, the documentation of the widespread pattern of fallout and the magnitude of thyroid doses provided by the NCI study lends considerable weight to public appeals for a public health response. In evaluating whether and how to provide such a response, government decision makers cannot avoid the historical and ethical context of these appeals. Not only are the health risks considerable, but the Government—by failing to warn and protect people from fallout exposures—bears direct responsibility for the ensuing injuries, even if it cannot be held legally accountable for them (Recommendation #6).

Assumptions about Access to Health Care

This brings us to the third point: the assumptions made about the relationships between individuals and the medical community. The assumptions that were made raise important ethical questions about the appropriateness of recommended follow-up actions. One reason that the IOM/NRC committees may have felt comfortable making the "semantic dodge" about the difference between symptomatic vs. asymptomatic individuals being tested for thyroid cancer is the emphasis they placed on what informed, concerned patients *should* do. In their opinion, first they should consult with their physicians:

> For concerned patients, read "anxious patients," who consult their physicians about screening for thyroid cancer, the decision about screening should be jointly made following a discussion of thyroid cancer risks and possible benefits and harms of screening...people need to be informed but they need to be discouraged from starting down that slippery slope [21].

ACERER members discussed the need for individuals and doctors to discuss together how to proceed when a patient was concerned about his or her risks. They also felt it would be best for individuals to consult with their health care providers about the potential benefits and harms of "starting down that slippery slope" of testing for thyroid cancer (sometimes referred to by members of the ACERER as "offer, but discourage"). So, here again, the ACERER and IOM/NRC were not far from agreement, except on some crucial normative assumptions having to do with distributional equity in health care.

Specifically, ACERER identified equity as a central ethical issue arising from the fact that many people in the United States are uninsured or underinsured. There is no guarantee that all individuals who had concerns about their risks from I-131 fallout exposures would have a doctor with whom they could consult in the way envisioned by the IOM/NRC committee [9, p. 8]. In fact, the IOM/NRC committee's opposition to thyroid cancer screening appears to be based in part on an assumption about the quality of routine care for *most* Americans: "There was no direct evidence that early detection of thyroid cancer through systematic screening rather than through *routine clinical care* improved survival or other health outcomes" [19, emphasis added]. Furthermore, as was observed by an ACERER member: the IOM/NRC report explicitly "opted out on that by saying that's not our mandate, and cost and effectiveness considerations were not our mandate, so we're not going to discuss it. But everybody is kind of walking a wide circle around this issue, which is central" [19, p. 162].

Because of the closed nature of IOM/NRC committees' deliberations, we do not know what kind of discussions they had about this issue, but we do know that it was raised on several occasions by ACERER members and SCA consultants. While the delivery of health care was also not formally within the mandate of the ACERER, its members did think it important enough to raise as an issue in Recommendation #6. Again, this was a product of their focus on the justice-related dimensions of the issues:

> Regrettably, the delays in releasing the information that the NCI did finally share with the public in the last year have only reinforced the cynicism of many citizens and exposed communities. It increases the burden that many federal agencies share in trying to overcome the suspicion that the Government is still unwilling to squarely acknowledge the harm caused by past policies and to commit resources to assist those who may have been injured as a result (Finding #4).

The IOM/NRC committees also assumed that people, "anxious people," should make decisions based on a rational consideration of the evidence provided to them by their doctors. They did acknowledge that fear might be an issue in individuals' responses, and there is evidence for such responses in some other situations [22].

In the end, however, the IOM/NRC revealed a patronizing assumption about what concerned or "anxious," members of the public *ought* to do. For example, they put much emphasis on the need to better understand peoples' risk perceptions so that people could be better managed and calmed about the possible risks of exposure to I-131 from fallout. Moreover, members of committees expressed surprise that "nonexpert" members of the public might elect to pursue medical tests viewed as inaccurate or high risk:

> We had in our workshop a presentation from an investigator at Dartmouth College who is very interested in the question of how many false positives in a screening program for mammography would women tolerate in order to have the reassurance of learning that their mammogram is either negative of that the false positive turned out to be an early cancer detected, and treated early, or a negative result. And we were staggered to see that something on the order of 40 percent of women were willing to tolerate up to several hundred false positives for every one true positive [19, pp. 20-21].

In the case of an informed population that may be fearful of involuntary exposures created by its own government, the IOM/NRC committees' message of "don't just do something, stand there" [19, p. 39] addresses the ethical principle of doing more good than harm, but it does not account for or acknowledge the desire people may have for reassurance about their health. Again, from ACERER's perspective, this was not a matter of choosing between a screening program for everyone (nationwide or regionally) or no screening program, or between cancer and noncancer disease. Rather, the recognition that people might want reassurance was part of the consideration of justice that should be addressed.

CONCLUSIONS

The public record of deliberations, reports, and meeting transcripts provides a view into the ways that two different groups of people addressed a complex public health issue. An important difference is related to the way that the ACERER emphasized social justice issues. It is not that ACERER members were smarter or had more experience with or care for community studies or that the IOM/NRC committees' members didn't care or were callous. Rather it had to do with the institutional context of the deliberations and challenges to a scientific orientation made by the public nature of the ACERER committee and its inclusion of public participants. Ultimately, the difference in the approaches and recommendations of the two groups had to do with how they each integrated scientific analysis with ethical concerns and applied ethical principles of beneficence and justice.

Scientific Objectivity and a Public Health Response

The ACERER was set up to enhance the *credibility* of a research program that had been shifted to the DHHS from the DOE. It was understood that credibility had both scientific and social dimensions *and* that these dimensions could reinforce each other. Its approach to the fallout issue is illustrative of the ways that the ACERER tackled many issues, including international studies in the former Soviet Union, the Hanford Medical Monitoring Program, Hanford Thyroid Disease Study, and proposals for "clinic-based research."

The ACERER adopted a normative framework that views science and values as intertwined. Steve Wing has referred to this as "strong objectivity [which] demands that scientists critically evaluate how the knowledge they create is shaped at every point by historical social forces" [23]. On the other hand, the IOM/NRC committees acted as if their judgments were evidence-based and scientific, divorced from the ethical and moral dimensions of the issue. Certain concerns and issues were not considered scientific. At the same time, in its consideration of the science, the IOM/NRC unavoidably came up against the need to make judgments about the meaning of uncertain, contradictory, or incomplete evidence. They were not successful in separating science from ethics. In fact, their conclusions were based on the following normative judgments:

- It is appropriate to base policy recommendations on consideration of "most" Americans, rather than those who were most susceptible to the exposures.
- The focus on possible public health responses should be on cancer and should exclude nonmalignant thyroid diseases.
- Lack of proof of harm or benefit means that there would be no harm or benefit.
- Individuals should only make decisions about possible follow-up in consultation with their doctors and should weigh risks and benefits in a "rational" way.
- The consequences of the I-131 exposures were similar in characteristics to other diseases that did not result from involuntary, government-caused (and covered-up) activities.
- Further studies and programs to test assumptions are not needed.

But as the evidence about thyroid cancer and nonmalignant thyroid disease screening suggest, other perspectives could be based on a rational and systematic interpretation of available evidence while being informed by the historical and sociopolitical context of exposures.

Balancing the Ethical Principles of Beneficence and Justice

Biomedical and public health research and practice adhere to a set of ethical principles that protect patients and research subjects [24]. Two such principles are beneficence and justice. Beneficence refers to the idea that one ought to act for the benefit of others and not in a way that causes or increases harm (this is often associated with the principle of non-maleficence.) Justice refers to the equitable distribution of burdens and benefits. Justice can also have a procedural dimension which refers to the ways that people can participate in decision making about issues that affect them [25].

The IOM/NRC committees, as discussed earlier, argued that evidence was lacking and that a thyroid cancer screening program would provide more benefits than harm. Moreover, they felt that there was a significant risk that some individuals might be harmed by such a program because it could result in unnecessary removal of thyroids in healthy people. Thus, they concluded that the appropriate response was "don't just do something, stand there" and to develop an education and outreach effort informing people that they may have been exposed and be at (a small) increased risk of thyroid cancer. Finally, they felt that the medical community was in the best position to guide patients' considerations of relative risks and benefits in noncancer disease evaluations (e.g., testing for hypothyroidism). In other words, the report of the IOM/NRC committees relies very strongly on beneficence and non-maleficence as principles to guide their recommendations. Furthermore, their report and public statements do not reflect as strong a concern for the principle of justice.

On the other hand, the ACERER developed its recommendations on the basis of beneficence and justice. The principle of justice was reflected in its strong concern for those who might be most vulnerable and their access to medical care. They tried to balance their concern for justice with the principle of beneficence, as suggested by their recommendation:

> In light of the IOM Committee's recommendations, and the substantive concerns about the negative consequences of implementing a large-scale screening program, the Committee recommends that DHHS look carefully at opportunities to implement screening efforts under circumstances that can reasonably be expected to promote more benefit than harm to those for whom the program would be available (Recommendation #6).

Moreover, deliberations within ACERER (and the SCA) meetings addressed the relative risks of thyroid cancer screening programs and the likelihood of false positives and false negatives. The ACERER did not recommend a national screening program but a narrowly targeted program for specific subpopulations defined by gender, age at time of exposure, and other limiting factors.

A difference in the ways that each group balanced the principles of beneficence and justice is also revealed in the ways that they interacted with members of the public. The IOM/NRC committees worked in an institutional context that kept public participants at a distance, although the NCI and NCEH requested that the committees operate in as open a way as possible, consistent with NAS procedures [26]. Typical of such committees well-known experts from a variety of relevant disciplines were asked to serve on the all-volunteer committees, guided by staff of the NRC and IOM. Because of the dual-committee structure in this study, some individuals served on both committees. Each committee held a series of meetings during 1997 and 1998; an intensive effort that required considerable effort on the part of committee members. Members of the public (of which I was one), the ACERER, and nongovernmental organizations (such as the Military Production Network, now the Alliance for Nuclear Accountability) asked the committees to make special efforts at openness because of the high levels of suspicion and distrust. In the end, the usual was done: some of the meetings were open public meetings, while others were for committee members and staff only. Open meetings (including a special workshop on Thyroid Cancer Screening and Health Implications of Exposure to Radioactive Iodine Fallout) were focused on "fact finding." Closed sessions were for consideration and deliberation of findings and recommendations. No members of the committees explicitly represented the concerns, knowledge, or experiences of potentially exposed populations or high-risk individuals. Rather, scientific, medical, and health policy experts talked about their beliefs about those experiences and concerns. As with all committees of the National Academy of Sciences, the conclusions and recommendations expressed in the report were approved by consensus of all members in both committees and the report went through an extensive peer-review process.

In contrast, ACERER members and, at least initially, agency staff were very concerned about including diverse perspectives and the social dimensions of public health research. For example, leading researchers in public health and advocates for community involvement in research were members of the ACERER. The ACERER used public involvement criteria to evaluate the health research agenda. In addition, the ACERER provided opportunities for community members and workers to participate directly in the ACERER's deliberations.

Involvement of "nonexperts"—those without traditional training and credentials of scientific expertise—provided important contributions to ACERER deliberations. First, they provided important information; this is widely recognized as a benefit of public participation in risk assessment and decision making [27]. The IOM/NRC committees made assumptions about what people would want and how they would act when provided with thyroid dose and risk information. The ACERER wanted to hear from people directly.

Second, participants such as SCA consultants helped to frame issues in terms of, for example, justice and prevention and invigorate ACERER attention to such issues. The ACERER's commitment to broader issues, such as social justice, was co-created by participation of consultants:

> It's not just doing the work well that's important. It's the kind of work that you do, right, that's important. And a lot of times good scientific work is done, it's just not addressing questions that are of interest in communities. And so I think one way around the credibility problem and around getting the answers that people like or don't like is to do good work on things that people want to know the answers to, not good work on things that Mallinckrodt wants to know the answer to, or Monsanto wants to know the answers to, or Battelle, or whatever. And I think the community advisory process is an important step in that direction. And we've had one incidence of it already at this meeting, which is [name of community consultant] pushing to have non-malignant thyroid disease, and [name of ACERER member] too, put on the research agenda. That's not something that came from IOM or NRC. It came—basically it's a community view. And it's an example of how the community can advance important research questions that can be attacked in a rigorous, coherent way that can enhance credibility [19, pp. 262-265].

Conflicts about what is the "right" process design can be hotly disputed. How they are resolved is important, especially in situations where there are no clear "right" answers that emerge from the scientific evidence. When outcomes must be based on subjective judgment (and values), procedural rules can be used to justify and legitimate decisions. Different beliefs are often grounded in different understandings of objectivity in scientific inquiry [28]. A preference for a process that limits public involvement to providing input that can be used to inform the deliberations of "experts" is grounded in the view that scientific analysis is a rational, objective enterprise that must be insulated from consideration of values, subjectivity, and social influence—what Wing has referred to as "naïve objectivity" [23]. On the other hand, a preference for a process that encourages the participation of a broad range of interested and affected parties in framing questions and lines of inquiry and deliberating about interpretations and recommendations reflects a different normative framework—what Wing has called "strong objectivity."

The clash of normative assumptions about the ability to separate science from values and ethics has been experienced in many settings. Many of these have involved risk management and policymaking about the health consequences of the U.S. nuclear weapons complex [18, pp. 50-57]. Increasingly, experience shows that in spite of their best efforts, those who attempt to construct a wall with science and rational decision making on the one side and values and ethics on the other often fail to adequately acknowledge how their own values inform their conclusions. Their decisions and recommendations may not reflect those whom they intend to help and may not garner the legitimacy needed for implementation.

Recent work by scholars of risk and environmental assessment and decision making suggests that it is better to integrate science and values—or analysis and deliberation—because assumptions are revealed and ethical and moral considerations are brought to the foreground [27]. This is where they ought to be when science cannot provide the "right" answer and judgments when important public health, social, political, and economic implications must be made.

NOTES

1. National Cancer Institute. 1997. *Estimated exposures and thyroid doses received by the American people from 131I in fallout following Nevada atmospheric nuclear bomb tests*, U.S. Department of Health and Human Services, National Institutes of Health, National Cancer Institute, NIH Publication No. 97-4264.
2. CDC. 2005. *Report on the feasibility of a study of the health consequences to the American population from nuclear weapons tests conducted by the United States and other nations*. Atlanta, GA: Radiation Studies Branch, National Center for Environmental Health, CDC, DHHS. Report available at www.cdc.gov/nceh/radiation/fallout/default.htm
3. Frohmberg, E., Goble, R., Sanchez, V., and Quigley, D. 2000. The assessment of radiation exposures in Native American communities from nuclear weapons testing in Nevada. *Risk Analysis* 20(1):101-111.
4. National Research Council. 1983. *Risk assessment in the federal government: Managing the process*. Washington, DC: National Academy Press.
5. See National Research Council. 1996. *Understanding risk: Informing decisions in a democratic society*. Washington, DC: National Academy Press; Shrader-Frechette, K. 1985. *Risk analysis and the scientific method*. Boston, MA: D. Reidel Publishing Company; Shrader-Frechette, K. 1991. *Risk and rationality*. Berkeley, CA: University of California Press; Functowitz, S., and Ravetz, J. 1992. Three types of risk assessment and the emergence of post-normal science. In *Social theories of risk*, eds. S. Krimsky and D. Golding, 251-274. Westport, CT: Praeger; and Wing, S. 2003. Objectivity and ethics in environmental health science. *Environmental Health Perspectives* 111(14):1809-1818.
6. See National Research Council. 1996. *Understanding risk: Informing decisions in a democratic society*. Washington, DC: National Academy Press; Renn, O., Webler, T., and Weidemann, P. 1995. *Fairness and competence in citizen participation*. Dordrecht, Netherlands: Kluwer Academic Publishers; Renn, O. 2008. *Risk governance: Coping with uncertainty in a complex world*. London: Earthscan; and Tuler, S., and Webler, T. 1999. Designing an analytic deliberative process for environmental health policy making in the U.S. nuclear weapons complex. *RISK: Health, Safety, and Environment* 10(1):65-87.
7. The way that the study was conducted and the release of the report also caused quite a stir. A hearing before the Senate Permanent Subcommittee on Investigations of the Committee on Governmental Affairs was held during September 1998 (Committee on Governmental Affairs 1998). Serious criticisms were leveled against the management and conduct of the study.

8. Rad (radiation absorbed dose) is a unit used to measure the amount of energy actually absorbed in some material, and is used for any type of radiation and material. The unit rad does not describe the biological effects of the different radiations.
9. National Research Council. 1999. *Exposure of the American people to iodine-131 from Nevada nuclear-bomb tests*. Washington, DC: National Academy Press.
10. By "screening" the IOM/NRC, quoting Eddy (1991), meant "the application of a test to detect a potential disease or condition in a person who has no known signs or symptoms of that condition at the time the test is done." This is a widely accepted definition and concerns the testing of *asymptomatic* people.
11. ACERER was established in 1992 after then-DOE Secretary Watkins appointed a panel to examine public and worker health studies conducted by DOE and its contractors at sites within the nuclear weapons complex. There was considerable criticism about the way that DOE conducted and interpreted epidemiologic studies of these groups, including the use of designs that produced inconclusive results and the treatment of scientists that spoke out about positive finding (e.g., Physicians for Social Responsibility. 1992. *Dead reckoning: A critical review of the Department of Energy's epidemiologic research*. Washington, DC: Physicians for Social Responsibility). The result of the review was to remove the conduct of the studies from DOE's responsibility because of conflicts of interest arising from DOE being the source of the problem and the evaluator of the problem. A Memorandum of Understanding (MOU) was approved in 1991 that gave responsibility for conducting the studies to the Department of Health and Human Services (i.e., CDC and NIOSH). Because of this context ACERER established scientific and public involvement criteria for making recommendations about a health research agenda and evaluating research conducted under the Memorandum Of Understanding (MOU) between DHHS and DOE. "Scientific criteria" were used to assess whether (1) a proposed study could reduce critical uncertainties of exposure, dose, or risk estimates, (2) the study had a high probability of success, and (3) clear risk-based criteria were applied to prioritize the need for the study. "Public involvement criteria" were used to assess whether (1) a proposed project would address worker and public concerns about potential exposures and/or health effects, (2) the project would involve public input, and (3) the project was supported by the public.
12. ACERER. 1998. Resolution of the Department of Health and Human Services' Advisory Committee for Energy-Related Epidemiologic Research (ACERER) with regard to exposures of the American People to fallout from the Nevada Test Site. Unanimously adopted at ACERER meeting, 24 September 1998.
13. The evidence for my observations about the IOM/NRC come from four sources. First, the texts of the 1999 IOM/NRC report and the 1998 ACERER recommendations themselves; what they say and how they say it. Second, the verbatim transcripts of two ACERER meetings, one of which included the presentation of the IOM/NRC chairs to the ACERER committee (meetings on 24 September, 1998 and 19 November 1998). Third, my notes of these meetings, as I was present as a consultant to the Subcommittee on Community Affairs. Fourth, emails circulated among ACERER members and SCA consultants about the IOM/NRC report and observations about the chairs' presentation to the ACERER.

14. Committee on Governmental Affairs. 1998. National Cancer Institute's management of radiation studies. Hearing before the Permanent Subcommittee on Investigations of the Committee on Governmental Affairs, 16 September 1998 (S. Hrg. 105-686). Washington, DC: U.S. Government Printing Office.
15. "Backyard cow" is used as shorthand to describe those who got their milk fresh from their own cows and goats or nearby farmers without the delays associated with commercially processed milk; National Research Council. 1999. *Exposure of the American people to iodine-131 from Nevada nuclear-bomb tests*. Washington, DC: National Academy Press.
16. In fact, the ATSDR reached the conclusion that screening could be beneficial for thyroid cancers in populations exposed to I-131 (ATSDR, 1997. *Hanford Medical Monitoring Program: Background consideration document and ATSDR decision.* Atlanta, GA: U.S. Department of Health and Human Services, Public Health Service, ATSDR). The ACERER noted with concern "that the interpretation of case studies and the reasoning offered by the IOM panel on the thyroid cancer screening issue is squarely at odds with that applied by the Agency for Toxic Substances and Disease Registry (ATSDR) in its July 1997 proposal for carrying out the Hanford Medical Monitoring Program (HMMP). The committee has not yet been able to fully evaluate the differences in the circumstances and reasoning as applied by the ATSDR at Hanford and by the IOM Committee to the Nevada Test Site exposures. We believe these differences warrant careful evaluation before final decisions are made about what medical screening responses are appropriate to address radioiodine exposures attributable to NTS fallout" (Recommendation #6).
17. Quotation from Recommendation #6 of the ACERER recommendations regarding fallout.
18. Connor, T. 1997. Burdens of proof. GA: Energy Research Foundation and Moore, L. 2005. Rocky Flats: The bait-and-switch clean up. *Bulletin of the Atomic Scientist* 6(1):58, 61.
19. ACERER. 1998. Verbatim transcript of the Advisory Committee for Energy-Related Epidemiologic Research (ACERER) meeting held in Washington, DC, 24 September 1998.
20. Rem (Roentgen Equivalent in Man) is the unit measuring the effective biological damage of an absorbed dose of radiation. To determine equivalent dose (rem) multiply the absorbed dose (measured in rads) by a quality factor that is unique to the type of radiation. For gamma and beta radiation one rem equals one rad. For alpha radiation one rad equals 20 rems.
21. In this context by "screening" the speaker was talking about a series of tests, not a screening *program*.
22. Decruyvenaere, M. et al. 1993. Perception of predictive testing for Huntington's disease by young women: Preferring uncertainty to certainty. *Journal of Medical Genetics* 30:557-561.
23. Wing, S. 2003. Objectivity and ethics in environmental health science. *Environmental Health Perspectives* 111(14):1809-1818.
24. Beauchamp, T. L., and Childress, J. F. 1994. *Principles of biomedical ethics.* Oxford, NY: Oxford University Press.

25. Abelson, J., Forest, P-G., Eyles, J., Smith, P., Martin, E., and Gauvin, F-P. 2003. Deliberations about deliberative methods: Issues in the design and evaluation of public participation processes. *Social Science and Medicine* 57:239-251; Chess, C. 2000. Improving public participation in solving environmental health problems. *Journal of Environmental Health* 63(1):24-27; Ledwidge, L., Moore, L., and Crawford, L. 2004. Stakeholder perspectives on radiation protection. *Health Physics* 87(3):293-299; Gillam, M. L., Fischbach, S., and Scott, R. 2005. Poisoned by poverty: A call to improve health outcomes for low-income and minority children. *Clearinghouse Review Journal of Poverty Law and Policy* May-June:4-12.
26. In fact, in one of its open sessions the committee discussed with NAS staff the Academy's position and its legal obligations with respect to the issue of the openness of the committee's deliberations.
27. NAS. 2008. *Public participation in environmental assessment and decision-making*. Washington, DC: National Academy Press.
28. Tuler, S., Webler, T., and Finson, R. 2005. Competing perspectives on public involvement: Planning for risk characterization and risk communication about radiological contamination from a national laboratory. *Health, Risk, and Society,* 7(3):247-266.

http://dx.doi.org/10.2190/TORC7

CHAPTER 7

Ethics of Uranium Mining Research and the Navajo People*†

Bindu Panikkar, Esther Yassie, and Doug Brugge

Uranium gained prominence in use in the 1940s with the growing sophistication of atomic research and the proliferating atomic nuclear interest at that time specifically to cater to the urgent need of developing atomic weaponry for national security reasons. In the United States, the Navajo lands became one of the prime targets for mining, contributing thirteen million tons of uranium ore from 1945 to 1988. Mining throughout the United States employed over 10,000 miners, of which approximately 3000 were Navajos [1-4].

Now there are at least one thousand abandoned and partially unreclaimed uranium mines within the Navajo Nation. During much of the peak years of mining from 1948 to 1969, no federal occupational standards kept miners safe from the harms of radiation and such intense mining. Apart from unrecorded accidents, health impairments and ailments, an estimated 500-600 out of thousands of uranium miners died of lung cancer over a period of 40 years;

*This report was funded by a grant from the National Institute of Health, National Heart, Lung and Blood Institute Grant Program for "Short Courses in Research Ethics" (T15HL069792). This collection of narratives does not necessarily reflect the views of the sponsors of this report: National institute of Health, Syracuse University, its affiliated departments, University of North Carolina, Chapel Hill, North Carolina or the collaborators of the Collaborative Initiative for Research Ethics and Environmental Health.

†Parts reprinted from Panikkar, B., and Brugge, D. 2007. The Ethical Issues in titanium mining research in the Navajo nation. *Accountability in Research* 14:121-153. Used with permission from Taylor & Francis, http://www.informaworld.com

a similar number is expected to die after 1990 [2-4]. Still the extent of health threats to the community, those exposed to the unreclaimed sites and drinking contaminated uranium water is unknown. Since mining ended the Navajo community is still struggling daily with high radiation and uranium exposures and many unknown environmental threats.

This chapter conducts a historical analysis of environmental and public health (epidemiological) research conducted in the Navajo Nation and questions the ethical breaches and harms in research conducted in the Navajo community.

THE NAVAJO URANIUM MINING HISTORY

The Navajo Nation stretches sixteen million acres across Arizona, Utah, and New Mexico. There are more than 250,000 enrolled members of the tribe, over 160,000 of whom reside on tribal land. This four-corners region is also where the largest quantities of uranium are found. Uranium mining in the Navajo region started in 1948, when the U.S. Atomic Energy Commission introduced a massive procurement program and announced that it would purchase all the uranium that was mined in the United States. Radium and vanadium were already mined at that time in the high plateaus of the Navajo lands. Expanding the operations to mining uranium was relatively simple, with its abundance discovered primarily in four regions of the reservation in Shiprock, New Mexico; Monument Valley, Utah; Churchrock, New Mexico and Kayenta, Arizona. Mining boomed in 1955-56 and became a flourishing occupation for many Navajo men, partially transforming the reservation from traditional grazing communities to a modern industrial wage economy [5] (see Appendix A and B).

The Navajo people, largely removed from the economic and social systems of the mainstream U.S. culture and possessing a different environmental and political consciousness, were unaware of the health effects associated with mining and had no understanding of the ionizing radiation properties of the ores being mined. While federal worker health requirements were established for companies that handled beryllium in the 1940s, such requirements were not established for uranium and few precautionary measures were undertaken in these mines [5, 6].

U.S. Public Health Service (PHS) research on occupational health effects of uranium mining started two years after the mining started, but ventilation requirements in mines were enforced only by the early 1960s. The first federally enforceable standard (0.3 working levels for radon and its daughters) in mines that supplied the federal government with uranium was announced only in 1967 by Secretary of Labor Willard Wirtz [5, 6]. By then, the federal contracts for uranium mining nearly ended in the Navajo Nation but private companies continued mining until 1988.

Community organizing around uranium mining started in the early 1960s. Harry Tome of Red Valley, a member of the Navajo Tribal Council, was one of their early advocates for a compensation system similar to the black lung benefits to disabled Appalachian coal miners in 1968 [5]. The efforts of Tome led to the first legislative bill filed in 1973 with the U.S. Congress to extend the black lung benefits to uranium miners [7], but the bill never passed.

It took two decades of organizing after the first legislative remedy was filed for the Radiation Exposure Compensation Act (RECA) to be passed in 1990. The RECA acknowledged that the U.S. Government historically mistreated the uranium miners and made provision for compassionate payment of up to $100,000 to underground uranium miners. It took another 10 years for the original law to be amended by the U.S. Congress to address the shortcomings in the original law [2].

METHODOLOGY FOR THIS CHAPTER

Community activism and scientific research collectively played roles in the passing of the 1990 RECA. Scientific research was the basis for determining safer mining conditions, legalizing appropriate levels of exposure and providing evidence to fight legally for better policies and regulations. Though the rigors of scientific investigations eventually helped uranium miners, it did come with a cost—the cost of ignoring warnings, the cost of delaying occupational safety measures until causality was determined, and the resultant harm to people, cultures, communities, and the environment.

In this research, we attempt a historical analysis of public health (epidemiological) research conducted in the Navajo lands since the inception of uranium mining. We track about 50 years of research from the 1950s until the end of the century. The analysis will be divided into (1) the "early" public health studies or series of studies that led to controlling radon exposures in mines in the 1960s, (2) the studies conducted between the 1970s and 1990, before the passing of the 1990 RECA, and (3) the studies conducted since 1990. This being the core of our analysis, we will conclude our study discussing the ethical breaches in research.

RESEARCH IN THE URANIUM MINING COMMUNITIES FROM THE 1940s TO THE 1960s

When the U.S. Government decided to start mining in 1948 it was developing a nuclear arsenal and was considering extending the technology to develop nuclear power. Though the Atomic Energy Act of 1946 did not allow for private commercial application of atomic energy, it did acknowledge in passing the potential "peaceful benefits" of atomic power. Entering "the nuclear power race" was considered by many government officials vital to maintaining dominance in the world scientific community and in maintaining international prestige [8].

By 1954, a broad political consensus was achieved and new legislation was passed permitting commercial use of atomic energy for power generation. At the same time, the act also instructed preparation of regulations that would protect public health and safety from commercial radiation hazards [6, 9].

The health effects of radiation, and uranium mining in particular, were known at the time the mining started from earlier studies conducted in Europe. In response to a lung disease called "Bergkrankheitr," long reported in detail in studies done in miners in Schneeberg and Joachimsthal in 1879, a ventilation project had been established in 1930 even if the causal agent was unknown [5, 10-13]. In 1942, Wilhelm Heuper, the founding director of the environmental cancer section of the National Cancer Institute (NCI), one of the National Institutes of Health, showed an excess occupational hazard of lung cancer in miners from exposure to radon gas [14]. Despite this scientific awareness, there was little thought given to public health and the safety measures in the work places when uranium mining started about a decade later.

The first wave of research studies on uranium mining in the United States started two years after mining began in 1948 with a study led by the U.S. Public Health Service (PHS) in conjunction with other state and federal agencies. The PHS study of Colorado plateau miners was started on the assumption that uranium mining would cause lung cancer [15, 16].

The PHS study involved an environmental study and an epidemiological study. Air samples and occupational histories were gathered to calculate exposure expressed in "working level months" (WLM).[1] Under the auspices of Colorado, Utah, New Mexico, and Arizona Health Departments, Duncan Holaday was recruited to direct the environmental study measuring radon levels in the mines. In a memo presented to the PHS Salt Lake City office in 1950, Holaday reported the levels of radon in the Navajo region to exceed expectations and concluded the results presented a rather serious picture and recommended that a control program be instituted as soon as possible [6]. In 1951, two researchers, William Bale [17] and John Harley (who was finishing his doctoral work) [18], showed that radon daughter isotopes attaching to dust can remain in the lungs and contribute to lung cancer. Following an internal meeting in 1951, both the PHS and Atomic Energy Commission (AEC) acknowledged that the levels of radon in these uranium mines were high enough to cause cancer and that ventilation was the way to abate the hazard [6].

However, this information was not shared with those at risk nor was there willingness on the part of the AEC to introduce relatively safe tolerance levels for radon in the mines. In 1952, a PHS interim report distributed on a restricted basis showed no evidence of health damage from radioactivity. Other health

[1] One WLM is equal to spending 170 hrs, or a month exposed to one WL, a concentration of radon decay products that will release 1.3 million electron volts per liter of air.

officials, such as Dr. Heuper, were asked to limit their speech on risks involved. Victor Archer, head of the PHS medical team, justified, "We did not want to rock the boat. . . . We had to take the position that we were neutral scientists trying to find out what the facts were, that we were not going to make any public announcements until the results of the study were published" [19, p. 46].

The PHS investigators did not warn the miners they recruited of the health risks of uranium mining, which was justified to be "out of fear that many miners would quit" [6]. This was not necessarily counter to the ethical standards of the time, as the Nuremberg standards required informed consent in *experimental* studies, while the uranium miner study was *observational.* A similar decision might well be made by researchers today based on the principle that subjects should be informed about risks due to participation in research with an *intervention* or with research tests, such as a blood draw, but not necessarily about risks they encounter in the course of work activities of daily living.

The environmental study ended in 1956 [6]. In 1957, a research report by Holaday and colleagues [20] on controlling radon in mines proposed a threshold exposure value of 1 WL [20]. By 1960, the states slowly started responding to the issue and adopted a guideline for radon exposure value of one working level (WL)[2]. And federal standards of 0.3 WL for radon and its daughters were set by 1969 [5, 6].

The epidemiological study was a prospective study and the miners were enrolled if they volunteered for at least one physical examination and provided social and occupational data in sufficient detail to allow follow-up. Not many miners were examined in 1950, 1951, and 1953. From 1954 onward, the study picked up and became a systematic epidemiological study and as many men that could be located and would cooperate were examined [9, 15]. This renewed interest and enthusiasm in the study may not be entirely coincidental, considering that the second Atomic Energy Act was also passed in the same year (1954), with its expressed commitment to the protection of health.

It is estimated that between 1957 and 1960, close to 90 percent of the men working in the industry were examined for their occupational history and level of exposure [9, 15]. Estimates of exposure were used when direct measurements were not possible. The total study group consisted of over 5,000 underground miners, uranium mill workers and other above-ground workers, including both white and non-white men. Despite the fact that the Navajo people represented about 30 percent of the uranium miners in the Colorado plateau, white miners (40 percent) were chosen for the primary research outcomes [9].

The analysis reported to the Federal Radiation Council (FRC) focused on a subgroup of 1,981 white male underground workers who started mining before

[2] Working level (WL) is the measure of the energy released by radon daughters. It is a physical measure that is closely related to the mechanism for biological damage.

1955. The analysis showed a clear association between exposure to radon daughters in mine air and a higher than expected likelihood of lung cancer deaths when the cumulative exposures were more than 1000 WLM [9, 15]. Subsequently, Wagoner reported a 10-fold excess in lung cancer in underground miners exposed over a longer period controlling for age, smoking, nativity, hereditary, urbanization, self-selection, diagnostic accuracy, prior mining exposure, or exposure to silica [21]. A mortality study that followed miners from the same data pool looked at 3,414 white underground miners in the region between 1950 and 1963. It substantiated these results with higher observed rates of deaths from violent deaths and malignant neoplasms of the respiratory system than expected. Cancer deaths markedly progressed with increasing exposure beginning in the range of 840-1,799 WLM. Smoking miners experienced cancer deaths 10 times greater than nonsmoking miners [22]. While these studies showed associations between uranium mining and lung cancer, lung cancer associations with smoking miners clouded the analysis leading to suggestions such as "uranium miners should not smoke" [22].

An important feature of these studies was the estimation of the relationship between dose and disease outcomes. This methodology, highly sophisticated for the time, was used to define the dose-response relationship. Stellaman [13] considered the occupational health study on uranium workers in his article on the history of epidemiology as on par with the other occupational health studies on chemical dye workers, bituminous coal workers, and smelting workers. He stated that these studies have been important sources of innovation in methodology and in development of logical reasoning leading to acceptance of causal relationships of occupational exposures that lead to respiratory diseases and cancer.

The fact that the research focused on establishing the dose-response curve rather than establishing a causal association per se, shows that this was a search for an acceptable risk, a scientifically sought acceptable level of exposure that could be applied to uranium mining. Possible preventive measures under these circumstances focused on estimating a certain safe level of risk, as stopping mining was not an option considered by the government until safer standards and ways of mining were developed. In this particular case however, the lowest level of risk was determined at the expense of many uranium miners, who became sick in the process and were not warned of the health risks, and at the time no system was set in place to see that those harmed were provided the needed care and assistance.

The issue of compensation for uranium miners reached the courts only in the late 1970s, but the courts did not see ethical violations. In the Begay decision the court found: "the epidemiological study and the conduct of the researchers were consistent with the medical, ethical and legal standards of the 1940s and 1950s" [23]. The researchers "were not experimenting on human beings. They were gathering data to be used for the establishment of enforceable maximum standards of radiation. . . . Thus, the court concluded, it was neither necessary nor proper for those physicians to advise the miners voluntarily appearing for examinations of potential hazards in uranium mines. . . . The government did not seek volunteers to work in the mines so that they could become part of the study group . . ." [6, Ch. 12, p. 11].

One argument could be that enforcing environmental and occupational regulations was not customary at the time. It could be that the PHS that undertook the study was not primarily an enforcing environmental agency, but a public health agency lost in the public health paradigm that intervened only when invited by the state officials and did little to push strong enforcement [24, 25]. Many efforts were initiated at the time to address the issue of setting standards. With respect to mining, a Federal Mining Bureau was set as early as 1865, but it did little to protect miner safety, nor did they inspect mines. A broader regulatory program to reduce injuries, fatalities and illness in mining was set only in 1978 under the federal Mine Safety and Health Administration [26].

With respect to setting precautions, voices for precautionary approaches were not uncommon at the time. A. W. Donaldson, in his 1969 article *The epidemiology of lung cancer among uranium miners* ends with a testimony by Dr. Abel Wolman, the major architect of Baltimore's water system, before a congressional committee in 1960 which is still timely:

> The development of criteria for the protection of health has invariably preceded full scientific understanding and acceptance. . . . The responsible health officer cannot wait upon perfect knowledge before interposing barriers between man and industrial poisons. He moves with the best at hand, always paying a price for over-estimating or underestimating hazard. . . . Criteria must rest upon public health protection and not cost . . . and by objectives of reducing diseases and fatality to a vanishing degree and not to a preconceived notion as to how many people we have a right to kill [12, pp. 568-569].

RESEARCH IN THE NAVAJO URANIUM MINING COMMUNITY 1980-1990

The early 1980s saw the second wave of research activities about the health effects of uranium mining. While the struggle for setting worker safety conditions and standards in the mines for uranium workers was slow, but ultimately victorious, the workers still did not have a compensation system. In the 1960s a compensation system for disabled workers was established for coal miners following a pitched struggle, but black lung benefits did not extend to uranium miners [7]. Scientifically, it was established by then that uranium mining caused lung cancer. But questions remained about the possibility that smoking could be a modifier of risk. One of the research initiatives in the 1980s was establishing that uranium mining caused lung cancer in non-smokers. Research on Navajo miners was prompted by the need to distinguish the effects of smoking and radon on induction of lung cancer. Navajo people with their low smoking rate and low lung cancer rates, fit the perfect picture for research to clarify the relationship of cigarettes and radon dangers.

The epidemiological studies from 1980 to 1990 focused on: (1) establishing that uranium mining caused lung cancer regardless of smoking status; (2) other ethnic groups with lower smoking rates, such as the Navajo uranium miners [27-31]; (3) causes of mortality among uranium miners in addition to lung cancer [22, 32, 33]; (4) meta-analyses of lung cancer among uranium miners across studies [34, 35]. This section will focus only on studies conducted in the Navajo Nation on Navajo men and will exempt the Colorado Cohort mortality study of white miners by Roscoe [32] which reported similar to those in the mortality study on Navajo men also conducted by Roscoe in 1995 [31].

Most of these studies were secondary analyses of data obtained from disease registries [27, 29, 31, 32]. Cancer registries have a short history. Development of hospital-based cancer registries initiated by the American College of Surgeons (ACoS) is as recent as 1956. Early hospital registries were, for the most part, inaccessible and used card files for data. More valuable information came with the development of large central registry systems such as the National Cancer Institute's Surveillance, Epidemiology, and End Results (SEER) Program in 1973 [36]. Also the advent of microcomputer registry systems in the 1980s opened a new window of opportunity to conduct research.

Some of the major studies in the Colorado Plateau benefited from the existence of these registries. Gilliland and Samet used the New Mexico Tumor registry, a member of SEER, to collect data and also drew from death certificates, abstracts of medical records, National Institute for Occupational Safety and Health (NIOSH) records and several uranium mining databases. Roscoe's mortality study used the PHS medical surveys conducted between 1950 and the 1960s, and the records of the Social Security Administration, Internal Revenue Service, National Death Index, and Health Care Financing Administration [31, 32].

These studies looked into periods between 1960 and 1993 and were published after 1982.[3] Most of the mines had been closed by then. Community-level organizing gained strength during this time. Phil Harrison a long-time advocate and educator on radiation and health (since 1975), was elected as the president of Uranium Radiation Victims Committee in 1982 and the Red Mesa/Mexican Water Four Corners Committee was established in 1985. Community organizing also had a part in assigning a pulmonary specialist, Leon S. Gottlieb at Indian Health Service (IHS), for the first time. He was the first physician to associate and document lung cancer and uranium mining among the Navajo people [37].

[3] Roscoe [31, 32] and Gilliland [29] are put under this section between 1980-1990 because they observe data between 1960 and 1963. Also because these studies are largely follow-up studies to their earlier counterparts to record the lung cancer incidence rates.

Gotlieb and Husen used health center records in the four corners area of New Mexico, Arizona, Utah, and Colorado to identify Navajo men who were admitted to the hospital between 1965 and 1979. They found that of a total of seventeen patients with lung cancer, sixteen had been uranium miners. The lowest WLM for disease induction was 58.8 WLM, and the lowest latency period for disease induction was five years while the longest was thirty years. Of sixteen cases, five developed lung cancer under the dose of 1,000 WLM, which was considered the threshold level at the time for disease induction.

Following Gottlieb's findings was Samet's case control study with a similar hypothesis but a larger population of lung cancer cases from the years 1969 to 1982. Of thirty-two cases and sixty-four controls, the relative risk for lung cancer was estimated to be fourteen times that of controls. Samet attributed the occupation of Navajo uranium miners as their primary risk factor for lung cancer [27]. A follow-up study, conducted by Gilliland, of lung cancer incidence in Navajo uranium miners over a period of twenty-four years from 1969 to 1993 concluded that 67 percent of lung cancer occurred in former uranium miners, suggesting that a majority of the lung cancers in the Navajo population were solely due to their occupation [29].

Biological Effects of Ionizing Radiation (BEIR) reports produced by the National Academy of Sciences had been summarizing scientific evidence of radiation risks with a particular focus on dose-response relationships. The history of the BEIR reports and their links with the AEC and DOE has long been seen by some as troubling. The BIER III report was particularly controversial for substantially lowering the estimated risk of low dose radiation [38]. However, the BEIR 1V [34] and later BEIR VI [35] were largely impartial meta-analyses of four and then eleven studies of uranium miners that assessed the dose-response relationship for radon exposure and lung cancer.

The BEIR studies arrived at several important conclusions, namely (1) there were substantial uncertainties in the actual doses received by miners in different mines; (2) the risk rises linearly with level of exposure; (3) the risk per WLM varies strongly by age, latency, mining cohort, and especially by dose rate or duration; (4) on average, more than half of the lung cancers among white miners and the Navajos in the Colorado plateau were caused by radon exposures; and (5) smoking and radon interacted in a greater than additive, but less than multiplicative manner.

Apart from lung cancer incidence studies in Navajo men, mortality studies in Navajo men were also conducted. Roscoe's mortality study in Navajo men from 1960 to 1990 found elevated risks for lung cancer, tuberculosis, pneumoconiosis, and other respiratory diseases and lowered ratios for heart disease, circulatory disease, and liver cirrhosis. In conclusion, Roscoe stated that light-smoking Navajo miners faced excess mortality risks from lung cancer and pneumoconiosis and other respiratory diseases [31].

These studies effectively proved that elevated radon exposures in uranium mines could cause high rates of lung cancer in non-smoking uranium miners. They also largely adhered to scenarios of occupational exposure and seldom addressed environmental exposures from open unremediated mines on community health. Also, the Navajo studies, like other uranium miner studies before them, relied on historical NIOSH and CDC records of radon levels in the mines to estimate WLMs for each miner.

While the early uranium studies have widely been judged to be unethical, the later studies met basic individual rights of study subjects and have not been, to our knowledge, subject to criticism. The ethical concerns with regard to individual rights for these studies were met through IRB regulation of the studies.

While the discipline of epidemiology depends heavily on data, some of it can now be obtained from the disease registries. With access to disease registries, there is little need for gathering input from the community. Perhaps ethical accountability to groups—families, communities—was an emerging concern. However community interest and engagement were seen through improved outreach and education to uranium miners in the 1970s and 1980s, which also led to the appointment of Gottlieb, a pulmonologist at the IHS.

DEVELOPMENTS IN URANIUM MINING IN THE NAVAJO AREA SINCE 1990

The 1990s were times of environmental justice movements and with them came the focus on affected communities and a realization of the existing/growing environmental calamities as the result of industrial pollution in one's neighborhood, and disparities in socio-demographic characteristics in such neighborhoods. With them also came federal dollars to affected communities and participatory research in order to solve local environmental health problems. The paradigm of community-based participatory research (CBPR) is not new but has had a long and successful history in the social sciences and international and rural development [39]. Moving beyond categorical approaches and emphasis on individual-level risk factors, CBPR has a positive model of health which recognizes the individual as "embedded within social, political, and economic systems that shape behaviors and access to resources necessary to maintain health" [40, p. 16].

The studies conducted from the 1990s onward deserve a special mention. Quite contrary to the studies initiated on uranium mining and lung cancer, these studies explored different diseases and facets of uranium mining and its exposures. Many studies from the 1990s onward looked into (1) disease etiology besides lung cancer, such as birth outcomes and renal disease; (2) outcomes on affected families as opposed to just miners; (3) environmental exposures as opposed to occupational exposures; and (4) research that was conducted based on community input and participation, rather than from disease registries.

Public health/environmental health research experimented with new styles of investigations including qualitative investigations, oral histories [41], in-depth case studies of lung cancer in a single miner [30], survey-based community outreach, education projects [42], and epidemiological studies of birth outcomes and chronic kidney disease [43, 44].

Dr. Lora M. Shields, a visiting professor at the Shiprock campus of Navajo Community College, initiated a twelve-year March of Dimes Birth Defect study looking into the birth outcomes from environmental radiation in Navajo babies born at the Public Health Service/Indian Health Service Hospital in the Shiprock, New Mexico, uranium mining area (1964-1981). A weak association between proximity to mining areas and birth defects was found [43].

Quite a variant from an epidemiological analysis is a single case study with the son of a 72-year-old Navajo male, nonsmoker, and teetotaler, who had worked for 17 years as an underground miner and developed lung cancer twenty-two years after leaving the industry [30]. Apart from epidemiological studies, a series of qualitative studies were conducted. Brugge and colleagues compiled a collection of oral histories of Navajo uranium miners containing twenty-five interviews with former uranium miners or family members of the Navajo Tribe, five video recordings, and a photographic collection of sceneries from the mines and the area where the miners lived, recording the health issues among Navajo uranium miners from prolonged exposure to radioactive uranium [41]. Markstrom and Charley studied the psychological impacts of Navajo uranium miners and observed psychological impacts from human losses and bereavement, environmental losses and contamination, feelings of betrayal by the government and the companies, fears about current and future effects and in offspring, and anxiety and depression [3]. Other studies have focused on advocacy and social work in health settings [37]. These reports contain a wealth of information about the suffering of the Navajo miners and their families.

Also shaping the new research in the Navajo Nation in the 1990s and protecting the interests of the Navajo people and their community was the establishment of the Navajo Nation Health Research Review Board in 1996. Though the Navajo Nation IRB is not substantially different from the Navajo Area IHS, IRB and following the traditional western framework, it does require pre-publication review of research and does not allow for exemptions, requiring full review of all proposed studies. It also reviews secondary scholarship that reports on the Navajo people and does not engage human participants directly. In 1999, the Navajo Nation also adopted a Navajo Nation Privacy and Access to Information Act to preserve the privacy interests of individuals and entities. The Navajo government views their regulation as a means to prevent harmful research that might stigmatize the Navajo people. The main requirement for community input is approval by affected local governmental units within the Navajo Nation called chapters [45].

ONGOING PROJECTS

A set of new studies have been initiated in the community and by the community to examine health threats apart from respiratory diseases. Setting good examples of community-based participatory research, three new community projects have been initiated in the Eastern Navajo Nation—the Church Rock Uranium Monitoring Project (CRUMP), Diné Network for Environmental Health (DiNEH), and Navajo Uranium Assessment and Kidney Health Project (NUAKHP) [42, 44].

The focus of these studies is environmental monitoring of the extent of environmental contamination, the levels of exposures in these communities and the prevalence of renal disease from contamination. By the late 1950s views had evolved that uranium may damage the kidney but it had not been the focus or research in the Navajo Nation [46, 47]. Though much research on Navajo lands until the 1990s focused on respiratory diseases, a series of studies on uranium ingestion through drinking water and changes in renal biomarkers were studied in Canada between 1982 and 1999 [48].

The CRUMP, primarily an environmental monitoring project, was initiated to address the possible impacts from abandoned mines in the Navajo community. Since 2003 the project has been monitoring environmental contaminants in water, land, and air in residential areas located near abandoned uranium operations in the community located northeast of Gallup, New Mexico. Having tested thirteen unregulated water wells for quality, gamma radiation levels along roads and near homes, and indoor levels in 139 homes, they have come to the conclusion that twelve wells had water quality that didn't satisfy federal standards, that the gamma radiation levels were ten times greater than the background next to homes within 1,200 feet of an unremediated uranium mine, and that thirty-four of the homes tested exceeded the USEPA action levels of 4.0 pCi/l [42, 44].

The DiNEH, funded by the National Institute of Environmental Health Sciences (NIEHS), is an educational and technical assistance project that started in the Eastern Navajo region in 2004. The purpose of the project is to research the capacity of twenty Navajo chapters in the Eastern Navajo area. The project administered water use surveys for four years from 2004 to 2008. They also surveyed unregulated water wells, windmills, and springs. At the end of their project the effort transitioned to the NUAKHP for testing associations between drinking water and high rates of kidney disease.

The NUAKHP, started in 2006, is an epidemiological study also funded by the National Institute of Environmental Health Sciences. It is an ambitious longitudinal surveillance study to assess kidney health through both standard clinical screening techniques and detailed biochemical analyses following a subset of patients for two years, drawing data heavily from the earlier CRUMP and DiNEH projects. In conducting these three studies, the Navajo community hopes to reduce uranium exposures and estimate relative risks for chronic kidney diseases from uranium in the eastern Navajo area.

The Navajo community has carefully planned and initiated these projects based on community-based participatory research models. The CRUMP, DiNEH, and NUKHP are collaborative projects that include both community groups, health agencies, academic institutions and such governmental agencies as the Eastern Navajo Health Board, the Crownpoint Services Unit, the University of New Mexico Community Environmental Health program, the Southwest Research and Information Center, NAIHS, Navajo Nation Water Resources Department, USEPA Region 6 and the USACE and Navajo Tribal Utility Authority.

RECENT DEVELOPMENTS IN URANIUM MINING IN THE NAVAJO AREA

Despite the long battle to bring justice to the issue of uranium mining and allot compensation to uranium miners, the issue of uranium mining is far from settled. Since 2001, there have been efforts to revive the nuclear power industry. With energy prices soaring in the United States, a new energy bill was passed in August 2005 providing subsidies for the development of nuclear power plants. There is a shortage of uranium worldwide; about twice as much of what is produced now is needed. The price of uranium in the world market has increased from $7 to $33. The western plains again are targeted for renewed mining, including mining proposals for Navajo lands that would use *in situ* leachate (ISL) methods that extract uranium by dissolving it and drawing it to the surface [4]. With *in situ* mining, oxygen and sodium bicarbonate are pumped into the rocks to leach uranium into the groundwater, yielding uranium concentrations 100,000 times higher than normally found in the groundwater. Some hydrologists predict that such mining is going to contaminate the drinking water wells in a matter of seven years destroying the only source of drinking water to about 15,000 people [49].

Mining resumed in parts of Colorado in 2004 and some of the neighboring states are following the lead. About 8,500 new mining claim permits have been issued in Colorado and Utah. About four mines in the Navajo mining area have been targeted to restart uranium mining. Hydro Resources Incorporated (HRI), a Texas-based company, has proposed to start mining at Crownpoint and Churchrock using the *in situ* leach mining process [49].

Policymakers have not addressed the reduction in working levels proposed by NIOSH in 1987 that would be one-fourth of the 1970 standard. The proposed standard was never enacted, leaving new workers who enter the profession today at substantial risk. However, the Navajo Nation council recently decided to prohibit mining on Navajo lands. The new community-based research on drinking water quality and renal health is vital to understanding how community health is impacted from drinking water contaminated with uranium.

The struggle in the Navajo lands over uranium is far from over. This historical analysis shows how the public/environmental health research has evolved over the years, shaped by the people and the ideologies of the time. It has broadened into a more encompassing, socially engaging, responsive and ethical science, and has shaped itself to be a vehicle for direct social change more powerful and more equipped to deal with challenges.

ETHICAL CONCERNS SPECIFIC TO THE URANIUM MINING RESEARCH IN THE NAVAJO COMMUNITY

Scientific research has shown to be an important player (1) as a key decision-making tool for setting standards and developing policies and regulations; (2) as a mechanism that informs our course of actions and habits in making informed decisions about our health; and (3) in preparing and responding to health risks, developing safer alternatives. Collectively it should help guide and serve the public interest to promote a healthy and safe workplace and environment.

Scientific research such as that on uranium mining carries with it a heavy social responsibility. It should be accountable to the public for providing just and ethical verdicts of scientific findings. In this analysis on the ethical issues in the epidemiological research conducted in the Navajo community, many issues stand forth in the early research as violating ethical standards of the times when the research was undertaken. The ACHRE report focused on one of the most important ethical violations in the PHS study conducted in the Colorado Plateau—the lack of informed consent,[4] a widely recognized problem with the early tier of studies. In this chapter we broadly discuss six topics of concern that are of relevance today and raise issues in the conduct of ethical research.

Assuming, that uranium mining was inevitable, what sort of research on uranium mining would have been ethical in the early mining period?

Evidence at the start of the U.S. mining program implicated radon daughter products as the causal agent in the development of lung cancer in miners. The obvious remedy was to install ventilation and dilute out particulates carrying radon daughters. It seems to us that a study of the efficacy of an early ventilation project would have been justified, provided that it granted full disclosure and informed consent to miners who voluntarily enrolled in the study. The point of the

[4] "Research participants are entitled to receive a thorough and understandable disclosure of the purpose of the research, the procedures to be administered, risks and potential benefits of research procedures and information regarding the voluntary nature of research participation, and the ability to withdraw from research" [50].

research would have been to assess the level of risk associated with the (lower) level of radon daughter products in ventilated mines and to make recommendations with respect to whether or not ventilation would need to be increased in order to meet politically agreed upon risk levels.

What level of proof is needed to initiate protective measures?

According to the ethical principles of nonmaleficence, beneficence, and avoiding exploitation, the research requires that the risk be favorable and not subject people knowingly to exposures that are harmful. Nonmaleficence requires not inflicting harm on others and minimizing risks. Beneficence requires acting for the benefit of others [50]. The early studies have violated these ethical standards. In considering a favorable exposure level, perhaps one could have been left with a question about what level of ventilation was needed, indeed that is still a point of some debate. In addition there is always the problem of what level of risk is considered "acceptable." There is no scientific answer to the question of acceptable risk because it depends heavily on the personal values of individuals and communities and various moderating factors, such as income and employment, that may be taken into consideration.

Is there an ethical responsibility to engage the affected population in research studies?

The studies of Navajo uranium miners unquestionably assisted in the eventual fight to gain compensation for the uranium miners with first the passage of and then the amendment of RECA. However, conventional epidemiological studies are hardly participatory. With the emerging paradigm of community-based participatory research, it is worth asking whether such studies have an obligation or could be improved if they engaged the affected communities actively during the research process rather than simply offering a public airing of their findings.

We would argue that there is not an explicit obligation to conduct community-based participatory research, even in cases such as this in which there are strong political campaigns and public policy consequences. However, we would also argue that there is a potential benefit both to the research and to the affected communities if CBPR methods are adopted. In particular, actively involving the community may assist with better aligning research questions with public policy needs. Further, recommendations have been made to use CBPR to reduce racial and ethnic disparities. CBPR sees research as increasing community capacity affecting social change by making research truly the responsibility of the community rather than seeing research as a mere process for increasing knowledge [50].

Do researchers have a responsibility beyond conducting technically valid studies?

Richard Rhodes, a historian on developing atomic weaponry, noted that many physicists allowed themselves to become assets of national security in exchange for the resources to pursue their dreams of unlocking nature's secrets [51]. There is something similar at work in the way that public health researchers were willing to conduct the early uranium mining studies without pressing very hard for alleviating the exposures to the miners. While some researchers, for example Duncan Holliday, did press for installing ventilation in the mines, even those efforts were limited to recommendations within a largely non-responsive system.

Scientific officials have a lot of power over decision-making and regulations, and they are directly or indirectly responsible for many occupational work standards, especially in cases such as uranium mining. The scientific verdict or silence of a scientist or the controlling officials has great consequences and repercussions that could cost or save lives. This is very evident from the thousands of lung cancer deaths that could have been prevented by the implementation of better ventilation standards in uranium mines.

At what point is it ethically incumbent upon researchers to "go public" or even commit civil disobedience by disobeying orders to protect the lives of affected workers? Today's whistleblower laws provide a modern pathway through which imminent serious dangers can be reported. Our personal and professional view is that researchers conducting studies of human health have an ethical obligation to publicly raise findings that appear to show risk. The manner in which such findings are made public could vary, but at a minimum, researchers must seek venues beyond academic journals to publicize their results and should prioritize reporting their findings to the affected populations through various means. Further, researchers must refuse to participate in studies that do not fully disclose risk to study participants or that are conducted such that known risks are allowed to persist unabated.

Science in private interest [52]: Corporate interest and public interest are not the same

Research ethics has become a major concern for communities affected by the onslaught of companies seeking to extract resources (hazardous or otherwise) while attempting to convince the general population that their extraction processes are harmless, and, in the long term, will benefit their communities. These companies often use the practice of "royalties" (small payments to show good faith), jobs, and other incentives to smooth the path to expropriation of these resources regardless of the disruption, disharmony, and imbalance of indigenous life in the process.

When a corporate industry walks into the neighborhood with their best researcher and scientifically presents a certain process, such as *in situ* leaching mining, to be safe, there is a potential that the research is skewed to justify the companies interest. This web of influence of the political and industrial restricts the beneficial application of science for public interest by withholding information. Mounting death and disease tolls are the perverse results of public-interest science with *distorted research priorities* that does not want to incur the displeasure of the industry or the influential committees [52]. Also a consequence of such research is reduced capacity to foresee and forestall calamities.

Is precaution an ideology or a target that can be attained to prevent conditions that are harmful: Acknowledging the inherent limitations in our scientific methodology?

Public/environmental health science has well-prescribed models to investigate disease etiologies, calculate disease incidences, and to understand disease patterns in the community, and interpret these many data layers. Still they often explain only the physicality of the problems, often proving what we already know. Comments such as, "the research just proved what we already know" are common statements with which we all are familiar. Still, at times, that same research becomes key in winning a compensation battle, a regulation that buys an extra breath of ventilation, or a tool that brought remediation for polluting lands and rivers.

While we have good diagnostic tools, we do not have good predictive tools. For public health or environmental health science to be effective, we need to have a good diagnostic system for early warning, or should be boldly proactive in adverse situations and be precautionary to prevent harm.

CONCLUSION

Research, as one of the key ways of solving and understanding our problems, needs new partnerships, collaborations, and voices to understand the ills and problems ailing our communities. Kemmis and McTaggart leave a view of research that is rooted in initiating direct change in one's community. They propose a research "where people want to make changes thoughtfully—that is after critical reflection. It emerges when people want to think realistically about where they are now, how things came to be that way, and, from these starting points, how, in practice, things might be changed" [50, p. 1]. We often forget that community building is not about capacity building and economic development but about building relationships, or as Ralph Nader puts it, it is about "building democracy as the central community problem solving process" [52].

APPENDIX A
A Personal Story
Esther Yazzie-Lewis

I recall growing up on the Navajo reservation with my parents only speaking Navajo. My first language was Navajo, and I began to learn English at age six after entering the Methodist boarding school in Farmington, New Mexico. I grew up as the youngest of ten children, herding sheep and farming, which taught me the practical side of sharing, and a much deeper appreciation for agrarian life. The Navajo clanship system edified the importance of family and community relationships. Interacting with neighboring ranchers and their families helped me to quickly build my Navajo social skills, and to communicate with Navajo community people on a much broader level. The ability to understand Navajo life and language helped me to become a professional interpreter.

In 1985, I was recruited to be a board member to the Tonantzin Land Institute, a nonprofit public interest organization advocating for human rights, land rights, and environmental justice. I was introduced to the injustice of uranium and its destruction of human life. I attended a world uranium victims conference in New York City. I met thousands of people who were fighting against the use of uranium. It was at this time I realized how much the world was affected by uranium and plutonium power plants in Japan. I gained a valuable perspective on the bombing of Hiroshima and Nagasaki where thousands of people died. I learned about the Navajo uranium miners and the relationship of uranium and nuclear power and war. I heard the people plea, "No more uranium mining" in Salzburg, Austria, at the world hearing in 1992.

Transcribing interviews of Navajo miners for Dr. Doug Brugge, Tufts University School of Medicine, Boston, Massachusetts. I learned that Navajo miners did not have knowledge about the dangers of uranium. They were never informed of the health hazards or long-term risk they were subjecting themselves and their families to. The children played at the sites and went down around the mine area with their father. The miners tracked the uranium dust into their camp among their wives and children. The wives and children were just as exposed to uranium as the workers. The miners did not know that the dust that covered their clothes was hazardous. Some of the miners talked about the cold water that ran down in the mines underground that they drank and that tasted so good. They never knew the water was contaminated with uranium. The water was cold, looked so clean, and tasted so good that they drank the water without hesitation. The company did not tell them the water was contaminated. The wives hand washed their husband's clothes not knowing the clothes they touched were full of uranium. They prepared food and dealt with their children not knowing the hazardous effects transmitted by mere contact.

At present, I am Board President of the Southwest Research and Information Center (SRIC). They are also a nonprofit public interest organization. SRIC is a multicultural organization with an objective to work and to promote the health of people and communities by protecting the natural resources, ensure citizen participation, and secure environmental and social justice now and for future generations. This organization is important to me with respect to helping the Eastern Navajos fight against uranium mining. I committed myself to SRIC on behalf of Navajo people who are victims of uranium mining. My participation has involved finding funding to hire a Navajo liaison to assist the Navajo people in developing and implementing Navajo legislation to *stop* uranium mining on Navajo land. I was raised taking care of livestock and I can sympathize and support the efforts of Eastern Navajo Diné Against Uranium Mining (ENDAUM) to protect the valuable resources for future generations. They have fought for years to prevent their land and water from being contaminated by the mining of uranium.

My work with Dr. Doug Brugge, Tufts University School of Medicine, Boston, Massachusetts, has further extended my involvement with the work and research studies on uranium miners and the injustices perpetrated against them by the uranium mining companies. The Navajo miners and their families have struggled strenuously for their compensation from the Federal Government for the damage done to their health. The majority of Navajo miners have not received any type of assistance from the federal government for long-term pain and suffering.

I am deeply honored to contribute to the establishment of the archive at the Navajo Nation Museum on Navajo uranium miners, and a part of the collective experience and effort to preserve this moment in time. I am also honored to be an instrument and voice of many Navajo people who have suffered through these painful experiences. The collective work has now been exhibited across the country in various universities to carry the message of the wrong done to Navajo miners. I am honored to have been a part in making that endeavor happen.

Through rendering my Navajo language skills, a valuable piece of history for many Navajo miners has been captured, recorded, and preserved. Therefore, I give my deepest appreciation to my mother and father who taught me how to speak Navajo with accuracy and distinct pronunciation. Needless to say, what has taken place over the years is history, but the pursuit of justice is an ongoing process. To this end I remain totally committed to producing more writing on Navajo uranium mining for the purpose of public education and the greater cause of achieving justice.

APPENDIX B
A Navajo Activist Perspective on Uranium Research Ethics

Esther Yazzie-Lewis

It is apparent that research studies conducted by the uranium companies did not include the community people. There was no inclusion of individuals who knew the language who worked with the companies to explain and educate the Navajo men on the dangers of uranium. Safety precautions were not preformed, such as using safety face masks and discarding work clothes and related contaminated garments. Any resource- extracting research, health-impact research, or communicable disease study that does not involve community representatives (for example, an oversight committee) is highly questionable and suspect. The research must be held to a certain standard of public health and safety when human lives are at risk. It has been proven time and time again that corporate interest and public interest are not one and the same. The questions are:

1. who has the *power and authority* to initiate research?
2. what is the *purpose* of the research?
3. who *benefits* from the outcome of the research?

There are the corporations who have an interest in uranium for various reasons to accommodate this country's industry and the military (Department of Defense, i.e., National Defense and Home Land Security). It is the corporations verses the community people. The corporations know about the dangers of the uranium. The federal government knows. The industry has a demand for uranium.

The Navajo people in this case took on the employment of mining uranium without fully understanding the health and safety risk involved. The need for income was the only reason. There are many of our rural (unsophisticated) communities that still remain vulnerable to the unethical research practices of corporate America. It must be said that these small rural communities cannot compete with corporate America's researchers who come into their communities armed with ulterior motives, unconfirmed data, and untested methods to convince these people that the corporations are actually looking out for their interest. In fact, they use uncorroborated scientific data (graphs, charts, bells and whistles), designed to confuse and exploit these people.

With respect to their research about health, for example, in Crownpoint, New Mexico, the company met with the Navajo people to inform them that the in-situ leach mining was safe. The company informed the people that they had developed a new way of mining uranium so that it would not contaminate their grazing land and water. *If the Navajo people allowed this, their ground water would be contaminated. Knowing the people are poor, companies dangle dollars in front of these community people to convince them it is economic development for them.*

The corporation knew, but did not inform the Navajo community people, of the dangers uranium may cause. The federal government knew, but did not ensure health and safety compliance for Navajo miners. By and large, the issue of uranium mining is driven by greed and super profits. The United States government is the official regulatory agency of all uranium mined and process in America. So, how complicit is the relationship between those that have the capital to invest in uranium mining, those researchers that are sent into the field to soften up the people with uncorroborated data, those that mine and process uranium, and those that supply uranium to industry (energy complexes), and the Department of Defense? These are critical questions that must be answered when we explore the relational dynamics on the question of *research ethics*.

What is ethical? Ethical is that which conforms to accepted principles of right and wrong that govern the conduct of a profession. There is health-related legislation enacted to protect the people of this country, but who are the people that are unprotected? There have been so many violations of the peoples' protection under the law that one can hardly keep up with the atrocities.

The federal government has developed basic principles that should guide researchers and established ethics review committees to oversee the research. These guidelines are supposed to give some moral standards to both parties in the research. However, corporations in most cases seem to have the upper hand with their high-tech scientists doing the research and intimidating the grassroots communities. The questions that must be asked include: Who were these regulations made for? What is fair about them?

The injustice of research and the decisions which derive from the research cause communities to take a defensive position to fight for their rights. For example, Crownpoint community people have come together to fight the in-situ leach (ISL) mining imposed on their land. The *community people* have formed an organization called the Eastern Navajo Diné Against Uranium Mining (ENDAUM) a nonprofit grassroots community-based public interest organization. ENDAUM fears the in-situ leach mining will contaminate their drinking water. This aquifer is the principal source of water in this area of the desert on Navajo land. ENDAUM has been fighting the mining company for over 10 years and they joined forces with the Southwest Research and Information Center (SRIC) in Albuquerque, New Mexico to strengthen their efforts. SRIC has provided technical research support to ENDAUM by supporting the organization in scientific geological knowledge, but also assisting the community's interest in stopping the mining.

Sometimes it would appear to be a never-ending battle, in spite of all their efforts and sometimes no encouragement from the people they represent. Nevertheless, their collaborative managed to sustain resistance by continuing to find ways to educate the community on the dangers of uranium. One important project in the initiative is the DiNEH project. As described above, its purpose is to document water quality in 20 Navajo chapters in the Eastern Navajo Area. A water-use survey of unregulated water wells, windmills, and springs will be conducted from 2004-2008. It is a long drawn-out process, however, they are determined to accomplish this research on their own without corporate or government interference.

The Navajo people in the Crownpoint area have become suspicious of corporate interests in new uranium mining. Hydro Resource, Inc. (HRI), the primary company promoting renewed mining, has continued to persevere for over seventeen years in their quest to open ISL mines in Church Rock and Crownpoint. SRIC hired a Navajo liaison to assist ENDAUM in their fight. The Navajo liaison, Harris Arthur, understood the grassroots people and asserted that the "Navajo legislation had to be changed." He met with the people and they put together the proposal for legislative change to ban uranium mining and processing, and with the help of Councilman George Arthur (the brother of the late Harris Arthur) sponsoring the legislation under the "Dine Natural Resource Act of 2005," the legislation was presented to the Navajo Nation Council and passed into law.

However, even with the Navajo ban on uranium mining, HRI continues to lobby the New Mexico Environment Department. The Navajo people, represented by ENDAUM, recently traveled to Washington. D.C. to lobby Congressmen to respect the Navajo ban on uranium. Navajo Nation President Joe Shirley, Jr. has taken a stand in support of the law and has been recognized around the world for banning uranium. Still the Eastern Navajos are not feeling secure. The fight goes on due to a lack of understanding by the federal government and state government as to why land and water is so important to the Navajo people. Navajo people believe by culture they are a part of nature. Land is what most indigenous people depend on to provide their existence. They are connected spiritually by being connected to every element, creature, and plant, even the rocks which have lived in some point in time. The land is the lifeblood of the people; a gift from the creator that provides all that is necessary to sustain life.

ACKNOWLEDGMENT

The first part of this chapter is reprinted from B. Panikkar, and D. Brugge. 2007. "The ethical issues in uranium mining research in the Navajo nation." *Accountability in Research* 14:121-153, with permission of the publisher, Taylor & Francis http://www.informaworld.com

REFERENCES

1. Eichstaedt, P. 1994. *If you poison us: Uranium and native Americans.* Santa Fe, NM: Red Crane Books.
2. Brugge, D., and Goble, R. 2003. The Radiation Exposure Compensation Act: What is fair? *New Solutions: A Journal of Environmental and Occupational Health Policy* 13:385-397.
3. Markstrom, C. A., and Charley, P. H. 2003. Psychological effects of human caused environmental disasters: Examination of the Navajo and uranium. *American Indian and Alaska Native Mental Health Research: The Journal of the National Center* 11:19-45.
4. Dawson, S. E., and Madsen, G. E. 2005. Safety concerns with resumption of uranium mining. *Salt Lake Tribune* (Utah), 23 October 2005.
5. Brugge, D., and Goble, R. 2002. The history of uranium mining and the Navajo people. *American Journal of Public Health* 92:1410-1419.

6. Advisory Committee on Human Radiation Experiments (ACHRE). 1995. Washington, D.C.: U.S. Government Printing Office.
7. Smith, B. E. 1987. *Digging our own graves: Coal miners and the struggle over black lung disease*. Philadelphia, PA: Temple University Press.
8. U.S. Nuclear Regulatory Commission. 2003. A short history of nuclear regulation 1946-1999. (NUREG/BR-0175, Rev. 1) June 23, 2003. http://www.nrc.gov/who-we-are/short-history.html
9. Federal Radiation Council. 1967. Report No. 8 Revised. Guidelines for the control of radiation hazards in uranium mining. Washington, D.C.: U.S. Government Printing Office.
10. Lorenz, F. E. 1944. Radioactivity and lung cancer: A critical review of lung cancer in the miners of Schneeberg and Joachimsthal. *Journal of the National Cancer Institute* 5:1-15.
11. Peller, S. 1939. Lung cancer among mine workers in Joachimsthal. *Human Biology* 11:130-143.
12. Donaldson, A. W. 1969. The epidemiology of lung cancer among uranium miners. *Health Physics* 16:563-569.
13. Stellman, S. D. 2003. Issues of causality in the history of occupational epidemiology. Series: History of Epidemiology. *Sozial- und Praventivmedizin* 48:151-160.
14. Hueper, W. C. 1942. *Occupational tumors and allied diseases*. Springfield, IL: Charles C. Thomas.
15. Archer, V. E., Magnuson, H. J., Holaday, D. A., and Lawrance, P. A. 1962. Hazards to the health in uranium mining and milling. *Journal of Occupational Medicine* 4:55-60.
16. Lundin, F. E., Wagoner, J. K., and Archer, V. E., 1971. Radon daughter exposure and respiratory cancer quantitative and temporal aspects. NIOSH-NIEHS Joint Monograph No. 1. U.S. Department of Health Education and Welfare.
17. Bale, W. F. 1980. Memorandum to the files, March 14, 1951: Hazards associated with radon and thoron. *Health Physics* 38:1062-1066.
18. Harley, J. H. 1980. Sampling and measurement of airborne daughter product of radon. (Reprinted) *Health Physics* 38:1067.
19. Ball, H. 1993. *Cancer factories: America's tragic quest for uranium self-sufficiency*. Westport, CT and London: Greenwood Press.
20. Holaday, D. A. 1969. History of the exposure of miners to radon. *Health Physics* 16:547-552.
21. Wagoner, J. K., Archer, V. E., Lundin, F. E., Holaday, D. A., and Lloyd, J. W. 1965. Radiation as the cause of lung cancer among uranium miners. *New England Journal of Medicine* 273:181-188.
22. Lundin, F. E., Lloyd, W., Smith, E. M., Archer, V. E., and Holaday, D. A. 1969. Mortality of uranium miners in relation to radiation exposure, hard-rock mining and cigarette smoking—1950 through September 1967. *Health Physics* 16:571-578.
23. *Begay vs. United States*, 591 F. Supp, 991, 1007. (Undated)
24. Lewis, J. 1998, March. Looking backward: A historical perspective on environmental regulations. *EPA Journal*. Available online at http://www.epa.gov/history/topics/regulate/01.htm
25. Ruckelshaus, W. D. 1998, March. Environmental regulation: The early days at EPA. *EPA Journal*. Available online at: http://www.epa.gov/history/administrators/ruckelshaus.htm

26. U.S. Mine Safety and Health Administration (MSHA). 2003. 25 years of safety and health values, United States Department of Labor. http://www.msha.gov/MSHAInfo/25Years/MSHA%2025%20Years.pdf
27. Samet, J. M., Kutvirt, B. A., Waxweiler, R. J., and Key, C. R. 1984. Uranium mining and lung cancer in Navajo men. *The New England Journal of Medicine* 310(23): 1481-1484.
28. Gottlieb, L. S., and Husen, L. A. 1982. Lung cancer among Navajo uranium miners. *Chest* 81:4.
29. Gilliland, F. D., Hunt, W. C., Pardilla, M., and Charles, R. 2000. Uranium mining and lung cancer among Navajo men in New Mexico and Arizona, 1969 to 1993. *Journal of Occupational and Environmental Medicine* 42(3):278-283.
30. Mulloy, K. B., James, D. S., Mohs, K., and Kornfeld, M. 2001. Lung cancer in a nonsmoking underground uranium miner. *Environmental Health Perspectives* 109(3): 305-309.
31. Roscoe, R. J., Deddens, J. A., Salvan, A., and Schnorr, T. M. 1995. Mortality among Navajo uranium miners. *American Journal of Public Health* 85:535-540.
32. Roscoe, R. J. 1997. An update of mortality from all causes among white miners from the Colorado plateau study group. *American Journal of Industrial Medicine* 31:211-222.
33. Waxweiler, R. J., Roscoe, R. J., Archer, V. E., Thun, M. J., Wagober, J. K., and Lundin, F. E., Jr. 1981. Mortality follow-up through 1977 of the white underground uranium miners cohort examined by the United States Public Health Service. In *Radiation hazards in mining. Society of Mining Engineers*, ed. M. Gomez, 823-930. AIME. Kingsport, TN: Kingport Press.
34. Committee on the Biological Effects of Ionizing Radiation. 1988. *Health risks of radon and other internally deposited alpha-emitters* (BEIR IV). Washington, D.C.: National Academy Press.
35. Committee on the Biological Effects of Ionizing Radiation. 1999. *Health effects of exposure to radon* (BEIR VI). Washington, D.C.: National Academy Press.
36. Surveillance Epidemiology and End Result (SEER). 2005. A brief history of cancer registration. National Cancer Institute. Accessed 2005 from http://training.seer.cancer.gov/module_cancer_registration/unit1_history.html
37. Dawson, S. E., Charley, P. H., and Harrison P. Jr. 1997. Advocacy and social action among Navajo uranium workers and their families. In *Social work in health settings: Practice in context* (2nd ed.), eds. T. S. Kerson and J. L. M. McLoyd, 391-407. New York and London: Haworth Press.
38. Nuclear Information and Resource Service (NIRS). 2005. *Controversial history of radiation epidemiology and risk estimation*. Accessed October, 2005 from http://www.nirs.org/mononline/appendixhisbeirletter1.htm
39. Agency for Health Care Research and Quality (AHRQ). 2001. *Community-based participatory research: Conference Summary Report,* 27-28 November 2001. U.S. Department of Health and Human Services.
40. Israel, B. A. 2001. Community-based participatory research: Principles, rationale and policy recommendations. (Keynote address) in *Successful models of community based participatory research.* Washington, D.C.: National Institute of Environmental Health Sciences (NIEHS) 29-31 March 2001.

41. Brugge, D., Benally, T., Harrison, P., Austin-Garrison, M., and Fasthorse-Begay, L. 1997. *Memories come to us in the rain and the wind: Oral histories and photographs of Navajo uranium miners and their families*. (Reprinted in 1999 and 2000). Boston, MA: Tufts University School of Medicine.
42. South West Research and Information Center (SRIC). 2004. Mitchell Capitan and eastern Navajo Dine against uranium mining: Take their message to the international stage. *Voices from the Earth* 5(3). Available online at http://www.sric.org/voices/2004/v5n3/capitan_5_3.html
43. Shields, L. M., Wiese, W. H., Skipper, B. J., Charley, B., and Benally, L. 1992. Navajo birth outcomes in the Shiprock uranium mining area. *Health Physics* 63: 542-551.
44. Lewis, J. 2006. On Navajo Uranium Assessment and Kidney Health Project NUAKHP, personal communications between March and June, 2006.
45. Brugge, D., and Missaghian, M. 2006. Protecting the Navajo people through tribal regulation of research. *Science and Engineering Ethics* 12:3.
46. Thun, M. J., Baker, D. B., Steenland, K., Smith, A. B., Halperin, W., and Berl, T. 1985. Renal toxicity in uranium mill workers. *Scandinavian Journal of Work Environment and Health* 11:83-90.
47. Leggett, R. W. 1989. The behavior and chemical toxicity of U in the kidney: A reassessment. *Health Physics* 57:365-383.
48. Zamora LM, Tracy BL, Zielinski JM, Meyerhof DP, and Moss MA. 1998. Chronic ingestion of uranium in drinking water: A study of kidney bioeffects in humans. *Toxicological Sciences* 43(1):68-77.
49. Eastern Navajo Dine Against Uranium Mining (ENDAUM). 2005. Interview with Rita and Mitchell Capitan. Homeland: Four portraits of Native Action (film).
50. Chen, D. T, Jones, L., and Gelberg, L. 2006. Ethics of clinical research within a community-academic partnered participatory framework. *Ethnicity & Disease* 16:118-135.
51. Overbye, D. 2005. Dr. Atomic: Unthinkable yet immortal. *New York Times*, 18 October.
52. Krimsky, S. 2003. *Science in private interest: Has the lure of profits corrupted biomedical research?* Lanham, MD: Rowman & Littlefield.

http://dx.doi.org/10.2190/TORC8

CHAPTER 8

Investigation of an Excess of Malignant Melanoma among Employees of the Lawrence Livermore National Laboratory

Donald F. Austin

RECOGNITION OF A POTENTIAL PROBLEM

From 1974 to 1988, I worked for the State of California, both as Chief of the California Tumor Registry (CTR) and principal investigator of one of the cancer-data collecting programs of the National Cancer Institute's Surveillance, Epidemiology, and End Results (SEER) Program. During that time, I received periodic requests for data from physicians, hospitals, or other local organizations, as well as questions or information from members of the medical community. The area for which we had complete cancer-incidence [1] data, dating back to 1972, included the five counties of the San Francisco-Oakland Metropolitan Statistical Area (SFO SMSA).

One day in late 1979, I received a telephone call from a San Francisco dermatologist, who informed me that the most recent five patients with malignant melanoma [2] seen in that office were all employees of the Lawrence Livermore Laboratories (subsequently named the Lawrence Livermore National Laboratories or LLNL). The LLNL is a high-technology research facility operated by the University of California as the nation's center for research on high-energy physics, including the development of nuclear weapons and other projects of interest to the U.S. Department of Energy (DOE). Upon receiving that news,

I recalled that several weeks earlier, we had filled a request for current incidence rates for malignant melanoma from the medical director of the LLNL, Dr. Max Biggs.

I retrieved my copy of the data we had provided to the LLNL and called for an appointment with Dr. Biggs. My purpose in meeting with Dr. Biggs was twofold. First, I wanted to determine whether there was any validity to the suspected cluster of malignant melanoma cases among LLNL workers and, if so, whether that possibly constituted any public health threat. My second purpose was to make sure that Dr. Biggs had both the necessary information and the experience to conduct an adequate assessment of the melanoma occurrence within the LLNL workforce. He was interested enough in the latter purpose to invite me, and a member of my staff, Peggy Reynolds (now Dr. Reynolds), to meet with him at the LLNL.

During that meeting, Dr. Biggs became convinced that he was unlikely to determine all of the cases of malignant melanoma among the workers, since they were under no obligation to share that information with the LLNL Medical Department. We, however, with an operating incidence system that identified all, or almost all, cases of invasive and *in situ* (preinvasive) cancer in the SFO area, had a much better chance of determining whether the LLNL was experiencing more malignant melanoma among its employees than one would expect. In addition, there were some epidemiologic analysis issues with which we were familiar that he was not and which we offered. What we needed, however, was a means by which we could identify which of our hundreds of cases of malignant melanoma collected over the five counties of the SFO SMSA were employees of the LLNL. The means by which we could tell who, among the reported melanoma cases, were LLNL employees and who were not, was by using their employee roster, and checking that against our cancer registry roster. Neither group could conduct an adequate investigation without the other. Thus, a collaboration between LLNL and the CTR was proposed.

COLLABORATION WITH THE LAB TO EVALUATE MELANOMA OCCURRENCE IN EMPLOYEES

The analysis plan was conceptually simple, but methodologically complex. Basically, we needed to accomplish two things. One was to establish an accurate count of how many cases of melanoma occurred among the LLNL workforce for each of the years for which we had complete data. The second was to accurately project how many cases would be expected to occur in that group, taking into consideration the number of employees and their age, sex, and race, and also taking into consideration the rates of melanoma among residents of the SMSA who were not LLNL employees. We operated under the initial hypothesis that the LLNL employees were no more likely to develop melanoma than anyone else of their age, race, sex, and neighborhood of residence. This latter factor was necessary because the SFO SMSA is a patchwork of different microenvironments, with different climates, temperatures, hours of sunlight, and levels of affluence among the residents. Up to that time, the only known risk factor for malignant melanoma was exposure to sunlight, and the city of Livermore, in which the laboratory is situated, is one of the warmest and sunniest areas of the SMSA.

In addition to the methodological challenges for the proposed study, there were administrative and political issues to be considered. Dr. Biggs needed approval from both the administration at the LLNL and UC Berkeley for our collaboration and to release the names of employees to an outside agency. We needed to be sure not to release the names of cancer patients reported to the state cancer registry to any outside agency without patient consent, and no patient contact was contemplated for this study. It had also become apparent that there were rumors of excesses of melanoma among employees. Some employees had formed a support group, a union had taken up the issue of radiation exposure hazards to employees, and an anti-war, anti-nuclear weapons activist group had learned of these rumors. If the lab management had wished to keep the subject under wraps, it was rapidly becoming apparent that it would not be possible. It was also clear that the lab did not have the means of adequately assessing those rumors by themselves.

Dr. Biggs ultimately received approval for the collaboration, with some strings attached. The assessment was to be considered a collaborative project, rather than an investigation of the state health agency of a possible health concern at the lab. Since I wanted to determine whether there was a real excess of melanoma, and whether there might be a public health hazard, I needed the cooperation of the lab. Being in a research facility, Dr. Biggs was receptive to a research project, but he didn't have the training or data to carry it out. I suspect the lab management was more receptive to describing the work as a collaboration because it avoided the public perception that the lab was being investigated by the State Health Department. The perception of a state investigation would have been bad public relations.

Another of the strings was that the CTR, an official state agency, would not release any information to the press, the public, or elected officials without a prior review by the lab. We could agree to this, providing that their review did not result in any substantive delay in making public any information that was clearly in the public's best interest to know. Furthermore, there was to be no lab oversight or censorship of the study or its results, but there were to be regular progress reports to the lab, and no surprises with respect to public disclosures. Several LLNL scientists were selected to be in the Melanoma Work Group, to assist Dr. Biggs in reviewing our results, when they became available.

Since the CTR work was clearly above and beyond the work our staff was budgeted to do, the LLNL agreed to provide some funds for an independent biostatistical consultant and for the time CTR staff spent on record linkage, resolving possible matches, cleaning data files, and conducting the necessary computations. It took the lab administration some time to arrange to pay for the time of LLNL employees spent on creating this file. Apparently, they sought and were eventually given approval by the DOE to expend some of their employee time on this project and also to support some CTR employee time. This resulted in a contract from the lab to the state, which gave the lab contract and project officer oversight of the CTR work.

COMPLETING THE INITIAL ASSESSMENT OF MELANOMA OCCURRENCE

For the CTR to perform the match between cancer cases and the LLNL employee roster, we needed to acquire from the lab an unduplicated electronic employee file, complete for each of the years of our study. This was a job that had to be carried out by LLNL administrative system computer personnel. Initially the computer staff at the LLNL claimed that to put together an unduplicated file, by year, of every LLNL employee and their address, was not possible. They may have made this claim because the request was not in their usual scope of work. They probably also viewed the project as a useless activity. Regardless, it took several months of working with them officially, and also with some employees unofficially, to establish that creating the necessary information files was indeed feasible. Ultimately we received the file containing the data we needed for our portion of the project, although the project suffered some delay.

We were very careful in conducting the agreed-upon analysis, realizing that all our decisions and computations would be examined and critiqued by a team of some of the top physics and chemistry scientists in the country. Our analysis showed that compared with people of the same age, race, and sex who lived in the same census tracts as the LLNL employees, there were four times as many cases of malignant melanoma occurring among lab employees for the time period 1972-1977.

There are two analytic strategies for determining the observed number of melanoma cases in comparison with the expected number, and they address slightly different research questions:

- Strategy A is the more conservative strategy, and it answers the question, "Does the LLNL workforce have more melanomas than expected, where the expected is based on a reference population that includes the LLNL workforce?" (This strategy includes the LLNL employees in the reference denominator and their melanomas in the reference numerator for computing the rate in the reference population.)

- Strategy B answers the question, "Does the LLNL workforce have more melanomas than expected, where the expected is based on a reference population that does *not* include the LLNL workforce?" (This basically compares the LLNL employees with the *rest* of the population.) Of course, if the rate of melanoma among the LLNL employees is substantially higher than the rest of the population, including them as part of the comparison group (as in Strategy A) raises the rate among the whole reference population. This has the effect of projecting a higher expected number among the employees, so that the observed number among the LLNL employees is not as different.

Even when using that more conservative strategy, it was apparent that the number of melanomas among the LLNL workforce was significantly higher than it should have been. Using Strategy A, the LLNL had three times the rate of melanoma as the reference population. Now that it was established through Strategy A that there was a higher occurrence of melanoma among the LLNL workforce, it was no longer appropriate to include them in the reference group. Strategy B could now be used to answer the question, "Just how much higher than 'normal' is the rate among the LLNL employees?" When the LLNL was not included in the reference population (because it had been established that the rate in the LLNL group was not "normal"), there was a fourfold excess seen among LLNL employees. The results, including both strategies, were ultimately published in *The Lancet* (with Max Biggs as a co-author). The LLNL, in all its publications and in public references to the study, always referred to a threefold excess, rather than a fourfold excess of melanoma in the population. The reason for this may have been because the larger the excess, the more difficult it is to attribute it to some error in the study. Also, it is politically worse for the LLNL to be responsible for the fourfold excess than for the threefold excess.

Prior to any public release of the LLNL study, we provided the study report to Dr. Biggs and to the Melanoma Work Group. We then met with the group to discuss the results and answer any questions. Drs. Peggy Reynolds and Harrison Stubbs (our biostatistical consultant) and I spent several hours explaining the methods and answering questions. We encountered considerable adversarial questioning by some members of the Melanoma Work Group, and responded to some statistical assertions that were incorrect. Others suggested that perhaps a combination of chance, bias, and confounding had served to create the impression of an increased risk of melanoma among the employees. Some of those possibilities could not be addressed with the data assembled in our analysis. However, when we completed the meeting, it was clear that there was no fatal flaw to our analysis, that the findings resulted from an acceptable epidemiologic research methodology, and that public release of the report was a responsible next step. Upon concluding that meeting, Dr. Mort Mendelsohn, the chair of the

Melanoma Work Group, commented, "Well, we'll take our lumps on this." It was clear that much of the motivation of the lab administration was to look good in the press, and not add fuel for anti-war, anti-nuclear groups.

POSITIVE RESULTS

It would have been a mistake for us or the lab to make the results public without having prepared a response to the question, "What are you going to do to address this excess rate of melanoma?" This question could be posed to either or both the LLNL and the CTR. Consequently, we advised the LLNL that we would prepare a proposal for further investigation of the melanoma associated with the lab. Rather than have us submit a proposal for investigation of melanoma to OSHA, NIOSH, or NCI, the LLNL suggested that we submit it to them, and that they could probably identify a means for funding a reasonable project.

The release of the study did capture considerable press and public attention. I was even asked to meet with the governor, who wanted my opinion as to whether his appropriate action would be to order the National Guard to shut the lab down for health reasons. I assured the governor that at this point we had not established that there was any hazard at the LLNL campus, and the logical next step would be to conduct a detailed investigation of the exposures and work conditions of those employees who did, and didn't, develop melanoma. The governor supported this conceptually.

FOLLOWING UP ON POSITIVE RESULTS

Our proposal for a two-year study employed a case-control design, with four controls selected for each case, and was based on a comprehensive questionnaire to be developed and administered by our research interviewers to an appropriately selected group of cases and controls among the lab employees. This proposal was ultimately approved for funding, with the extra funds for our study added to the DOE contract to the LLNL; again the CTR was a subcontractor to the lab.

The LLNL has several critical parts to play in the preparation for this study. Many parts of the lab campus were high security areas, and only people with special clearance could enter. Even the details of the actions and procedures of the workers in some of the areas were not open to discussion. Therefore, the lab management designated the Melanoma Work Group to help us identify chemicals, work locations, and projects that would be clearly recognized by LLNL employees, even though we may not have understood what they were. For example, we could ask "Are you now or have you ever in the past worked on the 'Alpha Big' project?" (a fictitious example) or "In your work do you ever handle radioactive isotopes?" or "Does your work require you to be in Building E?" but what was done in that building could be completely unknown to us.

Another role the lab needed to play was to provide for us a more detailed roster of employees, one that included the job classifications, the project assignments, and the employment history. We needed to select, for each melanoma case, four control employees of the same race (all the cases were white), age (within five years) and sex, who were employed at the LLNL at the time the case employee was diagnosed with melanoma. These had to be randomly selected from among the eligible employees, and we needed current contact information if they were no longer LLNL employees. We again encountered difficulty obtaining the necessary data files for our investigation, and though we eventually did receive what we needed from them, it delayed the project.

We needed to contact cases and controls and ask their consent for an interview. For current employees, Dr. Biggs provided a private place in the Medical Department if the employees wanted to be interviewed there, and LLNL administration approved work time for the interview. The lab did not know whom we had contacted with our request, but would know each person who elected to become interviewed at the lab on work time. Because only several case employees elected to be interviewed outside the LLNL environment, most cases and controls became known to the Melanoma Work Group, though most voluntarily informed the medical director of their melanoma anyway.

THE FRAGILITY OF THE FOLLOW-UP STUDY

The CTR case-control study, with support for part of Peggy Reynolds' time, some analyst time, interviewer, and interviewer supervisor time, was projected to take twenty-four months and cost approximately $400,000. This amount was funded by the DOE as a line item in the LLNL annual budget. We had some productive meetings with the Melanoma Work Group in obtaining proposed exposures, project names, and other types of information to collect in the study questionnaire. In addition, there were members of the melanoma support group, antiwar group, and union who asked to meet with us and offered us additional information about what might be fruitful topics to explore in the questionnaire. We completed the questionnaire design and tested it on some volunteer employees who were neither cases nor their matched controls. After a few adjustments to wording or format, we were ready to carry out the interviews.

There had been additional cases identified because of the time since the original record linkage and cases, and matched controls were selected and approached for interviews. We received excellent cooperation from most of the case and control subjects. Some resistance was encountered by senior scientists who had been randomly chosen to be controls, but overall, nearly all were interviewed. We then had the task of transferring all the information from paper documents to electronic media, of generating variables from the information gathered, and conducting a designed analysis. All this was scheduled for the second year.

Half-way through the project, I was invited to accompany several of the LLNL senior scientific management to Washington, D.C., to meet with the DOE representative responsible for their budget. Here I was informed that the LLNL was to experience a budget cut, and the second year of funding of this project was cut. This was devastating to the project since the data collected were not in any shape to analyze. Staff supported on LLNL contract funds had to be assigned to other projects or transferred out of the CTR. Some state-supported analytic staff were available to work on the project as their time permitted, but not much time was available. Peggy Reynolds, now working part-time while pursuing a PhD in epidemiology, was one of the staff with occasional small segments of available time.

COMPLETING THE FOLLOW-UP STUDY

In addition to the case-control study being conducted by the CTR, the LLNL undertook some studies of their own to address the melanoma issue. The LLNL hired a biostatistician who devoted his time, apparently exclusively, to finding alternative explanations for the excess at the lab. A number of different hypotheses relating to possible sources of bias or other sources of error were proposed and the lab funded their investigation. They obtained the services, as a consultant, of an internationally noted melanoma clinician and dermatopathologist from the University of California Medical Center in San Francisco. The lab tried to identify and recruit all of the employees who had developed melanoma and had the pathology slides of their malignancy collected, sent to the consultant, and independently reviewed. Employee patients were asked to be examined by this expert, at the lab's expense.

A study of the use of Kaiser facilities by LLNL staff was undertaken on the suspicion that because a greater portion of LLNL employees used that health system, and that system had a superior cancer surveillance and registry system and was likely to be more complete in reporting than the rest of the SFO SMSA, LLNL cases were more likely to be found and reported than the rest of the population covered by the local SEER program. If so, that would mean the measure of melanoma in the rest of the population was too low, and the computed expected number among the lab employees too low, creating a big disparity. Of course, to explain a fourfold increase, if the melanomas in the employees were 100% completely identified, only 25 percent of the melanomas in the comparison population could be reported, an implausible hypothesis. However, when the study was completed, there was some small difference caused by the bias stemming from differential completeness of melanoma ascertainment and reporting from different medical facilities. If applied to our results for the lab, the LLNL study suggested that the excess was slightly overstated. Even so, the LLNL argued in the press that since a higher proportion of their employees were Kaiser subscribers, melanoma in the lab employees was more completely reported and that partially explained their threefold (really fourfold) excess. In reality, it couldn't have explained more than a few percent.

A reanalysis of our data, with case findings among the lab going back in time a number of years was carried out. In that study, because the earlier years did not evidence an excess of melanoma, when averaged with the years of the study, the excess was smaller. Using the Method A comparison (a threefold excess), the lab study could demonstrate only about a twofold excess.

The strategy followed by the lab was similar to that successfully employed by the tobacco industry when evidence about the harmfulness of secondhand smoke was published. They created a "scientific controversy." The same strategy is used by some in considering global warming, and by defense attorneys in medical tort cases, using the Daubert ruling by the Supreme Court. The lab tried to generate as many studies as possible that cast some doubt on the accuracy of the findings.

What was particularly annoying was that the program of studies conceptualized and undertaken by the lab to discredit the CTR study suffered no shortage in funds. This clear disparity in access to support served as a strong motivator for those in the CTR to complete the study. Some professional and analytic staff actually donated their free time to help complete the project. Peggy Reynolds contributed, in my estimation, about 1,000 hours of her time as the lead analyst and epidemiologist on this project.

Eventually, about twelve months late, the analysis was completed. The study was conducted in a population of employees experiencing about a fourfold excess of melanoma. Our job was, through our analysis, to find factors within the laboratory or the employees that significantly predicted melanoma risk in cases as compared with other employees. Even though we had a relatively small number of study participants and a relatively large number of potential factors to sort out, some things became very clear.

One approach that I had hoped would be fruitful was to try to segregate the cases that would have happened anyway and look at the remaining cases. (In a fourfold excess, one fourth of the cases would be occurring under normal conditions, the other three fourths are the "extra" ones.) This was based on the presumption that what was causing the melanoma excess was not the same thing that caused melanoma usually. It quickly became clear that this presumption was incorrect. The cases were unusual in that most shared some personal characteristics that we concluded (and are now well known) were susceptibility factors for melanoma. They included familial history of skin cancer, the presence of large moles, and a poor ability to tan but a heightened susceptibility to sunburn. This raised the suspicion that perhaps the LLNL had inadvertently recruited a high proportion of highly susceptible employees. However, because of another study in an adjacent county, which surveyed a sample of residents, we were able to establish that the prevalence of the susceptibility in the LLNL white employees and white resident nonemployees were identical.

Similarly, we examined every possible alternative explanation we could imagine. Some of our analyses we shared with the Melanoma Work Group, as we completed them. It was interesting to me to observe the response to some of our findings. Some LLNL scientists approached the whole issue with the apparent conviction that because they were "good" people, that they couldn't be responsible for anything like cancer. Therefore, either the data were in error, or the investigators (us) were not "good" people. Some of their alternative explanations for the observed excess, we could address in our analysis, however. Since this was a unique episode, there could be no way to evaluate the consistency of the findings with other studies, although a similar study of the nuclear test site in New Mexico did not find an excess of melanoma. About this time, Dr. Biggs retired and a new medical director was hired, a former naval officer.

We drafted a final report and planned a public presentation of the findings and then provided the LLNL with copies of our draft final report. The final report concluded that some of the workplace variables that were significant predictors were causal, and recommended that a further investigation be conducted by an occupational physician to more explicitly define what we could only identify as workplaces and types of materials. The workplace variables were: (a) ever exposed to radioactive materials, (b) handling volatile photographic chemicals, (c) exposure to fumes from high explosives, (d) having a work reason to go to the off-campus nonnuclear detonation worksite, (e) working as a chemist (as opposed to having a job classification as a chemist), (f) and work assignments in certain buildings.

Before the public presentation, I was visited by the new medical director and a woman who was his assistant. He had reviewed the draft report and came to talk to me about the use of the word "causal." He complimented me on the analysis and the amount of work done, but advised me, as a senior professional, not to use the word "causal" since it would certainly harm my career. We discussed this issue at some length and while we each heard each other's point of view, no positions were changed. His last comment was that I shouldn't agree to the word "cause" unless I was right. I responded that I thought I was right. His assistant commented, "You could be dead right, you know." I must admit that comment did cause me some consternation. It could have been a harmless joke. However, because the reason for saying it was unclear, I kept mulling it over in my head, trying to decide whether it was really a threat. I couldn't believe it really was, but how else could it be interpreted? I had never had reason to doubt the professionalism of the lab management or scientists.

ATTEMPTS TO IMPEACH THE VALIDITY OF THE FOLLOW-UP STUDY RESULTS

The lab had two responses to our report. The first was to send the report out to a large number of local and national epidemiologists, researchers, and melanoma clinicians for review. Dr. Carl Shy was engaged to compile the reports into a summary peer review. The complete report of each reviewer was available in the compiled report, but a summary was prepared using excerpts from the obtained reviews. The summary of the results was critical of the conclusions of the project. However, reading the individual reviews, most were complimentary of the study. Almost all agreed with our recommendations.

The second response was to request that we make our data available to an independent investigator for confirmation of our results. If we would remove all personally identifying information from the research files, the independent investigator would start with the raw interviews and independently code the information, create variables, and do a completely independent analysis. This well-funded contract went to an academic team, headed by a national leader in regression analyses at the University of North Carolina School of Public Health, to duplicate what we had done mostly on our own time. We agreed to withhold submitting our results for publication in a scientific journal until the reanalysis was complete, and we offered to jointly publish the results with them.

The reanalysis team eventually completed their analysis and presumably reported their findings to the LLNL, though we did not learn of the outcome for several years. Their results were nearly identical to ours, although they did not offer any detailed interpretation of the results or offer recommendations. We elected to publish separately.

POSTSCRIPT

In our final report on this study, we recommended that the lab use our epidemiologic risk factors to those target workers for a special surveillance program of melanomas. Instead, they opened up their medical clinic for any employees who wanted to be screened for melanomas or their precursors and had their melanoma consultant do the skin exams.

We also recommended that a follow-up investigation be conducted by an independent expert in occupational hygiene and occupational disease investigations. We felt that our relationship with the lab was now compromised and work done in that atmosphere was likely to become even more adversarial and less productive. The lab did hire an occupational physician, but instead of following up on our findings, he participated with the previously hired biostatistician to do studies aimed at detecting bias or other alternative explanations for the excess we found. The lab biostatistician subsequently published several papers on melanoma, some coming to conclusions that were at least somewhat in conflict with our findings. Those papers were not published in peer-reviewed epidemiology journals and, in fact, had some basic epidemiologic errors.

There have been no other occupational or public health interventions outside the lab, and in view of the fact that there was no evidence of any related effect in the nonemployee population, that's probably appropriate. Both Dr. Reynolds and I have been contacted several times by others who found melanoma excesses in other occupational groups, but those studies also seem to be of unique situations and probably not related to our study or its findings.

NOTES

1. The incidence rate for a cancer is the number of new (i.e., incident) cases of that cancer, diagnosed in a year, per 100,000 population.
2. Malignant melanoma is a cancer of the pigmented cells of the skin, though rarely it can occur in other pigmented parts, like the eye.

http://dx.doi.org/10.2190/TORC9

CHAPTER 9

The Risks of Making Nuclear Weapons

Robert Alvarez

When I first met Dr. Thomas F. Mancuso in the fall of 1977, he was poring over computer print-outs in his small, cluttered L-shaped office at the University of Pittsburgh.

Spry, with a trim mustache and horn-rimmed glasses, Mancuso's passion for data collection often compelled him to bring his work home. Despite his efforts to transform his large spacious home into a research archive, Mancuso's wife, Rae, kept the place spotless. Occasionally, data would be strewn on the dining room table, but most of the records were kept in dozens of filing cabinets in the basement, like a highly guarded treasure.

Since 1945, he had mastered the art of assembling millions of bits of information into groundbreaking studies to determine long-term workplace health hazards. Before his pioneering research, "the major focus on workplace health dealt with on-the-job injuries," said Bernard Goldstein, Dean of the Pittsburgh University School of Public Health in 2004. Mancuso "developed techniques to look at the long-term health effects of working" [1].

Having given away his car to one of his children several years before, the bespectacled physician walked every day to his office in the somber Graduate School building, often stopping first to attend Catholic mass. In contrast to his contemplative side, Mancuso's temper was legendary. But his stubborn quest for perfection was more than offset by his loyalty and kind generosity. These qualities had served him well over the years, but now they were being sorely tested in a struggle over the effects of ionizing radiation on nuclear workers.

Conflict over his studies was nothing new. But it was the unprecedented ferocity of this assault against his research that surprised him. Now as he approached the closing years of his illustrious career, Mancuso had not expected that his tedious sorting of statistics would put him at odds with the U.S. nuclear weapons program, one of the most powerful scientific establishments in the world.

EARLY RADIATION EXPOSURE PROBLEMS

Since World War II, the amassing of nuclear arms resulted in the creation of one of the largest and potentially most dangerous industrial enterprises in the nation. At the outset, the hazardous magnitude of nuclear weapons work was recognized by the scientific members of the Manhattan Project. These concerns led to the creation of the Health Division of the Manhattan Project, led by Dr. Robert Stone, chairman of the Radiology Department at the University of California Medical School in San Francisco. According to Stone,

> It was estimated that the pieces of uranium that would have to be removed from the pile [reactor] after fission had occurred would contain materials far more radioactive than any that had been encountered in the radium industry. The chemical process of separating the plutonium from other extremely radioactive elements was recognized as another tremendously hazardous procedure. The effect that plutonium itself might have on workers was unknown [2].

During the war, Stone concluded that, "the whole clinical study of the personnel is one vast experiment" [2, p. 14]. Like Stone, other officials, such as John Wirth, Medical Director at the Oak Ridge, Tennessee, recognized that the health consequences to workers could result in "the unexpected appearance of dangerous changes months or years after exposure" [3, p. 55]. Wirth recounted problems where "minute invisible fragments might make an entire building uninhabitable. . . . It is always amazing what widespread contamination can be caused by a minute quantity of hot material once it has been allowed to get out of a container" [3, pp. 44-45].

The Manhattan Project had standard worker compensation insurance, which only covered illnesses or disabilities that appeared within 90 days of an accident or 30 days after leaving the project. But Cyril Stanley Smith, chief metallurgical chemist at Los Alamos, denounced it as "inhumane, unethical and unfair," as he and his fellow chemists refused to work without extra insurance. Bending to their wishes, the U.S. government set up a secret one million dollar fund for the plutonium chemists at Los Alamos [3, p. 62].

Ordinary workers in the Manhattan Project fared less well. Ted Lombard was an enlisted man in the U.S. Army assigned to work at the Los Alamos Laboratory during the war, who recalled less-than-ideal working conditions:

> We used to go to Fort Douglas, Utah in ambulances [to] pick up uranium and plutonium. We carried dosimeter badges in our pockets because you couldn't display them. . . . Then [after the badges were turned over to an officer] we would proceed to unload uranium and plutonium barehanded . . . the fumes and dust were constantly in the air; there was no ventilation system. The dust was on the floor. Uranium chips would be in your shoes that you continued to wear. You went to eat with the same clothes on. You went to the barracks with the same clothes and sat on the beds [4].

Given widespread exposure problems, concerns over financial and legal liabilities also influenced radiation protection decisions. An overriding concern according to Stafford Warren, medical advisor to General Leslie Groves, military chief of the Manhattan Project, was to protect "the government interests" against legal claims [3, p. 51].

By 1980, Ted Lombard was suffering from fibrosis of the lungs, severe bone marrow and blood-forming organ damage. Four of his five children born after working at Los Alamos had severe medical problems, including neuromuscular and blood disorders. When Lombard filed a claim with the U.S. Department of Veterans Affairs, he was denied repeatedly on the grounds that his medical and exposure records were missing.

Shortly after World War II and through the early 1960s, senior ranks of the DOE and its predecessors were informed that large numbers of workers were being overexposed at federal nuclear sites in New Mexico, Washington, New York, Kentucky, Ohio, Colorado, and Tennessee. In 1948, the Atomic Energy Commission Advisory Committee on Biology and Medicine (ACBM) was provided data and analysis regarding large occupational doses of radiation from leaking radiochemical facilities at the Hanford site in Washington. According to Hanford's chief health physicist, radioactive particles that deposited in areas containing thousands of construction workers on the site "can produce radiation damage" and that "the theoretical possibility of injury developing 10 to 15 years from now poses a serious problem" [5].

That same year, the AEC manager of the Oak Ridge site "submitted a report on radiation history of employees," which recommend that a terminating employee be informed if he or she was exposed to levels above official limits and that medical assistance be provided if that person believes he or she was made ill or injured by radiation [6]. However, the committee rejected this recommendation, and proposed instead that "a terminating employee should be advised at the exit interview as to the care that the AEC utilizes in protecting each employee" [6].

At the time, fears over liability and lack of public trust that might result from disclosure of workplace hazards was of dominant concern. In a memo regarding possible declassification of a study suggesting that occupational radiation exposure levels "may be too high," the head of the Insurance Branch of the AEC declared,

> We can see the possibility of a shattering effect on the morale of the employees if they become aware that there was substantial reason to question the standards of safety under which they are working. In the hands of labor unions the results of this study would add substance to demands for extra-hazardous pay . . . knowledge of the results of this study might increase the number of claims of occupational injury due to radiation [7].

By June 1949, the ACBM was informed of excessive exposure to workers in uranium processing plants [8]. Some workers were being exposed at levels 125 times greater than the default standard adopted in World War II [8]. By this time it was recognized that this standard was not protective against radiation hazards [8].

Dr. Ernest Goodpasture, Vice Chairman of the ACBM, made repeated efforts to convince the commission to conduct radiation-related cancer studies. In December 1951, he wrote to AEC Chairman, Gordon Dean, stating that, "Cancer is a significant industrial hazard of the Atomic energy business. . . . The Committee recommends the cancer program be pursued as a humanitarian duty to the nation" [9]. His plea went unheeded.

THE MANCUSO STUDY

Although high-ranking officials were aware of potentially serious health risks to workers and were urged by its advisors to conduct health studies, the Atomic Energy Commission did not initiate occupational epidemiological research until 1964. That year, Dr. Thomas F. Mancuso, Professor of Occupational Medicine at the University of Pittsburgh, was approached by staff of the AEC's Division of Biology and Medicine to undertake a feasibility study. According to Mancuso, the AEC staff asked him if there were sufficient data to "answer a basic question, that is, whether there were or were not any effects of low-level ionizing radiation" [10]. Based on a review of records at 14 AEC facilities, Mancuso concluded it was possible, and was awarded a five-year research contract in 1965.

By that time, Mancuso had established himself as a highly respected figure in the field of occupational epidemiology. While serving as chief of the Ohio Division of Industrial Hygiene between 1945 and 1962, Mancuso published a series of ground-breaking studies showing the toxicological and carcinogenic effects of cadmium, manganese, mercury, hydrogen sulfide, asbestos, aromatic amines, and chromate [11-13]. With the encouragement of his mentor, Wilhelm Huper, at the National Cancer Institute [14], Mancuso designed and published the first cohort mortality studies on occupational cohorts in the United States [13]. In doing so Mancuso invented a revolutionary methodology using Social Security death benefit claims that enabled researchers for the first time to follow exposed workers over the many years necessary to detect latent diseases such as cancer [15]. In 1961, he had been given a career award by the National Cancer Institute for his impressive body of work.

Mancuso was also known for his honesty and fierce independence. In the 1950s, Phillip Carey Corp., a manufacturer of asbestos insulation hired Mancuso with the expectation that he would provide evidence refuting compensation claims by workers dying from respiratory diseases following exposure to asbestos. Instead, Mancuso's research supported the worker's claims. He strongly advised the company that it had a responsibility to inform the workers of potential risks. Because Phillip Carey ignored Mancuso's warning throughout the 1960s, his research was subsequently used by claimants [16].

What motivated the AEC officials to approach Mancuso? A key factor was that the national security imperative to exercise control over radiation heath effects research was loosening as Cold War tensions reduced. Moreover, the AEC suffered a serious blow to its credibility in 1963, when the United States, Great Britain, and the Soviet Union ratified the Limited Nuclear Test Ban Treaty, which prohibited atmospheric nuclear weapons tests.

Beginning in the1950s, a major and often contentious debate was sparked by scientists, such as Nobel Prize winners Herman Mueller and Linus Pauling, who warned that radioactive fallout from testing was harming human health across the globe. The AEC and its scientists vigorously defended the tests claiming they posed little if no harm. "There developed what I consider to be a strange psychological frame of mind," Dr. Karl Z. Morgan, founder and director of the AEC's Oak Ridge Health Physics Lab reflected several years later. "It became unpatriotic and perhaps unscientific to suggest that atomic weapons testing might cause deaths throughout the world from fallout." Morgan found many of his AEC colleagues holding "onto untenable and extremely shallow arguments [and making] comparisons with medical and natural background exposures as if they were harmless" [17, p. 2]. Official repudiation of the AEC's claims about fallout came in 1997, when the National Cancer Institute (NCI) revealed that atmospheric nuclear weapons detonations at the Nevada Test Site resulted in significant radiological contamination of the nation's milk supplies. NCI researchers estimated that fallout exposure to Iodine–131 from Nevada tests might cause 11,000 to 212, 000 excess thyroid cancers in the United States [18].

Other factors included the curtailment of fissile material production for nuclear weapons and the emergence of the U.S. nuclear power industry. By 1964, the U.S. nuclear arsenal was shrinking as more accurate delivery systems were deployed. This in turn significantly reduced demand for plutonium and highly enriched uranium—leading to the closure of several large production reactors and radiochemical processing facilities.

Concurrently, dozens of new power reactors were now planned for construction in the United States. The AEC, which was responsible for commercializing nuclear energy, was gearing up to accommodate this major growth, while setting the stage for a new generation of reactors that would use plutonium as fuel. To pave the way for these developments, the AEC needed to strengthen its credibility. In particular, the formalization of occupational radiation protection standards in 1959, which limited annual external exposure to 5 rem [19] per year, provided a necessary framework for both the continuation of civilian and military nuclear energy activities.

AEC managers received assurances from its scientific advisors that Mancuso's work would not lead to unpleasant surprises. In his 1980 paper about the Mancuso affair, Theodore D. Sterling, public health professor at Simon Fraser University in Canada, explores this concern and concludes: "It was firmly believed by all scientific advisors and by management that the study design was not adequate to lead to [findings of adverse effects]. Rather, the study was implemented and supported for frankly admitted *political* reasons" (original emphasis) [20]. After initiating the study, some AEC officials referred to it as "Mancuso's folly" and openly viewed it as a public-relations sham [21]. The political need to have Mancuso continue this study is reflected in review comments made in November 1967, by Dr. Brian MacMahon, an AEC consultant from Harvard University:

> In my opinion this study does not have, and never (in any practical sense) will have any possibility of contributing to knowledge of radiation effects in man. I recognize that much of the motivation for starting this study arose from the "political" need for assurances that AEC employees are not suffering harmful effect [21].

MacMahon was seconded in November 1967 by Dr. William Schull, a geneticist who had worked on the Japanese Atomic Bomb Survivor study. Like previous advisors, Schull was interested in protecting the AEC against compensation claims:

> It seems highly improbable that if one went through the mechanics of calculating the kinds of radiation effects, which a study of the present magnitude might detect, one would be led to conclude that the undertaking is a hopeless one. However, as earlier recognized, it may have other merit in that it may provide a firmer basis for settlement of claims against the Atomic Energy Commission [21].

During the 1960s and early 1970s, Mancuso compiled data on workers at several facilities. He focused on the Hanford site in Washington State and the Oak Ridge site in Tennessee because they were the oldest and largest federal nuclear facilities. Throughout this period, AEC officials were eager for him to publish. "Repeatedly . . . I had been urged by [the AEC and its successor the

Energy Research and Development Administration—now the Department of Energy] to publish in scientific journals, the negative findings of the progress reports, and I refused to do so," stated Mancuso. "I believed that the findings would be misleading, no matter how well qualified in the presentation and could be misused" [10, p. 554].

By February 1973, Dr. Sidney Marks, Mancuso's AEC worker-study contract officer grew frustrated and suggested "early replacement of the contractor."

> Unless an immediate replacement [for Mancuso] is found, a public charge may be made that the AEC is stopping the program out of fear that positive findings may emerge. Overtures to possible candidates may be carried out in a clandestine atmosphere [10, p. 750].

Nonetheless, AEC officials tolerated Mancuso's reluctance to publish until the situation was abruptly transformed in late June of 1974. This is when Dr. Samuel Milham, an epidemiologist with the Washington State Department of Social and Health Services, met with AEC officials to report findings of a study he had just completed. Encompassing 300,000 deaths from 1950 to 1974, Milham compared the mortality of different occupations in the state and found that:

> Men who worked at the Atomic Energy Commission Hanford facility in Richland, Washington showed increased mortality from cancer, especially in men under age 64 at death. An excess was seen for cancer of the tongue, mouth, and pharynx, colon, pancreas, lung and bone. Excess mortality was also seen for aplastic anemia and amyotrophic lateral sclerosis [10, p. 495].

He concluded that, "since the Hanford facility is involved in the handling, fabrication, processing and storage of an array of radioactive materials, most of which are of proven carcinogenicity, I suggest that these materials are the most likely source for the observed cancer excess" [10]. At the meeting in Richland, Washington, Milham recalled that the atmosphere was "like a funeral, quiet, no smile. . . . The impression I got at the meeting with the AEC was that the release of my finding might cause concern and problems in the industry" [10]. After the meeting Milham decided to not to publish his findings, "because I was convinced that the appropriate population-based studies were in progress [under Mancuso's direction]. I felt that publication of my findings at this time might disturb the continuity of the study in progress and might cause undue concern in workers" [10].

Shortly after, Mancuso "was on the phone by the hour over a period of weeks" with AEC officials in the Division of Biology and Medicine. Dr. Sidney Marks, Mancuso's AEC contract officer, urged Mancuso to endorse a draft press release that stated "there is no evidence of cancer or other deaths attributable to ionizing radiation occurring more often among Hanford workers" [10, p. 559].

But Mancuso refused, explaining to Marks that Milham's findings could not be dismissed because they were based on more recent mortality data Mancuso had yet to obtain. Furthermore, Milham's study included construction workers at the Hanford site, which were not part of the AEC-sponsored study. Hanford construction workers, according to Mancuso, were "acknowledged to have more exposure" than operators, and his repeated attempts to have this group incorporated into his study over the years were denied [10, p. 531].

It was then that AEC officials started to end their relationship with Mancuso. In the summer of 1974, the AEC initiated a process to transfer a major portion of Mancuso's study to Oak Ridge Associated Universities (ORAU) in Tennessee. For several years the AEC, the National Aeronautics and Space Administration (NASA), and the Defense Department sponsored studies involving total body irradiation of animals and dozens of human patients in specially designed radiation chambers at ORAU, but funding for the research program was about to end. According to a 1975 report to NASA, ORAU study director, Dr. Clarence C. Lushbaugh, justified the experiments in part because, "unbiased clinical observations were sorely needed to defend existing environmental and occupational exposure constraints from attack by well-meaning but impractical theorists" [22].

Termination of this study was prompted in April 1974 by a critical extramural medical review, which gave it an "unfavorable rating." The panel reported that "the clinical facilities were substandard with respect to licensing and accreditation guidelines" [23]. In particular, the reviewers took issue with the clinical hematology program and sloppy research practices that may have endangered patients. Underneath the wood floor of one of the radiation chambers in which cancer patients were treated, researchers suspended cages of mice—creating sanitary hazards. According to the review,

> Animal caretakers enter the area twice a week to change the cages. . . . Dirty cages are taken through the patient area to an elevator and on to the cage washer. . . . This entire arrangement seems questionable because of the necessity of transporting animal, animal wastes and equipment through areas used by patients who frequently have compromised host defense mechanisms. Also this area would appear to be highly prone to severe infestations of vermin [23].

"In view of accepted therapeutic modalities," the reviewers reported, "*ethical questions were raised with respect to the protocol employed in these studies*" (emphasis added) [23].

Despite these problems, AEC officials appeared more interested in shoring up ORAU with new work. This was underscored by its decision to award ORAU with a large contract without the benefit of peer review, scientific protocol, principal investigator, and to an institution which had not performed epidemiological research before [25]. According to a memorandum prepared by the division of Biology and Medicine in January 1976, "Since ORAU medical division has been informed that, *if they developed the necessary expertise,* the health and mortality study will be transferred to ORAU and is to be phased in during the last year of Mancuso's contract which would begin in August 1, 1976" (emphasis added) [24, p. 533].

The AEC also took steps to move Mancuso's research to Battelle, which ran the Hanford laboratory. Dr. Ethyl Gilbert, a statistician working for Battelle at Hanford's Pacific Northwest was first tasked to review the Milham study. Around the summer of 1975, Gilbert submitted her analysis, in which she stated, "Our data exhibit no clear-cut relationship of death from cancer and radiation exposure" [24, p. 514]. A key table in her study, however, did show a relationship between radiation exposure and excess deaths [24, p. 516]. Alex Fremling, the AEC manager at the Hanford also reached a much different conclusion than Gilbert when he reported,

> There is a relationship between cancer as a cause of death and the total dose of external radiation received. . . . The message is clear that Battelle's data suggests that Hanford has a higher proportion of cancer deaths for those under 65 than the US. . . . Even more disturbing from our standpoint [is that] the analysis tends to show a much higher incidence of certain types of cancer [at doses below official limits]. . . . We hoped to get a good answer to the Milham report, and instead it looks like we have confirmed it [26].

The Battelle study remained buried until it was submitted into the record by Dr. Milham in 1978 at a hearing of the U.S. Congress [24, pp. 515-516].

In March 1975, the Energy Research and Development Administration (ERDA), the AEC's successor, informally notified Mancuso of its intentions when Marks asked him at a meeting, "You don't want to continue on with his project do you" [24]. Mancuso replied "clearly and definitively" that he wanted to devote the rest of his professional career to this research [24]. But Mancuso knew the die was cast after his colleagues approached Dr. James Liverman, Director of AEC's Division of Biology and Medicine, in 1975 and were told that an administrative decision to give the research to Oak Ridge Associated Universities and Battelle was already made. In January 1976, the University of Pittsburgh was formally notified by the Department of Energy, which succeeded ERDA, that it would not renew Mancuso's contract when it expired in 1977 [24, p. 554].

In March of 1976, Mancuso asked Dr. Alice M. Stewart and George Kneale, her statistician from the University of Birmingham in England, to analyze his data. Dr. Stewart, a member of Mancuso's advisory committee, was internationally recognized as establishing the link between fetal x-rays and childhood cancers. Since 1955, when she and her colleagues first reported this finding,

Stewart had constructed one of the world's largest epidemiological studies of low-dose ionizing radiation, the Oxford Survey of Childhood Cancers.

By the summer of 1976, Mancuso, Stewart, and Kneale produced a cohort analysis based on 3,710 deaths among Hanford workers collected up to 1973. They found a 5 to 7 percent excess in cancer deaths attributable to radiation. Workers exposed after the age of 45 showed higher sensitivity to cancer. Most significantly, the risk of dying from radiation-induced cancer appeared to be about ten times greater than current protection standards assumed. As soon as the analysis was finalized Mancuso and his colleagues briefed the Energy Department in October 1976 [27]. "They were clearly unhappy," Mancuso said. "They urged us not to publish. . . . My job in their eyes was simply to transfer the data to them" [28]. Present at the meeting was Sidney Marks. After helping to orchestrate Mancuso's firing, Marks left his government employment in June 1976 to administer the Hanford worker study at Battelle, where Ethyl Gilbert worked under his supervision [24].

By the fall of 1977, Mancuso's research funds had run out. In November, he published his paper in *Health Physics*, creating a firestorm of controversy. Though he continued to draw a salary from the University of Pittsburgh, Mancuso had no funds with which to continue his research. Though it was a bare fraction of what was needed, Mancuso began cutting into his personal retirement money to continue working on the Hanford study. Meanwhile the federal government persisted in its attempts to take the data away from him and most disturbingly, to destroy data Mancuso had collected.

Upon assuming control over the DOE worker study in 1977, Dr. Lushbaugh, Chief of Radiation Studies at ORAU, proceeded to shred and incinerate medical records from the Oak Ridge Hospital preserved by Mancuso [29]. All told, 21 out of 40 filing cabinets spanning the period 1952 to 1961 were destroyed. Mancuso took custody of the records after the old hospital, owned by the federal government, was transformed into the Methodist Medical Center. In November 1985, when allegations were made about the destruction, Lushbaugh claimed "we would never destroy these records" [30]. Several days later, ORAU officials conceded that the records were destroyed, and they were unaware they had been set aside by Mancuso. In his final report to the DOE in November 1977, Mancuso had clearly identified these records as part of his research program [31].

But in early 1978, the Department of Energy had come under Congressional scrutiny for its handling of Mancuso's contract. At the hearings before the House Energy and Commerce Subcommittee on Health and the Environment, it was brought out that the DOE had not informed Mancuso of the ostensible reason for his termination—that being his "imminent retirement" at age 62 from the University of Pittsburgh. Mancuso only learned of this reason in September 1977 in a letter from James Liverman to Karl Z. Morgan [32]. However, the AEC had not bothered to learn the university's policy, which set the mandatory retirement age at 70 years.

In his testimony to the subcommittee, Liverman backed away from the excuse of Mancuso's "imminent retirement." Instead, he charged that early peer reviews of Mancuso's work had been critical of him, when in fact they had lauded his capabilities and recommended that the study be continued under his control [32]. In the course of the hearings, Subcommittee Chair Paul Rogers (D-FL) concluded,

> It's the most disordered, unstructured mess that I have looked into some time. If our research programs are being carried out in this manner, where you just take a study from one scientist and give it to another group without knowing who the principal investigator will be or his qualifications, this is a very inefficient, poor way of managing a research program and is not a competent way to spend tax dollars [24, p. 783].

Congressmen Paul Rogers (D-FL.) and Tim Lee Carter (D-KY.) subsequently reported to Energy Secretary Schlesinger, that the justifications for the decision to fire Mancuso were "not supported" and the decision to transfer Mancuso's study to Oak Ridge was "highly questionable at best." The whole process, they said, reflected "serious mismanagement and is of highly questionable legality" [33].

In 1979, in response to Congressional hearings regarding the handling of Mancuso's contract and revelations about radiation exposure to military personnel and civilians from U.S. atmospheric nuclear weapons tests, a Federal Interagency Taskforce on Ionizing Radiation was convened by President Carter. The Taskforce, chaired by Health, Education, and Welfare Secretary, Joseph Califano, reported in 1980 that the Department of Energy maintained a virtual monopoly over the funding of radiation health effects research; and that the DOE had a potential conflict-of-interest between its missions of military and civilian nuclear energy development and assessing their health impacts. Califano proposed removing radiation health effects research from DOE's control and placing it in public health agencies [5]. Even so, Mancuso continued to face opposition. He managed to continue the study through private donations and his retirement money until labor unions pressured the National Institute of Occupational Safety and Health to reinstate the study in August 1979. This lasted until the spring of 1981—when the Reagan administration informed Mancuso his funding would once again be terminated.

Despite the difficulty in obtaining funding, Mancuso, Stewart, and Kneale persisted in their research and publications in the scientific literature [34]. By 1990, the Three Mile Island Public Health Fund, established as part of a legal settlement resulting from the Three-Mile Island nuclear accident in 1979, funded the continued work of Dr. Stewart and Kneale. While strongly supportive of their efforts, Dr. Mancuso had effectively withdrawn from the work, as a result of the difficult experience. However, in 1993, Mancuso published an analysis of Hanford workers, which clearly indicated that he had not given up the struggle:

> The search for the biological effects among worker cohorts has been mostly in terms of mortality experience. Yet it is well known that the primary and secondary causes of death on a death certificate do not reflect the diseases or illnesses which may have occurred prior to death. . . .The consequences have been the underestimation of the true nature and magnitude of occupational health effects when based solely on death certificates. . . . The death certificate provides a gross underestimate of the biological effects which may have occurred in that population [35].

THE AFTERMATH OF THE MANCUSO AFFAIR

The contract with Dr. Mancuso was in a sense a failed experiment by the federal nuclear program to enter the mainstream of public health. Most importantly, the Mancuso contract deviated from standard practices established by the nuclear weapons program in which a system of "in-house" contractors whose existence depended primarily on the federal nuclear program was fostered deliberately. By terminating Mancuso's study, the Department of Energy returned to business as usual. But as events unfolded, the federal nuclear program never truly recovered from the aftermath of this failed experiment.

In 1989, in response to Congressional pressure and a growing lack of public trust, Energy Secretary James Watkins convened the Secretarial Panel for the Evaluation of Epidemiologic Research Activities. The Panel reported that Energy's research lacked coordination and suffered from lack of peer review and competition for funding [36]. In 1990, the DOE entered into a formal agreement with the Department of Health and Human Services to manage and conduct DOE worker-health studies paid for by the Department of Energy. Since that time, these studies were obscured from public attention and went unappreciated. This all changed when the Secretary of Energy, Bill Richardson, announced on July 14, 1999 that the Clinton administration would seek to establish a federal compensation program for sick Energy Department contract employees.

In early 2000, the Department of Energy compiled a selected group of health studies of Department of Energy contractor employees from the most recent editions of published articles and unpublished technical reports. Additional recent published studies were obtained from peer-reviewed scientific journals. Based on the studies complied, this author analyzed twenty-seven studies of workers at DOE sites and nuclear sites in the United Kingdom and Canada.

All told, workers at fourteen DOE facilities were found to have increased risks of dying from various cancers and nonmalignant diseases [37-53]. The facilities include:

- Hanford nuclear materials production site in Washington
- Oak Ridge National Laboratory in Tennessee
- Oak Ridge Tennessee Eastman Electromagnetic Separation facility (TEC)

- Oak Ridge Y-12 weapons facility
- Oak Ridge K-25 Gaseous Diffusion Plant
- Feed Materials Production Center in Fernald, Ohio
- Los Alamos National Laboratory in New Mexico
- Linde Air Products uranium processing operation in New York
- Mallikrodt Chemical Works in Missouri
- Mound Laboratory in Ohio
- Rocky Flats facility in Colorado
- Savannah River Site in South Carolina
- Rocketdyne/Atomic International Facility in California
- Lawrence Livermore National Laboratory in California

By the end of the twentieth century, the Department of Energy occupational epidemiological studies constituted one of the world's largest and most extensive follow-ups of people exposed to low-level ionizing radiation and other substances. Dr. Mancuso had put in place a foundation that eventually provided a basis for the study of some 600,000 people who worked for federal contractors at industrial and research sites.

In December 2000, the United States enacted the Energy Employee Occupational Illness Compensation Act. The law represents the first time any nation has officially acknowledged that its workers were harmed from the production of nuclear weapons; and has established a entitlement program to compensate workers and their survivors. All told, some 700,000 people who worked at over 300 facilities in the United States can file for compensation. This unprecedented law would not have been possible without the pioneering work of Dr. Thomas F. Mancuso, who passed away on July 7, 2004, at the age of 92.

The groundbreaking contributions to occupational cancer epidemiology that Mancuso left behind remain today as primary sources used to protect the public and workers, as well as for compensation for illness and injury. "He was for a half century a leading light in occupational epidemiology," wrote public health physician Michael Gochfeld in 2005 [12]. While Dr. Mancuso may be most remembered for the controversy surrounding his last struggle to bring the risks of radiation in the nuclear workplace to light, his quest for the truth, and his deep respect for working people will serve as his lasting heritage.

NOTES

1. Taylor, M. 9 July 2004. Dr. Thomas Mancuso, long-time advocate for worker's health, Obituary, *San Francisco Chronicle.*
2. Stone, R. S. 1948. Health protection activities of the Manhattan Project. *Proceedings of the American Philosophy Society*. 90(1):11-19.
3. Haeker, B. C. 1987. *The Dragon's Tail: Radiation Safety in The Manhattan Project 1942-1946.* University of California Press, pp. 44-62.

4. Invisible Violence. 26 April 1980. Proceedings of the National Hearing on Radiation Victims. Environmental Policy Institute, Washington, DC.
5. U.S. Senate Committee on Governmental Affairs. December 1989. Early health problems of the U.S. nuclear weapons program and their implications for today. Majority Staff Report.
6. U.S. Atomic Energy Commission. 10-11 December 1948. Advisory Committee for Biology and Medicine. Thirteenth Meeting. U.S. Department of Energy Archives: 1947-1951. Secretariat Files. Box 1217, Folder 337. Germantown, MD. The report recommended:
   (1) a terminating employee be provided with a statement that he has not exceeded the permissible exposure to radiation, or *if he has exceeded the permissible exposure he be made aware of this fact by the physician giving the exit interview* [emphasis added];
   (2) that there be a clearer policy on release of information on radiation exposure records and other medical records to the contractor's insurance and life insurance companies;
   (3) that the terminating employee be advised that if he is to work with radiation in the future his new employer can make arrangements to procure his past radiation exposure history;
   (4) *that a group of qualified radiologists and physicians be available for consultation by any person who feels that he has been damaged by radiation at an AEC installation.* [emphasis added]
7. Report of the President's Advisory Committee on Human Radiation Experiments. Part II, Chapter 13. http://www.eh.doe.gov/ohre/roadmap/achre/ chap13_3.html
8. U.S. Atomic Energy Commission. 11 June 1949. Advisory Committee for Biology and Medicine. Sixteenth meeting. Transcript. U.S. Department of Energy Archives. AEC Division of Biology and Medicine Collection. Box 3218, Folder ACBM Meeting. Germantown, MD.
9. Goodpasture, E. W. 1 December 1951. Letter to Gordon Dean, Chairman of the Atomic Energy Commission. U.S. Department of Energy Archive. Germantown, MD.
10. Mancuso, T. F. 1978. Statement before the House Energy and Commerce Subcommittee on Health and the Environment Hearings. Effect of radiation on human health. U.S. Congress, House Committee on Interstate and Foreign Commerce, Subcommittee on Health and the Environment. 95th Cong., 2nd Sess., January 24-26, February 8, 9, 14, and 28, 1978, Serial No. 95-179, Vol. 1, p. 523.
11. Mancuso, T. F. 1949. Occupational cancer survey in Ohio. *Proceeding of the Public Health Cancer Association of America*, 50-60.
12. Gochfeld, M. 2005. Chronologic history of occupational medicine. *Journal of Occupational Medicine* 47(2):96-114.
13. Michaels, V. 2005. Comings and goings, Thomas Mancuso. NYCOSH. 8 July 2004. http://www.nycosh.org/UPDATE/printableArticle.php?articleid=454
14. Mancuso, T. F. Interview. 6 September 1980.
15. Mancuso, T. F. 1959. Methods of study of the relations of employment and long-term illness by cohort analysis. *American Journal of Public Health* 49:1525-1536.

16. United States Congress. 24 July 2000. House of Representatives, 106th Congress, 2nd Session. House Report 106-782–Asbestos Compensation Act of 2000. Available from http://thomas.loc.gov/cgi-bin/cpquery/T?&report=hr782&dbname=106&
17. Morgan, K. Z. December 1980. History of developments in nuclear safety and the development of international standards. Unpublished article submitted to Energy Department's Office of Consumer Affairs.
18. Simon, S. L., Bouville, A., and Land, C. E. 2006. Fallout from nuclear weapons tests and cancer risks. *American Scientists Online* 94(1):48.
19. Roentgen equivalent for man. A roentgen (an international unit of X- or gamma-radiation) adjusted for the atomic makeup of the human body.
20. Sperling, T. P. 1980. The health effects of low-dose radiation on atomic workers: A case study of employer directed research. *International Journal of Health Services* 10(1):37-47.
21. Mancuso, T. F. Interview. October 1980.
22. Oak Ridge Associated Universities. Studies relative to radiosensitivity of man: based on retrospective evaluations of therapeutic and accidental total-body irradiation. NASA-CR-144439. pp. 6-8.
23. U.S. Atomic Energy Commission. 16 April 1974. Extramural reviews of Oak Ridge Associated Universities, specific comments on LETBI and METBI Programs.
24. Mancuso, T. F. 1978. Effect of radiation on human health, p. 783. February 1978. Hearings before the U.S. House Energy and Subcommittee explored the process in which the contract Mancuso held was transferred. The questioning of DOE official, Dr. Walter Weyzen, and Dr. Sidney Marks, then at Battelle, by Subcommittee Chair, Rep. Paul Rogers is most revealing:

Mr. Rogers: So you didn't know the person who was going to be charge of the study, but you transferred it anyway?

Dr. Weyzen: It was transferred, yes, sir.

Mr. Rogers: And you did not know who would be the chief investigator would be?

Dr. Weyzen: Certainly, I didn't know at the time.

Mr. Rogers: Did you, Dr. Marks?

Dr. Marks: May I say that the decision to transfer would be contingent on proper staffing. The transfer was not made in March 1975. Discussions were held at the time in anticipation of the transfer on July 31, 1977 if proper staffing were developed.

Mr. Rogers: Then you told me before that the judgment was made to transfer the study back then, but you didn't even have a chief investigator. And now you come and divide it up again, where you have Dr. Marks at the meeting who is beneficiary from his corporation and you have Lushbaugh, who is a beneficiary. That group gets together and divides up a study, without any peer review.

Dr. Marks: Mr. Chairman, at the meeting of September of 1977?

Mr. Rogers: Yes.

Dr. Marks: The question of dividing up the study did not come up. The session was largely devoted to questions regarding the data base and the manner in which the study will be heard, carried forth in the future.

Mr. Rogers: Well now I thought Dr. Weyzen told us that it was on that basis that he made the judgment for separating the study.

Dr. Weyzen: That is correct, sir.

24. Mancuso, T. F. 1978. Effect of radiation on human health. p. 719.
Hearing Excerpt: Questioning of Dr. Sidney Marks by Congressman Paul Rogers
Mr. Rogers: When did you leave ERDA, Dr. Marks?
Dr. Marks: I left in June 1976.
Mr. Rogers: When were you hired by Battelle?
Dr. Marks: June 1976.
Mr. Rogers: Are you now doing part of the work that was originally covered in its contract in your organization?
Dr. Marks: I am assisting Dr. Gilbert. She is the principal investigator.
Mr. Rogers: Is it under your supervision?
Dr. Marks: Only in the sense that all environmental heath and safety work is under the supervision of—
Mr. Rogers: That is all I am asking. Is it under your office, as I understand it in Battelle?
Dr. Marks: Yes it is.
25. Milham, S. According to this table, workers who received the highest dose of 2.14 rems or more ten years prior to death showed elevated death rates for al cancers (27%) colon cancer (200%), pancreas (52%), lymphosarcoma (334%) and other lymphatic cancers (783%).
26. Fremling, A. 17 July 1975. Director, Atomic Energy Commission. Draft AEC Memorandum. Richland Operations Office.
27. Mancuso, T. F., Stewart, A. M., and Kneale, G. W. 1977, November. Radiation exposures of Hanford workers dying from cancer and other causes. *Health Physics Journal* 33(5):369-385.
28. Mancuso, T. F. Interview. 10 September 1980.
29. Lushbaugh, C. Interview. 3 June 1989.
30. Powellson, R. 1985. DOE health data destroyed, probers told. 15 November 1985. *Knoxville News–Sentinel.*
31. Powellson, R. Agency destroyed OR heath records. 21 November 1985. *Knoxville News–Sentinel.*
32. Liverman, J. Director of Division of Biology and Medicine, Atomic Energy Commission. 8 September 1977. Letter To: Karl Z. Morgan, Neeley Professor, Georgia Institute for Technology.
33. Rogers, P., and Carter, T. L. U.S. Representatives. 4 May 1978. Letter to James Schlesinger, Secretary, Department of Energy.
34. Mancuso, T. F. et al. 1978. A reanalysis of data relating to the Hanford study of the cancer risks of radiation workers. *International Atomic Agency Symposium Proceedings on the Late Biological Effects of Ionizing Radiation.* Vienna, Austria: IAEA-SM-224/510; Stewart, M. et al., 1980. Hanford IIb, The Hanford data—A reply to recent criticisms. *Ambio* 9; Hanford III, A cohort study of the cancer risks from radiation to workers at Hanford (1944 to 1977 deaths) by method of regression models in life-tables. *British Journal of Industrial Medicine* summer 1981.
35. Mancuso, T. F. 1993. Methodology in industrial health studies: Social security disability data and the medical care system. *American Journal of Industrial Medicine* 23:653-671.

36. Richardson, D. 25 September 1997. Low-dose radiation exposure. Public Meeting on Worker Health. Transcript http://www.sea-us.org.au/roxstop97/tdave3.htm
37. Mancuso, T. F., Stewart, A. M., and Kneale, G. W. 1977. Radiation exposures of Hanford workers dying from cancer and other causes. *Health Physics* 33: 369-385.
38. Gilbert, E. S., Omohundro, E., Buchanan, J. A., and Holter, N. A. 1993. Mortality of workers at the Hanford site. *Health Physics* 64:6:577-590.
39. Stewart, A. M., and Kneale, G. W. 1996. Relations between age at occupational exposure to ionizing radiation and cancer risk. *Occupational and Environmental Medicine* 53:225-230.
40. Richardson, D., and Wing, S. 1999. Radiation and mortality of workers at Oak Ridge National Laboratory: Positive associations for doses received at older ages. *Environmental Health Perspectives* 107:8 (Mortality study)
41. Wing, S., Shy, C. M., Wood, J., Wolf, S., Cragle, D., and Frome, E. L. 1991. Mortality among workers at Oak Ridge National Laboratory, evidence of radiation effects in follow-up through 1984. *Journal of the American Medical Association* 265: 1397-1402. (Mortality study)
42. Wing, S., Shy, C. M., Wood, J. L., Wolf, S., Cragle, D., Tankersley, W., and Frome, E. L. 1993. Job factors, radiation and cancer mortality at Oak Ridge National Laboratory: Follow-up through 1984. *American Journal of Industrial Medicine* 23: 265-279.
43. Loomis, D. P., and Wolfe, S. H. 1996. Mortality of workers at a nuclear materials production plant at Oak Ridge, Tennessee, 1947-1990. *American Journal of Medicine* 29:131-141.
44. Checkoway, H., Pierce, N., Crawford-Brown, D. J., and Cragle, D. 1998. Radiation doses and cause-specific mortality among workers at a nuclear materials fabrication plant. *American Journal of Epidemiology* 127(2):255-266.
45. Dupree, E. A., Wells, S. M., Watkins, J. P., Wallace, P. W., Davis, N. C. No date. Mortality among workers employed between 1945 and 1984 at a uranium gaseous diffusion facility. Draft Report. Oak Ridge Institute for Science and Education.
46. Cragle, D. L., Watkins, J. P., Ingle, J. N., Robertson-Demers, K., Tankersley, W. G., and West, C. M. No date. Mortality among a cohort of white male workers at a uranium processing plant: Fernald Feed Materials Production Center (FMPC). (Radiation research)
47. Wiggs, L. D., Johnson, E. R., Cox-DeVore, C. A., and Voelz, G. L. 1994. Mortality through 1990 among white male workers at the Los Alamos National Laboratory: Considering exposures to plutonium and external ionizing radiation. *Health Physics* 67:6:557-586.
48. DuPree, E. A., Cragle, D., McLain, R. W., Crawford-Brown, D., and Teta, M. J. 1987. Mortality among workers at a uranium processing facility, the Linde Air Products Company Ceramics Plant, 1943-49. *Scandinavian Journal of Worker and Environmental Health* 13:100-107.
49. DuPree E., Watkins, J. P., Ingle, J. N., and Phillips, J. A. No date. External radiation exposure and mortality among a cohort of uranium processing workers. Oak Ridge, TN: Oak Ridge Associated Universities. Unpublished report.

50. Wiggs, L. D., Cox-DeVore, C. A., and Voelz, G. 1991. Mortality among a cohort of workers monitored for polonium-210 exposure: 1944-1972. *Health Physics* 61(1):71-76.
51. Wilkinson, G. S., Teitjen, G. L. Wiggs, L. D., Gaike, W. A., Aquavella, J. F., Reyes, M., Voelz, G. L., and Waxweiler, R. J. 1987. Mortality among plutonium and other radiation workers at a plutonium weapons facility. *American Journal of Epidemiology* 125(2):231-250.
52. Cragle, D., Robertson-Demeyers, K., and Watkins, J. P. No date. Mortality among workers at a nuclear fuels production facility: The Savannah River site, 1952-1986. Oak Ridge Institute for Science and Education. Submitted manuscript.
53. Ritz, B., Morgenstern, H., Froines, J., and Batts, B. 1999. Effects to external ionizing radiation on cancer mortality in nuclear workers monitored for radiation at Rocketdyne/Atomics International. *American Journal of Industrial Medicine* 35: 21-31.

http://dx.doi.org/10.2190/TORC10

CHAPTER 10

Improving Community Research Protections for Communities Exposed to Cold War Nuclear Experiments

Dianne Quigley

Research ethics protections should be a major consideration in the conduct of community health studies in potentially politically charged research settings, such as nuclear weapons experiments, production activities and related health research on affected populations. Health assessments in these settings typically have higher levels of scientific uncertainty and "grey areas" in data modeling and data interpretation. Problems and complaints of research bias, incomplete assessments and statistical manipulations easily can surround studies with scientific uncertainty. Participatory research approaches, ethics guidelines and other field evidence can become critical resources for improving ethical approaches to these communities of study. The design and conduct of health studies around nuclear weapons facilities lacked substantial ethical guidance for protecting communities from negative research experiences and for ensuring community value and fairness in study designs, outcomes and publicity. Community consultation was developed for health studies but mostly for providing advice to researchers. More progressive models of community engagement, such as community-based research partnerships, were not considered. Additionally, the need to obtain community agreement or approval in the conduct of community health studies is a key area of development for the purposes of maximizing benefits and minimizing harm in these settings. Such ethical advice was not incorporated into the research approaches used around nuclear weapons facilities. In this chapter, I address ethical concerns related to community health research by detailing the advice of research ethics guidelines and new research approaches for community studies for their value in improving the ethical challenges that are dramatically expressed within the community and academic narratives. Advice from research ethics professionals who are trained in research ethics protections for communities of study could have helped to improve the beneficence of the health studies that were conducted. In this chapter the experiences of community members, health organizers, and researchers captured in the narratives here broaden an understanding of beneficence and nonmaleficence in research related to nuclear weapons activities. The narratives point to considerable work to be done in increasing our moral progress with these research ethics issues.

OVERVIEW OF ETHICAL CONCERNS

In his chapter, Krimsky reviews a set of ethical challenges that were evident in the conduct of health studies on community and worker populations around nuclear facilities [1, pp. 7-24, this volume]. I restate them here to create more understanding of the need for more ethical guidance with community health investigations:

- Pressures from national security/secrecy considerations that may impede the disclosure of harms to citizens;
- Forms of technical compartmentalization that would diminish understandings of interrelated risk impacts of nuclear weapons production (social, ethical, cultural, environmental, economic impacts);
- A dominant focus on technically-controlled risk-benefit calculations. This single focus can produce research activities and discourse decisions that are inaccessible to the communities-at-risk. The specialized and reductive nature of this scientific inquiry can exclude "quality of life" meanings and values for communities-at-risk;
- The ethical treatment of weaknesses in study designs (lack of adequate human and environmental exposure measures for specified time periods) and a lack of statistical power in epidemiological studies typically producing inconclusive/negative findings about health impacts of contamination;
- Public fears of scientific contrivance to minimize adverse health effects from contamination (types of scientific controversy, the termination or marginalization of scientists who produce positive findings from health risk impacts)
- The behavior of scientists and public health officials who become self-identified with a government agency to protect it against any claims of malfeasance; and
- The moral disengagement of researchers from valuable public health findings.

In addressing these ethical concerns, research teams would need to realize that research beneficence needs to achieve more than technical accuracy, particularly in light of the political, socio-economic and other contextual conditions of the affected communities. These challenges require the assistance of public health research ethicists to deal with the socially complex dimensions of the conduct of research around nuclear weapons experiments. A high reliance on risk assessments, epidemiological studies and dose assessments for understanding the health impacts of high risk technological activities can dwarf other considerations about research beneficence to affected community members. These technical approaches mostly focus on quantitative health assessments where researchers primarily strive for technical accuracy—only one area of research beneficence. Challenged by the demands for scientific rigor in these technical approaches, researchers often cannot work deeply with maximizing other benefits and minimizing harms to the community as the subject of research.

A Report from the Advisory Committee on Human Radiation Experiments (ACHRE) exposed critical areas of ethical improprieties in the actions of government researchers conducting scientific and Cold War experiments that led to individual and community harms [2]. These harms also extend to forms of cultural injustice to native, Polynesian and Black-American exposed groups, as discussed by ACHRE. An understanding of these problems regarding the ethical conduct of government researchers who conducted Cold War nuclear experiments is relevant to an assessment of the ethical conduct of the government researchers conducting health studies of these affected communities. ACHRE produced the findings below as the government community health studies were underway. It is not clear if the ACHRE findings were able to influence the conduct of these National Center of Environmental Health (NCEH) and DOE-funded studies of the affected communities/workers.

ACHRE Recommendations to the Human Radiation Interagency Working Group (Chapter 18, ACHRE Report)

- A practice of government secrecy led to a failure to disclose research harms from inadequate informed consent to research subjects to avoid potential liability and embarrassment (Chap. 18, Rec. 1-6:2). The rights, welfare and interests of citizens were violated in secret research leading to the abuses of individual rights and erosion of public trust in government.
- Inadequate record-keeping practices prevented research subjects from having exposure measurements from research experiments, which could have led to compensation for medical harms.
- Culturally-induced moral ignorance led to the unnecessary exposures of high-level radon daughters to Navajo uranium miners and their

subsequent respiratory cancers/deaths when ventilation measures could have been installed (Chap.18, Rec. 7-12:1).

- Cultural and health harms from radiation exposures from nuclear tests led to excess thyroid disease for the indigenous populations of the Marshall Islands. Inadequate communication (cultural incompetence) of the need for medical monitoring, tests, and follow-up to the Marshallese and the need for independent oversight of medical services to the Marshall Islands are still problematic areas.
- A lack of appreciation by researchers of the importance of the moral aspects of human subjects research and the value of institutional oversight was evident; including a lack of awareness of the Belmont Report, and many researchers saying "nobody told me." The need to elevate the importance of research ethics in science, the need to require competency in research ethics for researchers and require curricula for this in medical schools.
- The lack of a government mechanism for the continued interpretation and application of ethics rules and principles was also evident as ethical dilemmas in scientific research are never static.
- Problems with deference to authority, such as physicians and high-level scientists may have caused non-substantial autonomy in human subjects who volunteer for research.
- Silence and complacency was found among physicians and researchers in the nuclear weapons research establishment when it came to seeing colleagues who did not respect the autonomy of patients and research subjects.
- Moral inconsistency among "decent people" was brought out by the committee as so many physicians and researchers involved in human radiation experimentation claimed to be "decent people."

This history of outstanding ethical harms and concerns associated with scientific research and nuclear weapons activities demonstrates a need for more ethical protection for the populations (workers, communities, and military personnel) exposed then and now to nuclear weapons experiments and production activities.

APPLYING ETHICAL GUIDELINES AND PRINCIPLES TO IMPROVE RESEARCH PROTECTIONS

Compounding the ethical problems in radiation health research as it relates to government nuclear experiments is the lack of development and applied practices for ethical treatment of the "community as research subject," not solely individual human subjects. ACHRE made many substantial recommendations for improving informed consent practices that had failed to meet the requirements set forward in the Belmont Report, IRBs and other ethical oversight mechanisms. ACHRE also brought up the following key ethical principles important to the ethical review of human radiation experiments: "One ought not to treat people as means to an end;" "One ought not to deceive others;" "One ought not to inflict harm or risk from harm;" "One ought to promote welfare and prevent harm;" "One ought to treat people fairly and with equal respect;" and "One ought to respect the self-determination of others" (ACHRE, Chap. 4:1). All of these are derived from the common morality and the need to respect the autonomy of subjects.

In the past decade and continuing today, ethics committees have been deliberating on research protections for communities, groups and vulnerable populations [3]. Two critical ethical frameworks are available for promoting our moral progress when it comes to research ethics with community populations and workers: (1) the ethical principles of the Council for International Organization of Medical Sciences (CIOMS; 1991), and (2) the current ethical consensus regarding principles of Community-Based Participatory Research (CBPR) to promote partnership and collaboration among scientists and communities in research [4]. Although CIOMS guidelines were written to mitigate the exploitation of research subjects and communities in international settings, their specific recommended guidelines are useful for mitigating community research abuses in general.

CIOMS Guidelines (1991) and CBPR Principles are included in Tables 1 and 2 with the ethical provisions most relevant to the community research ethics issues that were discussed in the community narratives. Both sets of guidelines provide a new research ethics model that strives for the maximum protection, fairness and beneficence to the collective community as subject. These guidelines go well beyond common and standard IRB protections, such as a written consent for an individual subject or a brief researcher's perception of risks and benefits to the subject. Kahn warns that risks and benefits for the community separate from the individuals that make them up. In this context, informed consent issues with the community need to be thought about more broadly. We have to balance protection of individuals with protection of communities in our oversight processes [3, p. 919]. In these more protective models, the functions of informed consent: disclosure, comprehension, assessments of risks and benefits and voluntariness are applied to whole communities or whole groups and then require a more complex determination than that which a researcher normally considers.

The concepts of beneficence and nonmaleficence (minimizing harms) also need more expanded determinations, most importantly by engaging the community with setting these ethical goals as partners or collaborators in the research process. Both the CIOMS and CBPR principles provide advice for these considerations. There is a growing field of literature on implementing these ethical models in communities [5]. These new ethical principles could have been informative to overcoming what the community/academic writers perceived as research harms and inadequacies.

Table 1. CIOMS Guidelines for Ethical Review of Epidemiological Studies (1991)

Provisions for Community Protections

A. *Informed Consent – Community Agreement*

"When investigators work with communities, they will consider communal rights and protections as they would individual rights and protections."

Collective will of the community, how the community defines itself and who represents or speaks for the community, will need to be determined.

B. *Maximizing Benefits*

Investigators should seek to maximize benefits to the community from the research process. In particular, the committee recommends these provisions:

- Developing and implementing provisions for communication of study results
- Proving treatment or referral for health care needs
- Training local health personnel

C. *Minimizing Harm*

- Causing Harm and Doing Harm

Investigators should avoid transgressing values and exploiting scarce community resources; they should avoid risks of stigmatization or economic and social status losses. They should consider the potential risks of the withdrawal of services to the community and seek to minimize those risks. They should avoid harmful publicity to the community.

- Thorough analysis of risks versus burdens by researchers with the community.
- Cultural competence
  respect for social mores
  sensitivity to different cultures
  respect for ethical standards
- Protections of Confidentiality (linked and unlinked information)
- Conflicts of Interest

Investigators should disclose conflicts with government, labor, corporate, public interest groups, and others who may want to use findings to support a product or service or distort findings that may not be politically convenient.

In the following analysis, I review three ethical guidelines for their usefulness to community-based studies: (1) community agreement for community health investigations, (2) minimizing community harms, and (3) maximizing community benefits. These guidelines could have provided critical improvements in the moral response to these communities affected by Cold War nuclear experiments. For reference, Table 3 lists the health studies described in the community and academic narratives with their key findings and outcomes.

Table 2. Collective List of Research Ethics and CBPR Recommendations

Israel et al.(1998) sets out the basic tenets of community partnerships [16]:

- CBPR recognizes the community as a unit of identity be it geographic neighborhood or a dispersed geographic ethnic group or even overlapping communities in a defined area.
- CBPR builds on strengths and resources within the community.
- Facilitates collaborative partnership in all phases of the research: problem definition, data collection, interpretation of results, and application of results to address community concerns.
- Integrates knowledge and action for the mutual benefit of all partners.
- Promotes a co-learning and empowering process that attends to social inequalities; a reciprocal transfer of knowledge, skills, capacity, and power.

Quigley (2006) outlines a CBPR research process from a collection of CBPR case studies [17]:

- Preparation by Researchers for Community Health Research:
  Contacting community leaders about health research intentions
  Understanding community conditions; subcultural contexts, values, beliefs, socio-economics, geography, demographics, etc.
- Forming Collaborations or Partnerships:
  Recruiting Community Advisory Committees
  Administrative Arrangements between Researchers and Community Members
  Representation/Involvement of Community Members in All Stages of Research Process
  Community Agreements on Data Controls; interpretation of findings, dissemination of results, publications, and co-authorship
- Equity
  Reimbursement or Incentives for the Community for Involving the Community in the Research Execution; Capacity-building; Training, Resource Development for Research Needs
- Qualitative "Local" Knowledge Collection, Incorporation of Community Concerns, Knowledge Values in the Research Questions/Designs
- Research Sustainability; Long-term Commitment for Long-Term Problems

Table 3. Relevant Dosimetry/Health Study Findings

Hanford, WA Health Study Findings

- Radioactive-iodine atmospheric releases were estimated at 740,000 curies from 1944-1957.
- The Hanford Environment Dose Reconstruction (HEDR) reported that children exposed to radioactive iodine from the 1940s to 1950s received doses that were tens to hundreds of rads with a medium dose of 28 rad (Connor, 1997).
- Hanford Thyroid Disease Study reported that exposures at the level reported do not increase the risk of thyroid disease, "These results should consequently provide a substantial degree of reassurance to the population exposed to Hanford radiation that the exposures are not likely to have affected their thyroid or parathyroid health" (HTDS Executive Summary Draft, 1999).

Rocky Flats Dosimetry Study Findings

- Dosimetry study at Rocky Flats reported that the risks were inconsequential from 4.8-51.3 curies of off-site plutonium releases.

Fernald, OH Health Study Findings

- Fernald dosimetry study reported that it is possible that there could be some increase in lung cancer mortality from exposure to uranium, thorium, and radium. The Fernald Facility released 310,000 kg or airborne uranium dust into the atmosphere and 99,000 kg of uranium releases as liquid effluents into the Great Miami River and Paddy's Run Creek. Non-radiologic toxic substances also were released (chlorinated and nonchlorinated metal solvents).
- Fernald Risk Assessment Study made these worst case disease estimates: increase in lung cancer expected to be between 1-12% over a lifetime, with estimates of 4 additional kidney and 4 bone cancers, 3 additional female breast cancers, and 23 or fewer additional cases of leukemias, if well water is contaminated.
- Fernald site then had an "Assessment of the Feasibility of Conducting a Community-based Epidemiological Study for Lung Cancer and Offsite Exposure". This assessment concluded that with confounders (smoking histories) and low statistical power, it would be unlikely to detect an association between lung cancer and exposure to Fernald This study was not pursued, CDC no longer funded activities at Fernald after March 2000.
- Community requested follow-up of the groundwater pathway, measuring contaminants and estimating doses; they requested more follow up for bone, breast, and kidney cancers and leukemia. These requests were denied.
- Fernald ATSDR Health Assessment Study
  The study's initial findings in 2000 recommended further investigation of possible public health hazards from certain private wells and from inhalation of radon to off-site populations; these recommendations were removed in a 2004 final report: only if additional pertinent information becomes available should further follow-up occur.

Lawrence-Livermore Labs and Livermore, CA Health Study Findings

- Austin et al. reported that there was a threefold excess of melanoma in the worker population at Lawrence-Livermore Labs and that workplace variables were causally-related to this excess. The CA Health Department was not able to provide further public health assistance.
- ATSDR reported that the historical distribution of the plutonium sludge has no public health threat; the ACPACT committee under the CA Dept. of Health Services reported that the historic distribution of the sludge from LWRP processes poses an indeterminate health hazard due to a lack of data and recommended that DOE/LLNL provide more funding to Alameda County Health Dept. to implement a process to address the historic distribution of sludge. To this day, this funding has not been provided.

COMMUNITY AGREEMENT FOR COMMUNITY HEALTH INVESTIGATIONS

"When investigators work with communities, they should consider communal rights and protections, as they would individual rights" (CIOMS, 1991).

CIOMS guidelines strongly recommend "community agreement" with these ethical mandates:

- Community representatives should be chosen according to the nature, traditions and political philosophy of the community or group. If communal decision-making is customary, community leaders can express the collective will of the community.
- When people from the community are appointed by an outside agency or group, such as a department or government, to speak for members of the community, investigators and ethical review committees should consider how authentically these people speak for the community, and if necessary, they should seek the agreement of authentic community representatives. Members of a community may be in a position to design a research study and its ethical assessment.
- Investigators will be sensitive to how a community is constituted or defines itself, and will respect the rights of underprivileged groups. When members of a community are naturally conscious of its activities as a community and feel common interests with other members, the community exists, irrespective of the study proposal.

Community Agreement vs. Community Advice and Nuclear Weapons Sites Health Assessments

Community writers at three of the weapons sites (Hanford, Rocky Flats, and Fernald) reported that community representatives were nominated or recruited as part of a larger FACA (Federal Advisory Committee Act) or Advisory Panel committee with scientists and government and agency representatives. Collective will (consensus or majority views) of the community as partner or collaborator was not developed or implemented. Community members provided *advice* with other non-community representatives for selected activities of the research. This advice carried no official enforcement over research decisions.

For example, at Fernald, the National Center for Environmental Health (NCEH) set up the Fernald Health Effects Subcommittee. Yocum reports that the community and other members of the subcommittee were not involved in developing the operational guidelines of the committee [6, pp. 53-67, this volume]. The subcommittee was not exclusively community members but included scientists, government liaison representatives (Environmental Protection Agency, Ohio Dept of Health Services), labor representatives and local medical physicians. Current and former workers at Fernald were also members. The NCEH Executive Secretary set the agenda, conducted and facilitated the meetings. Yocum describes that the subcommittee received no training on the risks and benefits of health study methods, or any training for comprehending the methods enough to critically evaluate them.

> The public and Subcommittee would receive an explanation of the chosen health study, what research methods would be used, and its benefits during one meeting presentation. Most area residents would play a passive role as participants believed the researchers knew which research project would address their health concerns related to the Fernald site [6, p. 61].

The subcommittee formed work groups to make recommendations, primarily in the areas of community outreach and education. NCEH researchers could accept or reject these recommendations. Yocum reports that the subcommittee felt that the NCEH researchers believed the role of the subcommittee was to provide a consensus on the researchers' chosen health study. According to Edwa Yocum, some of the researchers resented reporting to the subcommittee due to their limited time getting the work done.

At Rocky Flats, a twelve-member oversight Health Advisory Panel was appointed by the Colorado Department of Health. LeRoy Moore said that these appointments included prominent scientists (not local), local public representatives, two Colorado Dept of Health (CDH) members (one that was the chair of the panel) [7, pp. 69-97, this volume]. The CDH held periodic meetings to involve the public. Moore commented that the public became reduced to spectators as the technical specialists mainly kept the discourse in risk assessment orthodoxy.

NCEH also set up the Hanford Health Effects Subcommittee which was reported in the Pritikin report [8, pp. 25-52, this volume]. This panel likely functioned in a similar way to the Fernald FACA where community members were appointed to give advice with other government, labor and technical members as the researchers had already chosen the study design and methods. It is likely that there was little development on assessing risks and benefits to the community and little attention to building critical evaluation skills in community members for comprehending the research agenda. I am aware that some community members who learned the study methods independently were able to ask more critical review questions.

In the Livermore Plutonium story, the California State Health Department set up the Alameda County Plutonium Action Taskforce (ACPACT) committee. This committee consisted mostly of community representatives who did come to consensus agreement on health assessment directions. This case study more truly represents the ethical process recommended by CIOMS, however the authors of the case study state that the Agency for Toxic Substances and Disease Registry

(ATSDR), as the government health study investigator, did not abide by the community recommendations. Also it is evident in the Tuler article that the Advisory Committee on Energy-Related Epidemiological Research (ACERER) committee, which had community representatives working with independent scientists for a national review of the National Cancer Institute (NCI) thyroid study, developed consensus recommendations [9, pp. 121-142, this volume]. These recommendations were the outcome of a model process for working with and establishing community agreement for a national study of affected communities from radioactive contamination events. However, these ACERER-developed recommendations still have had no attention from any involved federal agency.

For most of the conduct of the major uranium mining studies before 1990, few, if any efforts at any community agreement can be reviewed. Typically these studies have a completely technically-controlled research process. As Pannikar et al. have described, the Navajo Nation has since created a Navajo Health Research Review Board for the tribal regulation of research on the Navajo reservation [10, pp. 143-163, this volume]. This model now provides for tribal agreement on Navajo health studies.

Community-Driven Research Models

CBPR, as an emerging model for improving research processes with communities, especially communities with environmental contamination and health concerns, was not widely developed in the late 1980s and early 1990s when many of these studies were designed and set up with research contractors and NCEH researchers. From 1994 until today, funding agencies such as National Institute of Health (NIH), Centers or Disease Control (CDC) and Environmental Protection Agency (EPA) are requiring CBPR principles and arrangements in the Requests For Proposals. In those early years, there was a strong emphasis on public participation processes that included "advice" from the lay public. Recent partnership models of CBPR recommend much more engagement of the community members through community-based funding for the hiring and training of community research staff, the recruitment of advisory committees and in sharing decision-making authority. Considerations of community informed consent or approvals were not part of these research services to the communities. None of these large studies of the health effects of nuclear weapons plants allowed community-driven research agendas with stated CBPR principles. Primarily, these studies allowed for independent scientific and community review and advice under CDC, health department and DOE research agendas [11].

MINIMIZING COMMUNITY HARMS

CIOMS 1991 guidelines stress "minimizing harms" in community investigations. The rules for this principle involve (a) assessments of risks and burdens to the whole community, (b) assessments of the study's potential for beneficial change, and (c) avoiding harmful publicity.

Assessment of Risks and Burdens to the Community

The narratives here suggest that there was not a well-developed understanding of the risks from proposed risk assessment, dosimetry and epidemiological interventions. The narratives do not discuss any reports of a formal process in place for identifying risks with the community to conduct dosimetry, thyroid or risk assessment studies. There were some community and scientific opinions that dosimetry studies were too uncertain for identifying health risks to local populations and too expensive.

Assessment of risks and benefits to the community as research subject is not well developed generally for most environmental health studies. It may be evident that at all these research sites, a good development and process for assessing risks and burdens did not exist. Overall, this needs more work in environmental health and other forms of community research.

Foster et al. strongly advise researchers to work with the community to assess possible risks from research. Some types of risks, such as cultural risks, cannot be known by researchers unless there is a community deliberation on the possible consequences of study findings. Through a process of communal discourse, Foster et al. identified the risk of genetic research that might contradict stories of cultural origins [12, p. 1719]. Another strategy for assisting communities with assessing risks and benefits particularly for community epidemiological studies is to review a number of case studies where communities of study invested much effort with researchers to determine cause and effect relationships between environmental exposures and diseases. The case studies may point to some important advice for the community such as a need to modify research designs and methods to include other public health interventions that are not technically-driven and to guard against harms that may come from interpretations of findings by those with technical biases, conflicts of interests or political interests.

Assessment of the Potential for Beneficial Change

CIOMS recommends that ethical review committees should evaluate a study's potential for beneficial change. Investigators should not overestimate a study's benefits in case a community's agreement to participate is unduly influenced by its expectation of better health services.

There was a great deal of expectation among community members at the DOE health study sites for public health interventions that would assist them. Even with those expectations, a community-scientific process for evaluating a study's potential for beneficial change was not formally established. Again, this is likely not well developed in the field of community health research. For example, some basic criteria for beneficial change that could be served by a health study could be identified. A community advisory committee could rate the beneficence of certain study approaches, their methods and their potential findings to evaluate the potential for addressing health concerns. With studies that have the potential for large uncertainties in exposure estimates due to lack of source and exposure data to human and environmental pathways in the relevant historical time periods, and for studies that may have challenges reconstructing cohorts and finding potential cases and controls, a good, critical process is needed to evaluate both the conduct of these studies or the weight of their findings. An ethical review committee that could work with scientists and community members would be an important innovation to the challenge of creating beneficial change from health research investigations.

Dosimetry and HTDS Studies Posed Risks to Communities

Certain risks to the communities from the DOE health studies are suggested here. The Pritikin narrative indicates that at the Hanford site, federal funding was denied and services were withdrawn for proposed thyroid monitoring studies and long-term surveillance of an exposed cohort of children in the 1950s. The federal agencies could claim that this was justified since there were no compelling findings of harm that would require those follow-up services. However, many other scientists and community leaders were extremely critical of the overconfidence in the findings of the HTDS (see Pritikin narrative) [8].

Community and independent scientific recommendations for surveillance and health study follow up at Rocky Flats were denied. This seemed to be closely tied to the findings of the dosimetry study. Again, there is no critical assessment of how solid these dose reconstruction findings are or the legitimacy of discontinuing all other health assessments based on an interpretation of these findings. There were no prior agreements between the communities and the federal research agencies on what the weight or consequences of these study findings would be. Such agreements can provide critical guidance to dealing with all the potential for scientific uncertainties in the research process and who would bear the risks of those uncertainties. Without a fair process for assessment of risks and benefits and community agreement, the communities are at a disadvantage in the research process while the risks of these studies are primarily borne by community members.

The ACHRE warned in their report about the costs and conduct of exposure assessment studies that did not have good records for actual personal and environmental exposures. In the case of atomic veterans, they recommended that time and money spent on consultants and contractors for research administration in assessing health effects, particularly the cost and scientific credibility issues associated with dose reconstruction, may be better spent on relief and assistance to the victims (ACHRE, Rec. 1-6).

Dosimetry studies have been the focus of intense scientific interest. I do not find any evidence of an ethical review process in place that could have mediated the intense investment from the scientific community for these expensive, statistical modeling innovations and processes with the community's need to have positive outcomes that produced real closure for them or aided them with the ever-present concerns about risks to health and environment.

Avoiding Harmful Publicity

CIOMS guidelines (1991) include statements about the need to promote research protocols for communicating study results to communities to ensure fair communication of results and for mitigating other risks related to reporting results (see Table 1). They advise that researchers should assess the sensitivity of their findings to see if the findings have any potential for causing harmful results, such as loss of services or stigmatization. The guidelines recommend that data be interpreted and disclosed in a way that protects the interests of those that are at risk, and investigators should anticipate and avoid misinterpretation that might cause harm. CBPR involves community agreements on interpretation, dissemination and publication of study results. This guidance allows for a fair process for protecting the community from risks and harms from publicity and biased or unfair interpretations of findings.

In these cases, all study results and interpretations were primarily driven by technical researchers and federal agencies with little evidence of input from the community members about their communication, interpretation and dissemination. In these cases, key community advocates and FACA community representatives claimed unfairness in the interpretation and communication of study results; particularly in the Hanford and Rocky Flats narratives. I have not seen any evidence of protocols negotiated with these communities for managing study findings, dissemination, interpretations, publications and any potential harmful publicity. In an excerpt from two Macaulay papers, these authors discuss the need for protocols.

> The trickiest questions in full partnership surround ownership of the data and publication of results. . . . Researchers need to work within the political realities, fully disclose potential pitfalls at the beginning and listen to the advice of the community. This will of course take longer but the results will be more satisfying and the results will then help the community return to health, regain control and improve its self-esteem [13, pp. 1889-1890].

> There is continued sharing of power and control in the dissemination of results; including publication in scientific journals. In the case of a disagreement, the partner who disagrees with the interpretation of the data must be invited to communicate their own interpretation of the data as an addition to the main data, be it oral or written. All partners agree to withhold any information if the alternative interpretation cannot be added and distributed at the same time, providing the disagreeing partners do not unduly delay the distribution process [14].

> In the case of a disagreement, the partner who disagrees must be invited to communicate their own interpretation of the same data as an addition to the main communication, be it oral or written. All partners agree to withhold any information if the alternative interpretation cannot be added and distributed at the same time, providing the disagreeing partner(s) do not unduly delay the distribution process [14, p. 107].

These protections regarding communication of study results and avoiding harmful publicity could have reduced perceived harms by the community members.

MAXIMIZING BENEFITS IN COMMUNITY HEALTH RESEARCH

Developing Multiple Benefits for the Study Community

The CBPR research approach requires the development of local beneficence for the community of study in a research investigation. The NCEH, ATSDR, and DOE-sponsored studies did bring some educational and outreach services to the study communities. There was skills-building and training activities in public participation, research review, and radiation health effects. Particularly at Hanford, education programs were set up in many of the affected regions of Washington State and Oregon with hot-line telephone programs and other outreach activities. For affected tribes and state health departments, there were research development and infrastructure resources.

Community requests for short and long-term monitoring of contaminants however were not supported as elaborated on in the community narratives. Other needs were identified and could still be identified for improving health investigations, health services, oral history projects, and research ethics protections. As stated earlier, before the research begins, the community needs to develop research agreements on ways to ensure community value with the proposed study.

Identifying Beneficial Research Outcomes and Provisions for Long-Term Research Sustainability and Needs

A CBPR approach will promote identifying beneficial research outcomes and provisions for long-term research sustainability for research needs. The community narratives identify some indicators for developing the community's collective will for understanding/managing health risks from contaminants. This needed to be more formally established. In the Hanford, Rocky Flats, and Fernald cases, community members prioritized a number of research needs, including types of environmental monitoring, disease surveillance and monitoring programs, and case-control epidemiological studies. These were all requested but most requests for studies were denied. The findings of the dosimetry/HTDS studies appeared to overpower other sources of evidence about potential risks and ongoing exposures; leading to no further follow-up by the federal health agencies to date at these sites for any meaningful public health interventions.

The community narratives overall depict a strong disappointment from the communities about any positive outcomes of research investigations at their sites. As Krimsky has stated, there is no closure for these communities in terms of potential health impacts from the nuclear contamination at the sites. In terms of nuclear risk management, many community members feel abandoned by the federal health agencies for long-term health protection and research sustainability.

Community Ownership of Health and Environmental Problems

CBPR stresses community ownership of health and environmental problems. As we see with the Livermore plutonium story, the ACPACT committee has continued by itself to prioritize research needs and write grant proposals, only to have potential public agency sources of support deny these requests or refuse sponsorship of funds received for these requests. At Fernald, the FACA committee converted into a community-based research committee which prioritized its research agenda and sought funding support with University of Cincinnati in a CBPR partnership. Other DOE sites, including Hanford and Rocky Flats, have scientists and community leaders who have raised funds privately to fund small investigations that the communities have identified as priorities.

The CA State Health Department was unable to implement any protective preventive health services for the workers at Livermore Labs from the findings of worker risks in their health study. NCEH has indicated a low involvement with these sites, and have informed us in email correspondence that their priorities have now shifted to bioterrorism. As discussed in the Tuler article, the ACERER committee has disbanded with no possibility of follow-up on their consensus recommendations for the thyroid disease health risks indicated by the NCI study [9].

DISCUSSION AND SUMMARY

Since the initial design of the health studies conducted in these communities affected by Cold War nuclear experiments, public health research has encouraged more ethical treatment of communities in the research process. In this chapter,

CIOMS (1991) guidelines provided a template for expanding the Belmont Principles and their protections for individual human subjects to communities of study (see Table 1). CBPR guidelines will improve community involvement in research through authentic partnership, capacity-building for research infrastructure and training, and an action component that will strive to ensure beneficial change. Both sets of guidelines demonstrate that shortcomings existed in the government-funded, community health studies regarding the ethical protection of communities-at-risk. The most serious concerns focus on the need for community agreement; not just advice, but substantial, community aproval for the research investigation proposed by outside or federal researchers.

A critical concern in the community's approval for research designs is a process for a thorough disclosure and training for the community on the study's potential risks and benefits. A new innovation proposed is that the communities design with the researchers some criteria for beneficial change that the research design and methods can offer, and to rate various methods or public health interventions for their potential for creating beneficial change. From the narratives, community members have complained that the dosimetry and epidemiological studies created risks to the community that they did not adequately foresee nor try to resolve before having these studies conducted in their communities. Most important was how community members perceived that the decision by various government health agencies to conduct no further health studies was related to the negative findings of dose reconstruction or thyroid disease studies. Public health interventions that were targeted for some of these communities were terminated after the findings were released. A mistrust of federal health and academic research agencies was deepened in the Hanford region by a lack of protocol agreements between the communities and health researchers for the interpretation and dissemination of research findings. The existence of such protocol agreements was not evident in any of the health subcommittees.

It appears that there was very little public health ethics expertise in the research administration of these studies. The research processes described by the community, academic, and policy writers appear to be heavily-controlled by environmental risk researchers (dose reconstruction experts, epidemiologists, risk assessment professionals) with an abundance of technical risk discourse decisions where community members became marginalized due to a lack of technical expertise. In the community's role of only providing *advice,* there are no rigorous processes for providing equitable decision-making processes, allowing the community to organize and voice its collective will, and educating them on appropriate forms of research protections. Such a dominated technical process easily gives rise to all the ethical problems that Krimsky identified as potential ethical problems [1].

Moreno et al. wrote that "National reviews ought to be required for particularly sensitive research. . . . Science is a social enterprise . . . some kinds of research, especially those that involve special populations and novel interventions (human cloning) are so sensitive that some form of national review, perhaps conducted by a special panel, might be in order [15]. I would argue that populations exposed to environmental releases from sources such as military activities and other national security research experimentation deserve extra research ethics protections. Research in these settings becomes very politically-charged with economic and political risks to those sponsoring these experiments if their experiments cause health effects. This often causes political divisions in the local communities and states as public health protections bump up against the need for research experiments and their economic and national security benefits. Public health ethicists should be involved in every stage of the process, especially for a national research agenda of studies that total over 50 million dollars in ten years and affect multiple regions and communities.

In the ACHRE's Recommendation 11, the committee states that "No structure is in place for interpreting and elaborating the rules of research ethics, a process that is essential if research involving human subjects is to have an ethical framework responsive to changing times." This framework must be debated and adopted in public or it will fail to have the respect and support of the scientific community and the American public. Such a process is urgently needed for these communities as subjects of research experiments.

Working with Communities to Strengthen Community-Based Ethical Standards with Scientific Researchers

The experiences discussed in these narratives of community members give evidence to the need for affected communities to develop and strengthen their ethical standards with scientific researchers. In several narratives, community writers complain of the passive role that community members often fall into with technical researchers. A dominance of technical control with community impacts from contamination will continue to present ethical inequities when community members are bearing these risks. Communities of study need to have more research ethics discussions among their own members about moral meanings of contamination, such as: dealing with scientific uncertainties surrounding determining cause and effect of exposures and diseases; the long-term risks from contamination sources; the quality of interpersonal interactions (discourse, decision-making, etc.) among community members and the scientific, technical communities interfacing with them on contamination issues and other moral issues they determine are important.

With these ethics discussions, communities can develop sets of ethical standards for their interactions with the scientific-technical communities. They will be in a stronger position to demand actions from their collective will, to require fair research relationships, fair discourse and the need to respond to social justice issues. New public health research ethics initiatives and CBPR projects could facilitate this urgent task for these affected communities.

These narratives also identify the need for inter-cultural research standards in addition to community-based standards. The ACHRE cites two dramatic examples of cultural ignorance of the scientific community with Navajo populations and Marshall Islanders that contributed to continued harmful exposures of radiation that could have been averted. The culturally-diverse, Native American, Black-American, Marshall Islanders, and other cultural groups affected by radiation contamination and exposures could develop sets of culturally-appropriate ethical standards for their interactions with mainstream scientific researchers. Through their own internal community dialogues, these diverse community groups could require not only research agreements but a respect for and incorporation of cultural values on knowledge traditions, mutuality, intercultural approaches and other important cultural meanings that can be harmed or dismissed by mainstream researchers and their scientific experimental processes. Public health ethics or CBPR projects could assist with this development of intercultural research standards and cultural competence/humility training. The development of such standards also could also be used for training materials to scientists for providing them with cultural competence training in graduate school/medical school curricula. This was strongly recommended in the ACHRE report.

Continued Federal Support Needed

Lastly, there is a need to solicit more federal support and funding for resolving the health impacts to communities affected by Cold War nuclear experiments and current nuclear weapons research. The moral progress made with research ethics and CBPR approaches since the early 1990s demonstrates that new, community-based, public health initiatives could provide more beneficence and protections to the affected communities and nuclear workers than was provided by the technically-controlled research processes that are the subject of these narratives. A dynamic and community-based public health ethics field needs to be promoted and incorporated into these morally-challenging technical risk decisions.

NOTES

1. Krimsky, S. 2011. *Commentary on ethics and community-based research: Responsibility, precaution and transparency*. In this volume, pp. 7-24. New York: Baywood.
2. Advisory Committee on Human Radiation Experiments. 1995. Washington, D.C.: U.S. Government Printing Office.
3. Kahn, J. 2005. Informed consent in the context of communities. *The Journal of Nutrition* 135(4):918-920. Marshall, P. A. 2005. Human rights, cultural pluralism, and international health research. *Theoretical Medicine and Bioethics* 26(6):529-557. Strauss, R. P., and Sengupta, S. 2001. The role of community advisory boards: Involving communities in the informed consent process. *American Journal of Public Health* 91(12):1938-1943.

4. Council for International Organizations of Medical Sciences (CIOMS). 1991. International Guidelines for the Ethical Review of Epidemiological Studies. Geneva. CIOMS has updated these guidelines with a 2009 publication.
5. See www.researchethics.org folder on Annotated Bibliographies: "Community-Based Participatory Research" for references.
6. Yocum, E. 2011. *A community's experience with environmental health research ethics at the Fernald Feed Production Plant.* In this volume, pp. 53-67. New York: Baywood.
7. Moore, L. 2011. *Democracy and public health at Rocky Flats: The examples of Edward A. Martell and Carl J. Johnson.* In this volume, pp. 69-97. New York: Baywood.
8. Pritikin, T. 2011. *Insignificant and invisible: The human toll of the Hanford Thyroid Disease Study.* In this volume, pp. 25-52. New York: Baywood.
9. Tuler, S. 2011. *Institutional preferences for justice, avoiding harm, and expertise in public health policy making about the health consequences of iodine-131 nuclear weapons testing fallout.* In this volume, pp. 121-142. New York: Baywood.
10. Panikkar, B., Yazzie, E., and Brugge, D. 2011. *Ethics of uranium mining research and the Navajo people.* In this volume, pp. 143-163. New York: Baywood.
11. As an exception, in 1999, I was the project director for an NCEH-funded study that did allow for community-driven research with Native American tribes around the Nevada Test Site.
12. Foster, M. W., Sharp, R., Freeman, W., Chino, M., Bernsten, D., and Carter, T. 1999. The role of community review in evaluating the risks of human genetic variation research. *American Journal of Human Genetics* 64:1720.
13. Macaulay, A. 1994. Ethics of research in native communities. *Canadian Family Physician* 40:1888-1890.
14. Macaulay, A., Delormier, T., McComber, A., Cross, E., Porvin, L., Paradis, G., Kirvy, R., Saad-Haddad, C., and Desrosiers, S. 1998. *Canadian Journal of Public Health* March-April:105-108.
15. Moreno, J., Capian, A., Wolpe, P. R., et al. 1998. Updating protections for human subjects involved in research. *Journal of the American Medical Association* 280(22):1951-1958.
16. Israel, B., Schulz, A., Parker, E., and Becker, A. 1998. Review of community-based research: assessing partnership approaches to improve public health. *Annual Review of Public Health* 19:178.
17. Quigley, D. 2006. A review of ethical improvements to environmental/public health research: Case examples from native communities. *Journal of Health Education* 33(21):130-147.

http://dx.doi.org/10.2190/TORC11

CHAPTER 11

Ethical Review of Radiation Effect Narratives

Ernest Wallwork

The radiation health effect narratives in this collection implicitly raise a number of distinct moral issues. The aim of this chapter is to identify and to discuss the nine most important of these ethical aspects of the larger story of nuclear contamination and the government's response to it that these separate narratives reveal. Ethics is defined broadly here as critical reflection about "right" and "wrong" actions and "good" and "bad" character traits and other states of affairs (e.g., public health). Ethical interpretations differ from descriptive accounts in providing normative arguments about the actions and motivations of individuals and institutions.

Taken together, the nine distinct ethical dimensions of the narratives of radiation contamination examined here lead to a more comprehensive normative framework than that assumed in some other assessments, which focus more selectively on a few moral topics. The key questions are: How should we evaluate the actions and motivations of the main participants in narratives of nuclear radiation pollution from the mid-1940s to the present? What ethical lessons can we learn from these narratives? How should the government respond to individuals and communities who have been harmed by high levels of contamination? What should we do now to correct continuing problems?

I. NINE ETHICAL ASPECTS OF THE RADIATION EFFECTS NARRATIVES

1. First, the *rightness and wrongness of particular actions* initiated by key decision-makers (e.g., nuclear facility administrators, researchers, government officials, and their critics) can and should be evaluated in terms of such normative principles as nonmaleficence ("do no harm"), beneficence, truth-telling, equal respect for persons, informed consent, and various justice criteria. Violation of one or more of these widely acknowledged basic moral obligations lies at the core of the chief ethical complaints against the decision-makers and institutions involved in nuclear weapons research, development, and production. Although people disagree about the comparative weight to be assigned these basic principles when they are applied to nuclear activities and contamination, the validity of the basic principles are not in doubt. Partly constitutive of the common morality, these principles have been acknowledged for centuries, even millennia, in the West and, increasingly, elsewhere in the world as well. It is thus not inappropriate, as some suggest, to invoke these standards in judging the actions of moral agents as recently as sixty years ago.

2. A second ethical perspective emphasizes not the rightness or wrongness of the actions of various moral agents and institutions, but the *blameworthiness* (or praiseworthiness) of particular agents and institutions. It is one thing to say, in historical hindsight, that the distribution of free plutonium-contaminated sludge for gardening was morally wrong, because it risked harming residents of Livermore, California. It is a different issue entirely to blame specific officials at the Livermore Radiation Laboratory for this distribution, not only because it is hard to identify particular individuals, but, more importantly, because it is exceedingly difficult to know what they knew factually about the likely effects of plutonium in this form on public health and how these individuals evaluated what they knew within the worldview of the era. In the context of the times (the Cold War and naïve trust in scientific and governmental authorities), distributing plutonium sludge may not have been as morally irresponsible as it seems to us today.

3. A third ethical dimension of these radiation health effect narratives focuses on the *morally sanctioned psychosocial blinders*, such as the "culture of secrecy" [1]; deference to authority [2]; complacency resulting from "self-identification with a government agency" [1], fear of the costs of acknowledging responsibility, and self-serving ascription of virtues to colleagues ("good people can't do wrong"), that led managers of nuclear facilities and governmental agencies like the Atomic Energy Commission and the Department of Energy to refuse to study (and, later, to contest independent studies of) the elevated rates of cancer as well as thyroid and other diseases attributable to radiation exposures from plutonium and uranium.

4. A fourth aspect of these studies attends to the ethics of handling *uncertainty*, for example, what one ought to do when facts about risks of harm are unknown. The "precautionary principle" handles scientific uncertainty when great harm may result by advising that preventive measures be taken before cause-and-effect relationships are fully established scientifically.

5. A fifth perspective centers on the *injustice* of government agencies in a representative democracy violating the rights and liberties of their own citizens. For example, the rights of residents "downwind" of the Hanford nuclear site were violated in the name of "national security." Injustices occurred not only in the infringement of such rights as "life, liberty and the pursuit of happiness," but also in the unfair distribution of the burden, insofar as a very small segment of the total American population—those living near nuclear facilities—suffered disproportionately the costs of developing nuclear weapons to protect the entire nation.

6. A sixth ethical concern has to do with the value of *community involvement* in ferreting out information relevant to assessing the harms done to employees and to innocent neighbors of nuclear facilities as a result of nuclear weapons research, development and production. Without the voluntary associations organized around Livermore, California ("the Sludge Working Group"), the Hanford nuclear site, and elsewhere, we would not even know that some forms of contamination occurred, much less how they were covered up, understated by some investigative research designs and allowed to continue to pollute environments and damage health without remediation.

7. A seventh issue concerns the appropriate ethical responses of citizens to their government's malfeasance in risking serious harm to inhabitants and then concealing the actual harms that occurred.

8. An eighth issue is that of *remedial justice* raised by the question, "What is to be done now to rectify past moral wrongs?" Remedial justice seeks redress for the ill health effects of the government's failure to protect employees and the public from the risks of radiation contamination.

9. A related set of issues is raised by the question, "What is to be done now to lessen the likelihood of similar wrongdoing happening again?" This question is future oriented in contrast to the backward look of remedial justice: *what steps should the government now adopt to avoid repeating past wrong-doing in the future*?

II. ELABORATING ON THE ETHICAL ISSUES RAISED BY THE RADIATION EFFECTS NARRATIVE

1. The *rightness or wrongness of actions* is determined by applying widely accepted ethical principles, which minimally include these six principles: "One ought not to inflict harm or risks of harm." "One ought to prevent and remove harm and promote welfare." "One ought to treat people as equally worthy of

respect, as autonomous self-determining subjects, and never as mere means to the ends of others." "One ought not to deceive others." "One ought to keep one's promises." "One ought to treat people fairly and justly."[1] None of these principles is absolutely binding in the sense that they cannot be overridden by another principle under certain circumstances. Each principle is *prima facie* obligatory; that is to say, each principle is "on its face" or "theoretically" obligatory apart from particular circumstances. *Actual* obligations depend on which principle or principles are most salient in a particular situation. When principles conflict, the principle that overrides others is determined by weighing the relative importance of each principle as it relates to a unique situation. Discretion and wise judgment (*phronesis*, in Aristotle) are essential to evaluate the conflicting obligations and values present in a particular case and to arrive at a concluding judgment.

The most obvious moral wrongs chronicled in the radiation effects narratives are the significant *risks of harm* to the health of nearby residents and employees that eventually resulted in increased rates of various cancers, thyroid diseases, and other disorders. The many forms of environmental contamination that occurred at nuclear facilities over the decades, beginning in the mid-1940s, were morally wrong because they placed innocent people, including children, at risk of very serious harms to their health, risks that eventually resulted in enormous pain and suffering and early deaths for numerous innocent victims, who were never adequately warned of these dangers or encouraged to take appropriate steps to protect themselves. Those responsible failed to discharge their minimal moral duty to make sure safety measures (like fans in uranium mines) were in place to minimize known avoidable harms.

Ironically, these moral wrongs initially appear to have grown out of a *moral* commitment to "national security," which, unfortunately, ended up taking priority over the core moral beliefs for which this country stands, the rights of autonomous individuals to enjoy life, liberty, and the pursuit of happiness. As ACHRE puts it, "The moral justification would . . . be . . . that, in order to preserve the American way of life with its precious freedoms, some sacrifice of individual rights and interests would have to be made for the greater good." This cost-benefit calculation shares the familiar weakness of act-utilitarianism as a moral theory, namely, that patently immoral means, such as the sacrifice of innocent lives, can

[1] These principles are not offered as a comprehensive list of basic duties, but only those most relevant to evaluating nuclear contamination. The six principles are derived from Sir David Ross's list of prima facie duties, as modified by Beauchamp and Childress and the author [3]. The formulation of these principles in terms of "one ought" or "ought not" comes from the ACHRE Report [4]. However, I disagree with the ACHRE Report's characterization of some of these basic principles. For example, the ACHRE list fails to mention the duty to remove harm, which is very relevant to the ethics of dealing with nuclear contamination. The ACHRE Report also mistakenly creates two duties out of the single duty to respect another's autonomy, by adding a second, overlapping duty to "respect the self-determination of others." It is unclear what this adds to respect for autonomy, which encompasses self-determination ("autonomy" means self-rule, in Greek).

be justified by cost-benefit calculations, flagrantly disregarding the principle that one ought to treat people as equally worthy of respect as autonomous agents, and never as mere means to the ends of others. As critics of utilitarianism point out, cost-benefit moral reasoning needs to be limited by deontological side-constraints that protect the lives and health of individuals, respect their autonomy, and treat everyone equally and fairly.

Unconstrained cost-benefit calculations end up denigrating persons to mere means to the ends of others, as shown by the language of the declassified Atomic Energy Commission memo that refers to populations around nuclear weapons production sites as ". . . low use segment[s] of the population" living in "sacrifice zones" [5, citing 6, pp. xxiii and 109ff]. In this chilly, dehumanizing language, the rights guaranteed by the U.S. Constitution yield to scientific calculations of disposable human debris. No wonder managers acculturated to this dehumanizing language ended up subordinating the risks of harm to "downwinders' of the Hanford facility and Navajo uranium miners to the research and production goals of their employers.

Retrospective moral judgments holding that it was morally wrong to release large quantities of radiological contamination into the air (Hanford, Rocky Flats), soil (Livermore, Rocky Flats, and Crosby Township, Ohio), and groundwater of adjacent communities (Livermore, Crosby Township) without protecting the local population are sometimes contested on the grounds that those who supported these activities did not share our values. But whatever the changes in values that have occurred since the 1940s, such basic principles as nonmaleficence, beneficence, respect for autonomy, truth-telling, and promise-keeping were as familiar in the 1940s as they are today. Indeed, some would argue that these principles were more highly honored in the decades immediately following World War II than today. Mainstream American culture in the 1940s and 50s did not portray national security or the greatest good of the greatest number as justifying wanton violations of the rights and protections of ordinary Americans.

a. "One ought to prevent and remove harm and promote welfare." The obligation "to prevent and remove harm," as a minimalist interpretation of the general obligation to promote human welfare (beneficence), was broken repeatedly by those nuclear facility managers who, refusing to acknowledge the ever-increasing evidence of the dangers of radiation, continued to operate nuclear facilities as if nothing new had been learned about the risks to public health. For example, after the dangers to miners of radon levels in uranium mines had been well-documented and both the PHS and the Atomic Energy Commission had acknowledged that these levels were high enough to cause cancer and that ventilation should be used to reduce the hazard, nothing was done to reduce the level of radon in the mines to tolerance levels [4, 7]. Even when steps were taken to reduce the risks of contamination at nuclear facilities, the refusal to acknowledge past harms delayed informing those who were at risk so they could be monitored, diagnosed, and encouraged to seek early treatment.

The meager health insurance benefits for workers exposed to radiation at nuclear facilities provide another example of the widespread failure to observe the duty of beneficence. When the AEC manager of the Oak Ridge Site proposed that terminating workers be informed if they were exposed to excessive levels of radiation and that medical assistance be provide if they were made ill or injured by radiation, the recommendation was rejected and it was proposed, instead, that terminating employees should be advised "at the exit interview as to the care that the AEC utilizes in protecting each employee" [8]. Apparently, fears about liability, demands for extra-pay for working in hazardous conditions and increased insurance claims for occupational injuries attributable to radiation prevented the Atomic Energy Commission Advisory Committee from doing the right thing by its own employees [8].

b. "One ought not to deceive others." The injunction not to deceive was repeatedly disregarded at nuclear sites by policies and actions that were intended to keep secret from residents, employees and the public both the nature of the nuclear work taking place as well as the risks of contamination. Although justified initially as part of the secrecy surrounding the Manhattan Project, and, then, the arms race between the United States and the USSR during the Cold War, non-disclosure about radiation research and production continued after it was no longer necessary. This sometimes seemed to occur largely to protect administrators from criticism, to avoid cutbacks or closures that an alarmed public might have demanded, to minimize the costs of production and to avoid compensating workers and residents for radiation-induced illnesses [1, 8].

At times, administrative silence, in violation of the principle of truth-telling, resulted in outright lying—defined as intentionally withholding the truth or telling falsehoods in order to deceive. A clear example in the radiation effects literature is the PHS interim report of 1952 that lied about the lack of any evidence of health damage from radioactivity in uranium mines, even though, in the previous year, the PHS acknowledged in internal meeting records that levels of radon in uranium mines were high enough to cause cancer [7]. Victor Archer, head of the PHS medical team, justified this deception with the bureaucratic self-serving argument that "We did not want to rock the boat" [7]. Similarly, an Atomic Energy Commission officer, Dr. Sidney Marks, tried to counter Dr. Samuel Milham's finding that workers at the Hanford facility showed increased mortality from cancers of the tongue, mouth, pharynx, colon, pancreas, lung, and bones, by pressuring Dr. Mancuso to support a press release that stated "there is no evidence of cancer or other deaths attributable to ionizing radiation occurring more often among Hanford workers" [8]. The failure of the federal, state and local agencies to notify residents of Crosby Township, Ohio about the contamination of their wells by the Nuclear Feed Processing Plant is yet another potential case of deception serving primarily the narrow bureaucratic interests of the agencies involved, not national security.

Other forms of deception in the radiation effect reports that violate the *prima facie* obligation to tell the truth include: the intentional withholding of the dangers of uranium ore from Navajo uranium miners; misinforming neighbors of the Ohio facility that there were no risks; manipulating information about the extent of various forms of soil contamination around Rocky Flats, using highly technical language to obscure hazards, quibbling over the minutiae of research that was otherwise basically sound to discredit a report of contamination in its entirety. Even some reports of allegedly "scientific" reviews—like the critical peer reviews of Dr. Mancuso's work that James Liverman cited during his testimony to the House Energy and Commerce Subcommittee on Health and the Environment in defense of the DOE's termination of Mancuso's research contract—seem to reflect mostly the desire of their authors, and their institutional backers, to discredit sound scientific studies of radiation-induced illnesses rather than any genuine concern about the validity of the research. In fact, the peer reviews Liverman cited as justifying Mancuso's removal had actually lauded his capabilities and recommended that his research be continued under his control [8].

c. "One ought to treat people as equally worthy of respect, as autonomous self-determining subjects, and never as mere means to the ends of others." The importance of *informed consent* was widely discussed in 1947 in connection with the publication of the Nuremberg Code, which sought to avoid repetition of the horrors of the Nazi concentration experiments by setting forth the rights of research subjects to full knowledge of the nature and purpose of a research protocol and its attendant risks and discomforts to participants. Although the Nuremberg Code was not applied to the rights of employees, the core principle of informed consent was clear—namely, that the health and lives of individuals cannot be put at risk without their full knowledge and voluntary consent. According to the Nuremberg Code, the use of force, fraud, deceit, duress, over-reaching, or other ulterior form of constraint or coercion undermine the genuineness of informed voluntary consent.

The general practice in the radiation industry of not disclosing likely harms of exposure to nearby residents and employees violated their autonomy by manipulating them to do willingly what they would not otherwise do. By deliberately presenting plutonium sludge was safe, residents living near the Livermore nuclear laboratory were induced to solve a disposal problem by trucking away tons of plutonium sludge for their gardens and to consume, without question, contaminated water and local farm produce. The employment decisions of nuclear workers were similarly manipulated by withholding information that might have led them to consider less dangerous occupations or residential areas. Indeed, a stated goal of not warning nuclear workers was to keep them from quitting [4]. In the case of Navajo miners, deception easily exploited the cultural ignorance of the Navajo people about the properties of uranium ore. Deceptive practices like these became widespread throughout the nuclear industry because, by treating human beings as means rather than ends, they successfully prevented unfavorable publicity, avoided costly legal suits, and helped maintain a compliant, cheap workforce.

An interesting attempt was made in 1979 by the federal Department of Housing and Urban Development to provide potential off-site residents near Rocky Flats, Colorado, with the equivalent of informed consent by requiring anyone seeking federal mortgage insurance to sign the "Rocky Flats Advisory Notice" that would notify them of plutonium contamination of the soil and the "Emergency Response Plan" that would be implemented in the event of "an accidental release of radioactive materials" from Rocky Flats [9]. This proposal for informed consent was abruptly terminated shortly after Ronald Reagan took office in January, 1981, apparently because it was opposed by powerful local real estate interests [9].[2]

2. The issue of whether particular individuals and/or institutions are *blameworthy* or *praiseworthy* is different from the question of whether or not their actions are morally wrong. In retrospect, it was morally wrong to harm people by releasing radiation into the soil, air, and water around nuclear facilities; nonetheless, the guilt of those who were responsible for doing so may be mitigated by the pervasive influence of culturally induced ignorance. The perpetrators are not fully responsible, this line of reasoning contends, because they were not fully aware of the consequences of what they were doing or their awareness was blunted by its cultural interpretation.

The matter of blameworthiness lies behind such questions as: What were people thinking when they exposed Navajo miners to unsafe doses of radiation, Livermore gardeners and their families to plutonium sludge, and Rocky Flats residents to dangerous concentrations of plutonium in the soil? Did they assume that small amounts of radioactivity were safe, like the amounts emitted by the foot x-ray machines that were commonplace in shoe stores in the 1940s, until they were shown to be highly dangerous and withdrawn? How one answers these questions affects what one thinks about such issues as: Was the distribution of plutonium sludge an honest mistake or a devious, immoral way for the Livermore Water Reclamation Plant to get rid of radioactive sludge cheaply? Was the construction of the public garden lined with sludge intended to deceive the public or does it reveal naïve beliefs about the probable dangers?

Trisha Thompson Pritikin argues against the excuses offered by nuclear facility officials and their defenders at Hanford that "the large radiation releases from Hanford were allowed due to incomplete understanding among early Hanford scientists of the dangers from radiation" [5]. She points out that Hanford officials

[2] A similar manipulation of purchasers of land near the Rocky Flats nuclear bomb factory occurred when the Department of Energy colluded with local contractors to conceal studies of nuclear contamination by sealing court records so the public was denied information relevant to the safety of residential areas [9].

considered the possibility of radiation harm to workers and surroundings communities sufficiently serious to established guidelines for the amount of radiation that could be released safely, and yet these "guidelines were routinely ignored from the beginning of plutonium separation in December 1944 into the early fifties" [5]. Moreover, awareness of the dangers of radiation were sufficiently well-known by the late 1940s for the Atomic Energy Commission, Department of Defense, and the National Institute of Health (NIH) to require investigators to obtain prior group review of the risks of research using radioisotopes (and, at the NIH, for all hazardous procedures). No explicit government policies at the time stated that national security concerns might justify violating the rights of American citizens in the context of environmental contamination. No policies bared government agencies from informing the public that potentially harmful radioactive substances were being released into the environment.

Even if the early distributions of plutonium sludge and the radiation releases into the environment at Hanford and Crosby Township, Ohio, were due to innocent mistakes, the risks of serious harm to public health became increasingly obvious as the adverse effects of radiation exposure became increasingly clear in the decades following the 1940s. The failure of officials at Hanford, Crosby, Livermore, Rocky Flats, and elsewhere to take corrective action once the harmful effects of radiation were widely known indicates that at least some later administrators were morally blameworthy. In some cases, like the Ohio Department of Health's (ODH) testing of well water around the Fernald uranium ore processing facility, officials appear to have lied—when, for example, they told residents that the ODH was sampling to measure bacteria (when they were really testing for radiation) [10]. Those officials responsible for repeatedly and deviously attempting to discredit evidence of radiation in the environment around nuclear facilities, such as the Atomic Energy Commission's hiring of their own specialist to dispute Martell's evidence at Rocky Flats, are morally blameworthy not only for obfuscating the truth, but for putting the off-site population at risk of various cancers from carcinogens released from the soil in the encroaching suburbs. The mystery of the missing Livermore "log-book" with the names and addresses of the households that received the plutonium-sludge smells of the sort of mendacity that Big Daddy sniffs out in Tennessee Williams' *Cat on a Hot Tin Roof.*

Nonetheless, the acts of a few officials at nuclear facilities are praiseworthy. For example, Dr. Biggs, the medical director of the Livermore facility (LLNL), courageously bucked the culture of secrecy at Livermore when he decided in 1979 to cooperate with Donald Austin to conduct a scientifically accurate investigation of the malignant melanoma occurrences within the LLNL workforce. The study identified a causal connection between working conditions at the lab and melanoma and, thus, the need for continued health monitoring as well as identification and compensation for those employees who were injured. Subsequent administrators at the LLNL appear to be morally culpable for going out of their way, at considerable expense, to contest the evidence that LLNL workers were developing melanoma at threefold or fourfold rates over controls as a result of their working conditions. LLNL's obstructive actions prevented timely monitoring of LLNL workers and provision of health care for those with melanoma attributable to their employment (measured in terms of the degree of their on-the-job risk).

The most morally praiseworthy individuals in these narratives were those who, like Jacqueline Cabasso, Peggy Reynolds, Edward Martell, Carl J Johnson, and Thomas Mancuso, persevered against great odds, sometimes at considerable personal cost, to investigate the facts, to publicize them, and to press for corrective action on behalf of the public's health.

Jacqueline Cabasso was the Executive Director of Western State Legal Foundation, who closely tracked the environmental record of Livermore's nuclear weapons laboratory for fifteen years and first urged California Department of Health Services researchers to "look into the sludge issue." Peggy Reynolds donated about 600 hours of her time as the lead epidemiologist to continue a study of malignant melanoma cases among LLNL workers after funding of the California Tumor Registry study was eliminated by LLNL officials and resources were reallocated at LLNL to hire investigations to refute evidence of a fourfold excess of malignant melanoma occurring among lab employees from 1972 to 1977 [11].

Edward A. Martell, a radiochemist with the National Center for Atmospheric Research located in Boulder, Colorado, was the first to obtain hard evidence of plutonium deposits in the soil near Rocky Flats [9] and to alert the public to the risks of radiation-induced health effects. For his courageous work, Martell would apear to have been punished by loss of his lab and almost his job. His activities also seem to have cost him promotion to the rank of Senior Scientist, despite three decades of original radiochemical research at the National Center for Atmospheric Research.

Carl J. Johnson, Director of the Health Department of Jefferson County, Colorado, stood alone for years as an innovative investigator and advocate for people with public health concerns related to contamination released from the Rocky Flats site. For this activism, he was vilified and forced from office by a combination of nuclear interests and promoters of urban sprawl [9].

Dr. Thomas Mancuso, Professor of Occupational Medicine at the University of Pittsburgh, persevered in studying whether Atomic Energy Commission employees were suffering harmful radiation effects despite the unprecedented ferocity of an assault against his research. After his funding was cut off by the Atomic Energy Commission, Mancuso drew upon his personal retirement money and fought to protect his data in order to continue groundbreaking epidemiological studies that proved crucial for establishing the magnitude of health effects on workers at various nuclear sites.[3] These studies provided essential data for compensation claims by victims [8].

3. The *institutional obstacles* to acknowledging the extent of nuclear contamination and its seriousness, like the "culture of secrecy" in weapons labs that inhibited conversations about the effects of radiation, are ethically significant because they interfere with knowing important truths about potentially harmful activities and timely preventive steps that might limit ongoing harms. A culture of secrecy and strategies of compartmentalization that prevent workers from knowing what others are doing function like defense mechanisms in individuals; they help to diminish guilt and other moral emotions by disavowing the meanings of some painful realities. Explicit or implicit denial is an integral aspect of all defensive strategies within institutions and individuals. People behave as if there is no danger, say, from nuclear radiation or terrorism. To help efface accurate perceptions of reality, partial truths are used to obscure unwelcomed facts. For example, "we are contributing to a worthy patriotic cause" obfuscates the equally true statement that "we are endangering the health of our neighbors and their children by polluting the environment." Blaming critics and/or depreciating or humiliating them is a familiar tactic in institutional efforts to circle the wagons against the dangers of admitting the accuracy (or partial accuracy) of a critic's accusations. The perpetrator preserves belief in the goodness of his/her own strivings, against evidence to the contrary, by depreciating and demeaning critics—like Martell, Johnson, and Mancuso.

A familiar feature of these and other defenses is that nagging doubts are quickly rendered innocuous. Institutional defenses, like intrapsychic ones, aim at silencing reservations as they are beginning to be formed, as, for example, when a scientist's budding worries about his findings regarding increased mortality among nuclear workers are silenced on the grounds that they "might cause undue concern in workers" [8]. Powerful self-interests, like keeping one's job and avoiding the disapproval of employers and neighbors, both of which sustained the culture of secrecy in nuclear facilities, keep the conscious mind from acknowledging challenges to local conventional opinion. When defensively motivated words and actions of bureaucrats persist in the face of overwhelming empirical evidence to the contrary, outsiders start asking the question that the reader of these narratives often does: "What could they possibly have been thinking?"

The narratives under review here do not provide access to the shared psychic mechanisms that enabled highly educated scientists and administrators at nuclear facilities to engage in patently self-serving attempts to disavow the

[3] When 21 of 40 filing cabinets of his data were intentionally destroyed, Mancuso took custody of the remaining records, storing them in his own basement, where he continued to use them to prove the increased risks of exposed employees dying from radiation-induced cancers [8].

well-established causal relationship between radiation exposure and lung cancer, thyroid cancer, and thyroid disease, to mention only a few ill-effects of exposure to plutonium and uranium. Robert Jay Lifton's studies suggest that an investigation of the defenses employed unconsciously by scientists and administrators at nuclear facilities would include "psychic numbing" and "doubling." *Numbing*, a diminished capacity or inclination to feel emotions, is produced by "divesting oneself from the actuality of what one is part of, not experiencing it as 'real'" [12, p. 442]. A key function of numbing, which is commonly enhanced in groups by heavy drinking, is to avoid feelings of guilt about harming others. "*Doubling* involves an unconscious splitting of the self that enables a second self to perform "dirty work" [12, p. 419, italics added]. Doubling is like the "compartmentalization" described by Pritikin as part of the culture of secrecy at the Hanford facility. But, whereas Pritikin uses "compartmentalization" to refer to institutional arrangements whereby workers were only told what was necessary to perform their jobs, psychic compartmentalization or doubling allows the same person to sequester morally unacceptable conduct at work from the general sense that she/he is a good person in the rest of her/his life. By keeping what is known from being fully known, doubling allows a person—a nuclear facility official—to avoid dealing affectively with the guilt that would otherwise be aroused by acknowledging the deleterious effects of his/her actions, for example, poisoning one's neighbors.

Typically, the harmful psychological effects of defensive denial on the victims of wrongdoing are also denied, with the result that perpetrators commonly appear devoid of natural human empathy. The reader senses this in Trisha Pritikin's powerful report on the human toll on those who lived downwind of the Hanford nuclear site. One source of "downwinder" suffering has been the relentless denial by Hanford officials of the damaging effects of radiation releases. Her report discusses what might be described as the re-traumatizing of Hanford residents, who felt themselves obliterated from a research study's myopic conclusions that no harm had occurred. As the Hanford Health Information Network put it "[t]he HTDS actually inflicted a good deal of harm on those whom the study was intended to serve." The harm was the denial of the experiential reality of their pain and suffering:

> Suddenly, HTDS and its results, released after months of hushed and restrictive secrecy, reflected, not life as it was for those of us who grew up in the Hanford downwind area during release years, but as a funhouse mirror, distorting our lives, denying our experience. I felt myself becoming deeply angered. They needed to understand that too many of us, too many of the people I had grown up with, now had thyroid disease, and/or thyroid cancer. They needed to know that I, and *we*, were *not* reassured by HTDS' purported "no harm" findings. It was up to us to let the world know that this epidemiologic study, for some reason, did not reflect our reality. This study had made us insignificant and invisible [5].

4. The evidence in these narratives that some nuclear administrators used scientific *uncertainties* about the effects of radiation to justify taking risks with the public's health raises the ethical issue of what ought to be done when key facts are unknown about potentially significant harms. From the outset, the scientific members of the Manhattan Project recognized the extremely hazardous magnitude of nuclear weapons work, even though at the time the precise effects, for example, that "plutonium itself might have on workers was unknown" [8, 13]. By at least 1948, Dr. Robert Stone, head of the Health Division of the Manhattan Project and chairman of the Radiology Department at the University of California Medical School in San Francisco, recognized that it might take months or years after exposure for workers to experience serious health problems [8]. Yet, instead of the enormity of the potential harms spurring great caution and continual study as well as vigilance regarding the probable need for corrective and/or remedial action, the opposite appears to have occurred. Scientific uncertainty was used repeatedly as a cover for continuing ongoing radiation contamination and denial of its ill effects. One particularly disturbing tactic was to hire and to direct scientists to design studies aimed at disputing the growing evidence of the serious health effects of nuclear pollution—e.g., by diluting soil samples of airborne radiation by digging deeper.

Ethically, the rule-of-thumb guideline for acting in situations of uncertainty, where great harm can result, is "precaution," not denial. The "precautionary principle" holds that where there are scientific reasons to suspect a causal relationship (as with the causal role of radiation in the development of various cancers) precautionary measures should be taken before cause and effect relationships have been fully established scientifically [14].

The moral wrongness of the nuclear industry's response to evidence of environmental contamination is highlighted by the implicit strategy that seems to have guided the industry's actions in a wide range of very diverse situations of uncertainty, a strategy that might be dubbed the "anti-cautionary" policy. The aim of an "anti-cautionary policy" is to preserve the status quo ante by contesting any evidence of a causal link by using all available means to undermine the scientific legitimacy of studies that identify such a link or, barring that, the integrity of the researchers. For example, at Rocky Flats, when plutonium contamination of the soil was shown to exceed established standards, sampling methods were adopted that eschewed sampling soil at specific sites, some of which were presumably hot spots, in favor of compositing all the soil collected from all samples, thereby diluting particularly high readings by averaging them with lower ones [9]. Similarly, by taking soil samplings at increasingly greater depths, the false impression was created that the quantity of plutonium in the soil was steadily decreasing. When Carl Johnson first presented his findings in 1979 about the dangers of residing near Rocky Flats, the Department of Energy sought to undermine public acceptance of his findings by paying a bonus to its contractor, Rockwell, for persuading the *Denver Post* to publish an editorial questioning Johnson's evidence. Later, uncertainty about Rocky Flats contamination was sustained by preventing any direct health study of people living in areas contaminated with plutonium released from Rocky Flats, despite the fact that epidemiological data indicated excessive incidences of lung and bone cancers in areas near Rocky Flats [9].

At other facilities, the Department of Energy, the Atomic Energy Commission, the CDC, and specific nuclear facilities have managed to keep the public uncertain about the nature and degree of radiation contamination by such maneuvers as:

- minimizing, ignoring or covering up evidence of the adverse effects of human exposure to radiation [9, 14];
- failing to study plutonium releases [14];
- adversarial questioning of independent scientific findings about the effects of environmental radiation near nuclear facilities [11];
- hiring scientists and biostatisticians to conduct studies aimed at detecting bias or identifying alternative explanations for empirical findings linking nuclear contamination to various diseases [9];
- discrediting undesired scientific findings by selecting biased sampling techniques and interpretations of empirical data [9];
- terminating funding for independent data collection [11];
- firing scientists who have demonstrated their independence [8, 9];
- sealing [sequestering] crucial scientific data and information about wrongdoing in court records [9];
- publishing overly critical, unbalanced evaluations of research reports that diverged from the findings desired by the nuclear establishment;
- thwarting new studies from being conducted [9].

Taken together, these tactics have worked too well to insulate the nuclear establishment from the full weight of ethical criticism.

5. A central ethical issue when government agencies act contrary to the health interests of their citizens lies with the anti-democratic nature of such actions. Since these institutions are ultimately the agents of citizens in democratic societies, they undermine their own *raison d'etre* to the degree that they infringe on the rights, liberties, and welfare of citizens. Ironically, the rationale nuclear facilities administrators offered for their hazardous activities—defense of our democratic institutions—was belied by their own actions when, in the name of national security, they risked serious harm to the very citizens whose interests they were supposed to serve. The residents of the Fernald Communities were thus justifiably "outraged by the fact that the local, state and federal agencies formed to protect the public continued to stay in the background and not communicate with the affected community" [about the effects of contamination]. Injustice here consists not only in the violation through environmental contamination of such

rights as "life, liberty, and the pursuit of happiness," but also in the hidden unfair distribution of the burden, insofar as a very small segment of the total population living near nuclear facilities has borne a burden unlike that of any other group of citizens. The justification for their exposure was usually couched in terms of cost-benefit analysis [9] that violate individual human rights by calculations of costs that end up consigning "some to disease, deformity, and premature death, whether in the near term or in the wholly unknown long term" [9]. As Moore puts it, "the [current] system [of representative democracy] fails because of the fundamental conflict between the democracy professed on the one hand and denied on the other. Nuclear weapons that supposedly protect our democracy destroy it, when utilization calculations are employed to override basic human rights" [9].

6. The value of grassroots environmental groups, including community sponsored research partnerships, is particularly salient where radiation contamination is feared.[4] Volunteer environmental groups, like the Fernald Residents for Environmental Safety and Health" (F.R.E.S.H.) enable local populations to find ways of breaking through the fog of secrecy surrounding the environmental effects of nuclear production on public health by gathering data, educating themselves and the community, even launching research studies the nuclear establishment have tried to block. F.R.E.S.H. began by asking the uncomfortable question that established institutions and their leaders had avoided: "What is the health risk of being exposed to radionuclide and toxic chemicals released from the Nuclear Feed Material Production Center?" Voluntary associations like F.R.E.S.H. are more likely than individual initiatives to attract the attention of the media and potential independent researchers and to muster effective political support to pressure state and federal agencies, like the National Center for Environmental Health, to address local health concerns. F.R.E.S.H.'s success with Ohio Senator John Glenn and with persuading Congress to request that the NCEH conduct an epidemiological study in the Fernald community is an impressive example of this kind of community clout.

Several virtues of community research partnerships, as contributors to public discourse and to civil society, are highlighted in the narratives. One is the value of local experience in sparking interest in investigating unusually elevated rates of cancers, thyroid diseases, and other disorders in residential areas near nuclear facilities. Local knowledge of elevated rates in particular may help direct the search for causes, like the elevated thyroid cancer rates among the "downwinders" of the Hanford facility. Residents of a community are also motivated in ways others are not to push for certain kinds of research that would not otherwise be undertaken; sometimes, because the nuclear establishment has a stake in discouraging it. Additionally, community partnerships are

[4] For analysis of ethical justifications of community-research partnerships [15].

able to bring information to the attention of investigators—for example, the location of abandoned dairies—that may be of assistance in formulating hypotheses, investigating data, and interpreting results. As Krimsky points out, neglect of local knowledge may result in researchers missing important causal connections or misinterpreting their findings. Additionally, inclusion of community members in a study that addresses widespread fears of nuclear contamination is important in countering the suspicion and mistrust of research findings, especially when they deviate from what the community expects. When done well, the results and recommendations of a study that includes community members are more likely to be accepted, and, eventually, to lead to closure and peace of mind.

However, the primary impression left by these narratives about community efforts to study radiation contamination is that their well-intentioned efforts were often undercut by the better-organized, well-funded, politically powerful nuclear industry. As Dianne Quigley points out in her contribution, community groups pushed for research but failed to anticipate the hostile response of technical-risk experts hired by the nuclear establishment. The interests of vulnerable communities were rarely presented with sufficient clarity in setting research goals and interpreting them. In the absence of effective community research partnerships in which community interests in research were represented, affected communities were usually reduced to the role of spectators of technical specialists who ignored valuable investigative leads provided by community members as well as alternative interpretations of data made possible by local knowledge.

7. A somewhat different ethical dimension raised by these narratives concerns the reader's response, especially that of those citizens who learn of their government's role in harming fellow-citizens and concealing. One need not have been a participant in the events described in these narratives to ask: What should we, as citizens, learn from these narratives? And how should this information affect our thinking and acting as informed citizens?

What we learn, in a nutshell, is:

- that nuclear facility administrators and government officials in positions of public trust appear to have morally wronged employees of nuclear facilities as well as unsuspecting nearby residents by exposing them without their knowledge or consent to significant doses of radiation that risked serious damage to their health;
- that federal, state, and local governments failed to inform American citizens about radiation exposures and contaminations in a timely way and, in so doing, deprived those affected of their right to decide for themselves whether or not to expose themselves to risks of harm and/or to take protective actions;

- that for years, a number of government supported institutions engaged in elaborate forms of concealment to keep the facts about the risks and actual effects of harmful radiation exposures from coming to light;
- that these deceptive practices often included harmful attacks on the reputations of those scientists and community leaders who tried to study the extent of radiation contamination scientifically and to inform the public;
- that good research studies on the effects of radiation that address communal concerns are still wanting;
- that the harmful consequences of nuclear contamination have affected not only individuals, but families and communities, whose lives have been diminished by the loss of relatives and neighbors as well as fears about the intergenerational transmission of health problems and the continuing effect of environmental contamination; and
- that voluntary associations of concerned citizens have often been stymied in their efforts to address these wrongs by the economic and political power of corporations, the nuclear establishment and local, state, and federal governments.

8. What do we do now? When ethicists and legal theorists discuss appropriate responses to past moral wrongs, they speak in terms of what is just and fair. The concepts of just "reparations" or "remedial justice" deal with what perpetrators of injustice owe their victims in order to right past wrongs. Aristotle captures a key idea of reparative justice: restoration of the state of affairs that existed prior to the injustice. Exodus 22:14-15 expresses a similar idea: "If a man borrows anything of his neighbor, and it is hurt or dies, the owner not being with it, he shall make full restitution" (RSV). The problem with defining "reparations" in terms of full restoration is that it works best when the cause-effect relationship is undeniable and the loss is calculable in financial terms that can be set right by paying the exact amount of the original loss.

Unfortunately, some moral wrongs, like those that generate increase risks with difficult-to-determine cause-effect relationships among multiple variables cannot be traced back, in particular instances, to specific actions and agents. For example, a specific case of lung cancer may be due in part to radiation exposure in the environment that has caused an increase in lung-cancer rates in the geographical area, but maybe not; the main causes may be smoking and/or genetic predisposition. The exact contribution of multiple causal factors cannot be determined for a particular individual. The best one can do is to show that certain actions increased the proportion of those suffering from certain causally related diseases, like lung cancer and thyroid diseases. Additionally, there is no precise way of calculating some of the main deleterious effects, such as the subjective costs of years of ill-health and an early death on a victim and his/her family. In such cases, precise causal responsibility is somewhat murky and the original state of affairs (or what it would be if contamination had not occurred) is difficult to determine, and, in the cases of terminal illnesses, the original state can never be restored. Under these circumstances, the concept of just reparations has to be interpreted in a broader sense of remediation, that is to say, the perpetrators of injustice have a *prima facie* duty to make amends, symbolic as well as financial, for the consequences of their wrong-doing in proportion to their contribution to the deleterious effects suffered by the population of those affected.[5]

A problem with seeking remedial justice years after a harmful event or series of events, like radiation releases, is that of identifying the moral agents who were responsible. Most of the officials responsible for nuclear contamination are now dead. However, the culpable institutions, such as the nuclear facilities and local, state, and federal governments, remain and they can be held accountable across generations. There is precedent for this, in cases of governments and other ongoing institutions. For example, Swiss banks have paid reparations for their long-past wrongdoings during the Holocaust. To the objection that government reparations unfairly penalize contemporary citizens by making them pay for wrongs they did not commit, one persuasive response is that citizens today inherit the benefits as well as the burdens (including liabilities for previous wrongful actions) of their governments.

Since remedial justice can take a variety of forms, one question is, what kind of remediation is appropriate for radiation contamination that mostly occurred decades ago and that contributed in some indeterminate way to the ill-health and early death of individuals? And what is owed, if anything, to those individual family members who have not suffered ill-health by radiation poisoning, but who have been deleteriously affected by the loss of family members, anxieties about their own health, and concerns about their offspring as well as contamination of their environment?

An apology from the federal government and some state and local governments as well as ongoing nuclear facilities, like those at Livermore and Hanford, for their specific role(s) in allowing the radiation contamination of employees and fellow-citizens is obviously important, as part of a process of taking full public responsibility for past moral wrongs. An apology is an expression of remorse for having wronged and injured another. But for an apology to be sincere, it needs to be more than a "feel good" gesture. It needs to demonstrate clearly and persuasively that the institution and its representatives intend to behave differently in the future (for discussion, see Section 9).

Compensation in the form of lump sum financial settlements and the provision of health benefits for those individuals who can be identified as having been harmed by radiation is another appropriate form of reparations. Unfortunately,

[5] For a useful discussion of the problem of reparations, including symbolic reparations, in connection with the claims of African Americans for the legacy of slavery, see [16].

the language of the Radiation Exposure Compensation Act, 42 U.S.C. P 2210 that compensates "individuals who have contracted certain cancers and other serious diseases as a result of their exposure to radiation during above-ground nuclear weapons tests or as a result of employment" evades the just claims of others equally wronged and harmed by their government. Additionally, the reference in the Act to compensation as "compassionate" misconstrues as beneficence a matter of justice reparations owed for acts of injustice. "Compensation" is an appropriate term, as long as it is understood in the context of making amends for wrongs done and damages and/or losses suffered as a result.

The population of those who qualify for benefits under the Radiation Exposure Compensation Act unfairly excludes whole classes of justified individual claimants, such as the "downwinders" at Hanford, who have as good a case against the government as those identified for compensation under the Act. The Radiation Exposure Compensation Act also limits compensation too narrowly to monetary compensation alone. Not only is a financial settlement of $50,000 to $100,000 woefully inadequate, given the pain and suffering of some of those affected, it fails to address appropriately some of their specific needs, such as health insurance and specialized medical care, which should also be provided as part of a comprehensive compensation package.

The problems facing those individuals who were exposed to radiation but whose cancers and thyroid diseases cannot be shown conclusively to have been caused by radiation because the requisite data about their exposure is unavailable or their diseases could be due to other causes, like smoking, suggest some sliding-scale compensation system. Again, health insurance coverage or its equivalent should be included. In areas adjacent to nuclear facilities, compensation for those who can prove they were residents in areas affected by radiation releases initially might best be provided in the form of free monitoring and free medical care for diseases traceable to radiation, whether or not direct causation from a nuclear facility can be proved.

The individualistic focus of current thinking about compensation programs needs to be corrected by greater appreciation of the lasting harm that radiation releases have caused families and communities over time. Radiation releases, the narratives about Navajo uranium miners and the "downwinders" of the Hanford nuclear site make it clear that not only were individuals harmed, but also family lines. Descendants of individual victims suffer anxieties about their own health and that of their children and their children's children. Their lives are blighted by a history of being treated shamefully by their own government and thwarted in their efforts to understand what really happened. Depression, anger, and hopelessness are common among surviving family members. Their suffering calls for a remedy that includes a public apology for their ordeal as well as medical care that responds to their real needs.

Some whole communities that remain intact, like the Navajo, now have new stories dating from the uranium mines and nuclear fallout to add to older narratives about the wrongs done to their ancestors and living communities by the U.S. Government. These stories clearly damage self-esteem, depress confidence and hope for the future. They also require some sort of effective remedial response to community needs, such as education and employment, that go beyond financial settlements with individual claimants. Similarly, the continuing environmental concerns of less cohesive communities, like residents living near Livermore and Rocky Flats, need to be addressed by clean-up efforts and free monitoring programs.

9. The federal government needs to demonstrate, alongside its apology and remedial actions, its intention to learn from its mistakes by designing and implementing public policy changes aimed at *preventing repetition of the offending practices in the future*. This is especially urgent currently, as nuclear power gains popularity again as a source of energy. The government needs to insure the basic human right that people ought not to be unknowingly exposed to serious health risks. Congress might look again at the statement that the Military Production Network (the forerunner to the Alliance for Nuclear Accountability) drafted and circulated to Congress in 1989 entitled, "Democracy and Weaponry, A Bill of Rights for Citizens in the Shadows of America's Nuclear Weapons Production Facilities."

Policy directives should also seek to facilitate better ethical reflection by governmental agencies and those receiving government contracts by requiring mechanisms like a local IRB review of high-risk technological activities that are likely to impact deleteriously the health of employees or the public. As Dianne Quigley observes in her contribution to this volume, "it is . . . crucial to have more ethical oversight in potentially politically-charged research settings, such as nuclear weapons experiments, production activities and related health research on the affected populations" [2]. For ethical oversight to become part of high-risk technological activities, scientists, engineers, technicians, and community representatives will need better training in ethics throughout their careers—a goal the present collection seeks to advance with cases that encourage dialogue about what went wrong as well as what needs to be done to prevent or correct similar wrongdoing in the future.

NOTES

1. Krimsky, S. 2011. *Commentary on ethics and community-based research: Responsibility, precaution, and transparency.* In this volume, pp. 7-24. Amityville, NY: Baywood.
2. Quigley, D. 2011. *Improving community research protections for communities exposed to Cold War nuclear experiments.* In this volume, pp. 199-218. Amityville, NY: Baywood.
3. Beauchamp, T. L., and Childress, J. F. 2001. *Principles of biomedical ethics* (5th ed.). New York: Oxford University Press.

4. Advisory Committee on Human Radiation Experiments (ACHRE). 1995. Washington, D.C.: U.S. Government Printing Office.
5. Pritikin, T. T. 2011. *Insignificant and invisible: The human toll of the Hanford Thyroid Disease Study.* In this volume, pp. 25-52. Amityville, NY: Baywood.
6. Gallagher, C. 1993. *American ground zero: The secret nuclear war.* Cambridge, MA: MIT Press, pp. xxiii and 109ff.
7. Panikkar, B., Yazzie, E., and Brugge, D. 2011. *Ethics of uranium mining research and the Navajo people.* In this volume, pp. 143-163. Amityville, NY: Baywood.
8. Alvarez, R. 2011. *The risks of making nuclear weapons.* In this volume, pp. 181-198. Amityville, NY: Baywood.
9. Moore, L. 2011. *Democracy and public health at Rocky Flats: The examples of Edward A. Martell and C. J. Johnson.* In this volume, pp. 69-97. Amityville, NY: Baywood.
10. Yocum, E. 2011. *A community's experience with environmental health research at the Fernald Feed Production Plant.* In this volume, pp. 53-67. Amityville, NY: Baywood.
11. Austin, D. F. 2011. *Investigation of an excess of malignant melanoma among employees of the Lawrence Livermore National Laboratory.* In this volume, pp. 169-180. Amityville, NY: Baywood.
12. Lifton, R. J. 1986. *The Nazi doctors: Medical killing and the psychology of genocide.* New York: Basic Books, Inc.
13. Stone, R. S. 1948. Health protection activities of the Manhattan Project. *Proceedings of the American Philosophy Society* 90(1):11-19.
14. Sutton, P., Cabasso, J., Barreau, T., and Kelley, M. 2011. *A collaborative effort to address the distribution of plutonium-contaminated sludge in Livermore, California.* In this volume, pp. 99-119. Amityville, NY: Baywood.
15. Wallwork, E. 2007. Ethical analysis of research partnerships with communities. *Kennedy Institute of Ethics Journal.* Forthcoming.
16. Thompson, J. 2005. *Repairing the past: Confronting the legacies of slavery, genocide, and caste.* Proceedings of the Seventh Annual Gilder Lehrman Center International Conference at Yale University, October 27-29, 2005. www.yale.edu/glc/wwwjustice/thompson.pdf

Postscript

Some final comments are provided from Tim Connor, former research director of Hanford Education Action League, Spokane, Washington, journalist and longtime activist on nuclear weapons health-risk issues who spearheaded many public involvement efforts for resolving health concerns about nuclear contamination from weapons production. Mr. Connor reviewed these narratives and offered these comments.

The wealth of information that Trisha Pritikin [1] brings together to show the broad disconnect between the inherent and introduced flaws in the HTDS and the cock-suredness of the conclusion that there were no health consequences of the Hanford emissions is very impressive. I've always thought that the finding reported on the remarkably high gross incidence of thyroid disease found in the medical screening part of the HTDS—was a conspicuous and plainly visible rebuttal to the HTDS conclusions of no observable effect from Hanford exposures. It actually gets to the heart of the confusion and weakness of the HTDS. And that was its reliance on dose-response analysis in a situation where the dose information was badly compromised. This gets to an important ethical issue. Whose fault was it that the dose information was so poor? Which gets to my next point.

The responsibility for the badly compromised dose information was the federal government and its contractors who, for nearly four decades, kept the Hanford radioiodine releases secret. The only purpose for the secrecy was to avoid the political consequences of disclosure. And it had devastating consequences. The only way a dose-base study like HTDS can work is if there is a high level of quality and confidence in the dosimetry. Dose response is a two-way street. Whether you have one health effect or thousands, you can't do a dose-response study like HTDS without good information on doses. And yet, because of the forty-year lapse in disclosure, the dose reconstruction project was forced to rely, heavily, on personal recollection of source and dietary habits going back to early childhood. As Ms. Pritikin notes, this is what escalates the uncertainty over the doses that reviewers identified before the HTDS results were made public. Given the inherent uncertainty on the individual doses, it's hard to escape the conclusion that the main reason the government escaped accountability for the Hanford exposures is that it managed a successful cover up for so long. And yet none of this was acknowledged by the HTDS researchers and CDC. In my book, that was unethical.

Dr. Seth Tuler [2], in his ethical review of the NCI Iodine-131 study and follow-up, poses an important question in his conclusion, as to what explains the differences in the approaches and recommendations between IOM/NRC and ACERER, and "how they integrate scientific analysis with ethical and moral concerns and how they applied ethical principles of beneficence and justice differently." I've given interviews on this recently and have reread much of the record on this dispute. My conclusion is that ACERER conducted itself in a more intellectually honest manner than did IOM/NRC. We had a better process and we reached a more technically defensible result as a consequence. And, yet, IOM/NRC prevailed because it was a more prestigious institution and because it rendered an answer—essentially, do nothing—that was welcome news to the government. This debate also has to consider the findings from other studies that physicians and scientists really expect to have the power of their credentials at hand in their relationships with patients and the public at-large. I can't discern whether it was intellectual or class elitism that governed their behavior in this instance. All I'm sure of is that they got it wrong.

REGARDING THE PANIKKAR ET AL. NAVAJO URANIUM MINING ETHICAL ISSUES

Whatever else this is, it's a powerful indictment of the PHS and the government because of what it reflects about the absence of any moral and social compact between the American government and the Navajo people and the individual miners. In that sense, it transforms research ethics into a larger human rights violation, and can really only be approached within that context. And that's the connection I think is missing from the Conclusion. There may be good lessons here for building relationships, building community, and building democracy, but the narrative thread between the gross human rights violations and the role of science and scientific research in building democracy, community, relationships has been short-circuited in the conclusion, and that's a shortcoming. There's so much good material here to learn from, and the broader lessons can still be harvested with a conclusion that brings it all together.

REGARDING THE QUIGLEY ARTICLE CONCERNING ETHICAL IMPROVEMENTS TO HEALTH STUDIES

I would certainly underscore the issue advanced by ACHRE about the trade-off between the funds necessary to do dose reconstruction and other scientific studies on populations and the acts of actually providing "relief and assistance to the victims." Actually, it's *the* most importing point I made in 1995 speech/paper presented at the annual meeting of the National Council on Radiological Protections and Measurements, entitled "Public Interest and Expectations in Dose Reconstruction." Here's how I put it then:

> The final point I'd like to make is exemplified by the Hanford experience but is applicable to the broader efforts at DOE facilities to address health concerns. The fact that we're now entering the tenth year since the disclosures of the extraordinary radioiodine emissions from Hanford and haven't done a thing for the citizens exposed to those releases is a travesty. Forget the pending lawsuits, forget where we put the decimal points on the radiation doses, and forget the outcome of the Hanford Thyroid Disease Study. The fact is we knew enough in the spring of 1986 to know that taking care of the people exposed to these emissions was the right thing to do. A plan for medical monitoring should have been put in place, a compact to provide medical care for potentially exposed people now suffering from thyroid and thyroid-related diseases should have been signed and sealed. Given the fundamental breach of trust involved—where the government exposed people and simply tried to ignore it for decades—such a response was and still is morally justified.

Given the debacle of the Hanford Thyroid Disease Study, I would use even stronger language today. After the HTDS came out, I publicly apologized to the people of my state for being one of the primary advocates for Congressional funding of the study. I felt and my organization felt, in 1986, that a health study would be a stepping stone to getting needed medical care to people. But it turned out to be, instead, something of a massive federal assistance program for scientists and epidemiologists who, instead of helping to bring assistance to those exposed, wound up insulting their intelligence while giving Congress and the agencies a basis for not going ahead with medical assistance. Just when the Hanford Medical Monitoring Program was about to be implemented the flawed HTDS study became the basis for pulling the plug on it. This despite the fact (as Trisha Pritikin [1] noted in her chapter in this volume, pp. 25-52) that the HTDS clinical results found an extraordinarily high incidence of thyroid disease.

Tim Connor

NOTES

1. Pritikin, T. T. 2011. *Insignificant and invisible: The human toll of the Hanford Thyroid Disease Study*. In this volume, pp. 25-52. Amityville, NY: Baywood.
2. Tuler, S. 2011. *Institutional preferences for justice, avoiding harm, and expertise in public health policy making about the health consequences of Iodine-131 nuclear weapons testing fallout*. In this volume, pp. 121-142. Amityville, NY: Baywood.

Contributors

BOB ALVAREZ is a Senior Scholar at the Institute for Policy Studies in Washington, DC, where he is currently focused on nuclear disarmament as well as environmental and energy policies.

DON AUSTIN, PhD, teaches epidemiology as Emeritus Professor at Oregon Health Sciences University (OHSU) and participates in research at the VA Medical Center in Portland. His career spans both research and public health in state and federal health agencies, and academia. He has developed cancer surveillance systems, conducted and interpreted epidemiologic research, and applied his experience to the curriculum for medical students, residents, and MPH students.

TRACY BARREAU is an environmental scientist with the California Department of Health Services, Environmental Health Investigations Branch. She has worked for the past 11 years evaluating health impacts to communities living near hazardous waste sites. In collaboration with citizen groups, community members, the City of Livermore, and Alameda County, she conducted an investigation into the historic distribution of plutonium-contaminated sewage in Livermore.

DOUGLAS M. BRUGGE, PhD, MS, has a PhD from Harvard University and an MS from the Harvard School of Public Health. He is currently associate professor in the Department of Public Health and Family Medicine at Tufts University School of Medicine. He is director of the Navajo Uranium Miner Project and the Tufts Community Research Center. He has published over 100 papers and is co-editor (with Pat Hynes) of a book from Ashgate Publishing Group (UK) on community research in environmental health and co-editor (with Esther Yazzie-Lewis and Timothy Benally) of *The Navajo People and Uranium Mining* (University of New Mexico Press, 2006).

JACQUELINE CABASSO has served as executive director of the nonprofit Western States Legal Foundation (WSLF) in Oakland, California, since 1984. Founded in 1982, with a local focus on the Livermore Nuclear Weapons Laboratory, WSLF seeks to abolish nuclear weapons as an essential step in making possible a more secure, just, and environmentally sustainable world.

Cabasso has extensive experience with community education and outreach and speaks frequently in local, national, and international settings. She is also a published author. www.wslfweb.org

MARYLIA KELLEY is Executive Director of the Livermore, California-based Tri-Valley CAREs. Marylia brings to Tri-Valley CAREs' program 23 years of in-depth research, writing and facilitating public participation in decisions regarding Livermore Lab and nuclear weapons, waste, and cleanup. She serves on the "Community Work Group" (since 1989) to advise the federal Environmental Protection Agency, state agencies, and the community on the Superfund cleanup of Livermore Lab. She has provided input to the National Academy of Sciences, including on the nuclear proliferation risks of the National Ignition Facility and on toxic and radioactive pollution at the Livermore Lab's main site and site 300. She can often be found speaking at diverse venues, from local city council meetings to international conferences in Russia and Japan. Marylia has written for numerous publications, including the Bulletin of the Atomic Scientists. She also serves as editor for Citizen's Watch, Tri-Valley CAREs' monthly newsletter. Her work with Tri-Valley CAREs has garnered numerous awards over the years, and, in 2002, she was named to the Alameda County Women's Hall of Fame. Marylia has a background in journalism and humanities, and graduated summa cum laude from John F. Kennedy University in 1984. She has lived in Livermore since 1976. marylia@trivalleycares.org

SHELDON KRIMSKY, PhD, is professor of Urban & Environmental Policy & Planning in the School of Arts & Sciences and adjunct professor in Public Health and Family Medicine in the School of Medicine at Tufts University. He received his bachelors and masters degrees in physics from Brooklyn College, CUNY, and Purdue University respectively, and a masters and doctorate in philosophy from Boston University. Professor Krimsky has been elected Fellow of the American Association for the Advancement of Science for "seminal scholarship exploring the normative dimensions and moral implications of science in its social context."

AMY LOWMAN, MPH, is a project manager and research associate at the University of North Carolina School of Public Health. For the last several years she has worked on CBPR studies of the health effects of polluting industries on surrounding communities. She has also participated in the development of a protocol for the surveillance and investigation of residents complaints related to the land application of sewage sludges.

LEROY MOORE, PhD, a founder of the Rocky Mountain Peace and Justice Center of Boulder, Colorado, and has worked on issues related to Rocky Flats since 1979. He served on several bodies set up to advise the DOE and the regulators on cleanup of the Rocky Flats site. Author of the *Citizen's Guide to Rocky Flats* (1992), "Rocky Flats: Bait and Switch Cleanup," the Bulletin of the Atomic Scientists (January/February 2005), and numerous other writings, he served on the board of the Alliance for Nuclear Accountability and was the token outsider on two committees of the National Council on Radiation Protection and Measurement.

BINDU PANIKKAR is a doctoral student in Environmental Health at Tufts University. Her current areas of focus are occupational health issues, immigrant health, environmental history, environmental hormones, ethics in research, and community-based participatory research. She is one of the board members at Tufts Community Research Center. She is also a recipient of the National Institute of Occupational Safety and Health Student Research Award for her doctoral work on "Assessing and Controlling Occupational Risks Among Immigrants in Somerville, MA." She has an MA in Urban and Environmental Policy and Planning and an MS in Environmental Health from Tufts University.

TRISHA THOMPSON PRITIKIN was born in Richland, Washington, adjacent to the Hanford nuclear weapons facility in southeastern Washington State, during years of off-site radioactive emissions from the plant. Over many years she has volunteered her time as a member of the Hanford Health Information Network (HHIN) advisory board and served for consecutive terms as a citizen representative on the Hanford Health Effects Subcommittee. As a result of her work, she was appointed to the Subcommittee for Community Affairs to the federal Advisory Committee on Energy Related Epidemiologic Research and served as co-chair of that committee. Trisha's mother and father died from aggressive cancers, which she believes were more than likely caused by exposure to fallout from the Hanford facility. Trisha herself has health problems that she attributes to *in utero* and childhood exposures to Hanford's radiation. It is her goal to secure medical and other help for people who, like herself and her family, have suffered harm due to U.S. nuclear weapons production and testing programs.

DIANNE QUIGLEY, PhD, is an ethics researcher and adjunct assistant professor at Brown University's Center for Environmental Studies and lecturer at UMASS–Dartmouth. Ms. Quigley was the principal investigator of a grant from the National Institute on Health titled "Collaborative Initiative for Research Ethics in Environmental Health" (2000-2007). She was also a principal investigator on several major NIH grants for "Nuclear Risk Management to Native Communities" (1994–2000) and executive director of the Childhood Cancer Research Institute (1987-2000). Ms. Quigley continues to develop ethics training projects and research from the CIREEH with Brown and Syracuse Universities. She holds a masters degree from Clark University, Worcester, Massachusetts, in the Environment, Science, and Policy Program.

PATRICE SUTTON, MPH, is a research scientist with 20 years of experience in occupational and environmental health research, public health practice and policy development, and professional- and community-based public health advocacy. She has published over two dozen peer-reviewed scientific articles and government technical reports and has also co-authored chapters on nuclear weapons in *War and Public Health* (Oxford University Press, in press, 2007) and radiologic and nuclear weapons in *Terrorism and Public Health* (Oxford University Press, 2002). Ms. Sutton was a member of the Board of Western States Legal Foundation between 1992 and 2002, and has been an active member of the American Public Health Association since 1986.

SETH TULER, PhD, has extensive research experience on hazard management, public involvement in environmental and risk assessment and decision making, and program evaluation. Over the last decade, he has been involved with a variety of projects to facilitate environmental health education, training, and public participation with community residents affected by contamination from U.S. nuclear weapons production and related facilities.

ERNEST WALLWORK, PhD, is Professor of Ethics at Syracuse University and a psychoanalyst in private practice. His books include *Durkheim: Morality and Milieu* and *Psychoanalysis and Ethics*. He has been the D.R. Sharpe Lecturer on Social Ethics at the University of Chicago; a Fellow at the Kennedy Institute of Ethics, Georgetown; Bioethicist at NIH; and a Fellow at the Woodrow Wilson International Center.

STEVE WING, PhD, teaches epidemiology at the University of North Carolina School of Public Health and conducts research on occupational and environmental health. Recent work has focused on the health impacts of ionizing radiation, industrial animal production, and environmental injustice. He is a founding member of the North Carolina Environmental Justice Network.

ESTHER YAZZIE is a board member and board president of the Southwest Research and Information Center, Albuquerque, New Mexico, working on nuclear risk issues in New Mexico. She worked with Total Benefits Communication in Atlanta, Georgia, in presenting the Navajo Nation 401(k) to the Navajo Nation employees with the assistance of the Navajo Nation Retirement Office, Window Rock, Arizona. Ms. Yazzie was a faculty member to the Native American Alliances Foundation-Native Americans on "The Healing and Wellness Courts" across the country. She is a member on the Diversity Advisory Committee with the Federal Judicial Center, Washington, DC. She is a member of the Justice and Women of Color Committee, National Consortium of Task Forces and Commissions on Racial and Ethnic Bias in the Courts with the National Center of State Courts. Ms. Yazzie serves as a peer review consultant to the National Institute of Justice through the Technical Assistance and Support Program in Washington, DC. She was an advisory committee member to the "All My Relations" project for First Nations and Health Source, Albuquerque, New Mexico.

EDWA YOCUM is a community leader for Fernald Residents for Environmental Safety and Health (FRESH), Inc. and Fernald-Community Health Effects Committee, Inc. From 1984 to the present time, she has been the officer and health chairperson for FRESH. She created the FRESH Cancer Incidence Map. From 2001 to the present, she was a research assistant for the Fernald Community Health Effects Committee (F-CHEC) working with the University of Cincinnati on a CBPR research project related to the Fernald contamination. Ms. Yocum lives one-and-a-half-miles south of the former Fernald Nuclear Weapons Plant, located 18 miles northwest of Cincinnati, Ohio.

Index